Inflammatory Bowel Disease

A Clinicians' Guide

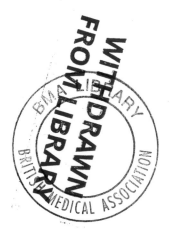

Inflammatory Bowel Disease

A Clinicians' Guide

SECOND EDITION

Alastair Forbes BSc MD FRCP
St Mark's Hospital for Intestinal and Colorectal
Disorders, London, UK

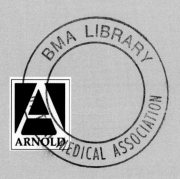

A member of the Hodder Headline Group
LONDON • NEW YORK • NEW DELHI

First published in Great Britain in 2001 by
Arnold, a member of the Hodder Headline Group,
338 Euston Road, London NW1 3BH

http://www.arnoldpublishers.com

Distributed in the USA by
Oxford University Press Inc.,
198 Madison Avenue, New York, NY10016
Oxford is a registered trademark of Oxford University Press

British Library Cataloguing in Publication Data
A catalogue record for this book is available from the British Library

Library of Congress Cataloging-in-Publication Data
A catalog record for this book is available from the Library of Congress

ISBN 0 340 80727 X

1 2 3 4 5 6 7 8 9 10

Commissioning Editor: Nick Dunton
Production Editor: Wendy Rooke
Production Controller: Martin Kerans

Typeset in 11 on 13 pt Garamond by Cambrian Typesetters, Frimley, Surrey
Printed and bound in Great Britain by The Bath Press, Bath

What do you think about this book? Or any other Arnold title?
Please send your comments to feedback.arnold@hodder.co.uk

Contents

Preface to the second edition

I was very pleased to discover that the first edition of the *Clinicians' Guide to Inflammatory Bowel Disease* appeared to fill a niche. Its appearance prompted several generous reviews and a second print-run was required. I was taken to task for using data presented only in abstract form, but I believe I have been vindicated by this approach as only in a few relatively minor areas have conclusions drawn on this basis had to be revised, and the book remained 'fresh' for that bit longer.

Nonetheless, the field is an active one and the information collected in 1996 and early 1997 has now been superseded in many important areas, not least in the therapeutic application of biological immunomodulators. I have accordingly been encouraged to produce a second edition. I have revised the book in its entirety. Several of the chapters have been completely rewritten, and all have been extensively updated, but in what I hope will remain a familiar style. The previously used abstract data have been replaced by reference to full papers where they exist and deleted in the few cases where they do not. New information available now only in abstract form is, however, included. I have continued to give special attention to topics less well covered in the major textbooks, and these areas also have been revised carefully. I have been able to extend the list of contacts for organizations with an interest in inflammatory bowel disease, and there are additional suggestions for advice on support material for patients.

My hoped-for readership is fundamentally the same group of professionals as for the first edition, and I hope that you will appreciate that the book, though modified, is not significantly longer or heavier than before.

Alastair Forbes
February 2001

Introduction and causation

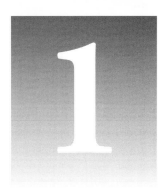

There are a number of inflammatory bowel diseases to be considered, but for the most part this account will concentrate on ulcerative colitis and Crohn's disease. It is still debated whether these idiopathic diseases are truly distinct or merely different ends of an inflammatory spectrum. The relevant sections of this book will illustrate such differences as in their biochemical and immunological behaviour, their clinical, radiological and histological features, their complications and disease associations, and in their responses to therapy. Compelling circumstantial data such as these cannot, however, quite answer the question. The elucidation of the function of the human genome will perhaps permit a clear distinction, but until we have more certain aetiological information about inflammatory bowel disease there can be no authoritative conclusion. As there are so many differences it will be assumed that it is legitimate to describe two diseases, but with the proviso that, if this is proved incorrect, much of the information collected here will nevertheless remain pertinent.

Ulcerative colitis was first described in forms clearly recognizable to the present-day reader in the mid nineteenth century with a compelling account of a fatal case and a subsequent small series reported by Wilks in 1859. It is probable that the disease was well established long before then and that recognition was obscured by incomplete distinction from infectious diarrhoea and dysentery.[1] Crohn's disease had to wait until 1912 for the clear description of non-tuberculous granulomatous ileitis by Dalziel,[2] eponymized by Crohn (of Crohn, Ginzberg, Oppenheimer and Berg) only in 1932.[3] While it is probable that 1907 and 1908 accounts of inflammatory tumours of the bowel were Crohn's disease, the extraordinary account of the ultimately fatal metre-long tight stricture of the lower ileum reported by Coombe and Saunders in 1806 may genuinely have been the first description.[4]

Epidemiology

On the whole, ulcerative colitis and Crohn's disease are found in the same populations,[5] both conditions becoming more prevalent with improving socioeconomic status. It is a general observation that increases in ulcerative colitis occur before those in Crohn's disease, with a lag period of 15–20 years.[6] Most studies have a small excess of females with Crohn's disease and of males with ulcerative colitis,[6,7] although males with Crohn's disease as well as with ulcerative colitis may also be over-represented in studies from lower incidence areas.[8] The male excess in ulcerative colitis is more striking with increasing age. This was shown most obviously in a large southern European study ($n = 1255$), still only available in abstract, in which there was a 2:1 male excess in those with ulcerative colitis presenting over the age of 65 ($n = 114$), compared with a more usual nearly equal frequency in those under 25.[9] Intermediate ratios of 1.4 and 1.7 were found in the 26–35 and

36–50 years groups. Similar findings from the Mayo Clinic[10] and in a collaborative pan-European study indicate that this is a real phenomenon,[7] but whether it is a cohort effect from an influence operating much earlier in life is unclear.

ULCERATIVE COLITIS

Reasonable data on the incidence and prevalence of ulcerative colitis exist for most developed nations. There has been considered to be an annual incidence of around 7 per 100 000 population, but higher figures are seen in regions more distant from the equator. Moum *et al.* record an incidence of 12.8 per 100 000 in southern Norway,[11] and Bernstein *et al.*, 14.3 per 100 000 for Manitoba in Canada.[12] During 1991–93, 10.4 new cases per 100 000 were found in the 15–64 year age range for 20 disparate European centres,[7] including 24.5 per 100 000 in Iceland, and 1.6 per 100 000 in Portugal, which are, respectively, the highest and one of the lowest rates yet documented; the incidence in the indigenous population in Leicester was 9.2 per 100 000.

Within individual population groups in northern Europe and America, the incidence of ulcerative colitis is now considered to be relatively constant over time.[13] The South Wales study, which examined 357 incident cases in a stable population over the period 1968–87,[14] found that although the range of annual incidence was wide (between 3 and 9 per 100 000 for individual years) the mean annual incidence for the entire period was 6.3 per 100 000, and showed neither an upward nor a downward trend. The very detailed Mayo Clinic analysis covering the period 1940–1993 yielded an overall incidence of 7.6 per 100 000, rising from under 6 between 1940 and 1963 to peak at 9.4 between 1974 and 1983 before slipping back to 8.3 for 1984–93.[10] This is very similar to the trends of the Swedish study which also reached an apparent peak about 1980.[6]

In Italy (which appears representative of southern Europe), it is probable that the annual incidence is still slowly rising. The Lombardia survey of 1990–94 revealed an average of 7.0 cases of ulcerative colitis per 100 000,[15] and the pan-European study of 1991–93 yielded 10 per 100 000 for Milan; these are the highest figures yet recorded in Italy. It is possible that a component of this increase is from improved case ascertainment, but unlikely that this is the complete explanation; sequential long-term observation of stable populations is needed to clarify this.

The prevalence of ulcerative colitis is in line with incidence, but in most reports prevalence is only a little above 10 times the incidence, even in northern centres (e.g. Bernstein *et al.* quote 170 per 100 000)[12]. Despite Logan's comments about ascertainment bias and confusion introduced by the various forms of self-limiting colitis,[13] for this to be so for a disease that has its onset in young adulthood and is cured only by surgery suggests that the true incidence is still rising. Only the most recently published prevalence, from Olmsted County, of 229 per 100 000 (27.5 times the related incidence) begins to refute this, equating to a plausible 'survival with disease' of 27.5 years, which implies death or colectomy on average at the age of 62, given the median age of 34.5 at onset of colitis in their recent patients.[10]

CROHN'S DISEASE

The incidence of Crohn's disease has generally been lower than that of ulcerative colitis, but has risen to approach it in most of the regions in which it has been studied sequentially.[13] Studies from Europe and North America mostly yielded annual incidences for Crohn's of below 4 per 100 000 until around 1970, and of about 5 per 100 000 in the 1970s and early 1980s.[16–18] The later 1980s and early 1990s figures are generally higher still. Again, there is a trend for the frequency to increase with greater distance from the equator. In

Norway (1990–93), the incidence was 5.8 per 100 000,[19] and the pan-European study performed in 1991–93 demonstrated an overall incidence of 5.6 per 100 000 in those aged 15–64, which ranged from only 0.9 in north-west Greece, to 9.2 in the Netherlands;[7] the incidence was 3.8 per 100 000 in the indigenous population of Leicester.

Virtually every study that has been able to measure changes in incidence of Crohn's disease has shown an increase with passing decades, but it is unlikely that this continues indefinitely. The initial rise is probably explained in part by better case ascertainment, and by assignment of a Crohn's disease diagnosis to some colitic patients who would previously have been considered to have ulcerative colitis. It is, however, unlikely that either of these factors is sufficient to account for the magnitude of the increase recorded by some centres, especially since the incidence of ulcerative colitis has remained broadly constant. In Copenhagen County, for example, the incidence recorded for 1979–87 of 4.1 per 100 000 was sixfold higher than in the early 1960s.[17] The clinical features in these incident patients were relatively constant over time and did not appear to be less severe in later years; it is accordingly probable that changes in case ascertainment were at most of minor impact. The English study based on Blackpool Victoria Hospital confirmed the general upward trend, but suggested that it had ceased after 1980, with standard age-adjusted incidence figures for 1971–75, 1976–80, 1981–85 and 1986–90 of 3.6, 6.0, 6.4 and 6.5 per 100 000.[20] There is a little anxiety about the veracity of a hospital-based rather than community-based study, but this is unlikely to influence this observation greatly, unless more cases are being managed by general practitioners without hospital support. As the condition is better recognized and more widely discussed, this is a possible but improbable explanation. The Swedish and Mayo Clinic data are concordant with a view that incidence rates rise to reach a ceiling beyond which no

further increase occurs. The Crohn's disease incidence remained between 5 and 7 per 100 000 from 1965 to 1983 in one Swedish series[6] and stabilized, having risen to a mean of 4.6 per 100 000 after 1970 in another.[21] The Olmsted County survey yielded an adjusted annual incidence of under 3 per 100 000 before 1964, but after a peak of 7.8 per 100 000 in 1974–83 the incidence has slipped back to 6.9 per 100 000 for 1984–93.[18] Nonetheless, increases are still occurring in high incidence areas such as Denmark.[22,23]

The increase in frequency of Crohn's disease seems particularly obvious to paediatric gastroenterologists. In the under-16s in South Wales, the incidence of Crohn's disease rose from a mean of 1.3 cases per 100 000 from 1983 to 1988, to 3.1 over the period 1989–93.[24] There is a resultant prevalence of Crohn's disease in the under-16s of 16.6 per 100 000, now considerably exceeding that of ulcerative colitis in the same age group (3.4 per 100 000). This may in part reflect the earlier diagnosis of young adults who thus fall into a paediatric classification, as is strongly suggested by the Stockholm study which recorded increases in incidence in the under-15s but a drop in those aged 15–19.[21] The ongoing study of inflammatory bowel disease in all those under 20 by the British Paediatric Surveillance Unit and the British Society of Gastroenterology should clarify this point. A prospective study performed in children aged under 16 in southern Norway, still only available as an abstract,[25] yielded an annual incidence of 2.0 per 100 000 for Crohn's disease, rising with age, inflammatory bowel disease being a rare diagnosis in the under-10s. This is similar to figures previously reported for Scandinavia and points away from a rising incidence in this already high-incidence region. There are, moreover, data from several centres that indicate that the median age at presentation is actually increasing overall.[21–23]

The prevalence of Crohn's disease is in line with that of an incurable non-fatal disease, which has incurred the observed changes in incidence over the past half-century. The Olmsted County study reported a prevalence of 144 per 100 000 in 1991;[18] this will inevitably increase even if incidence peaks have been reached.

RACE AND ETHNICITY

The influence of race and ethnicity is discussed further in relation to the aetiopathogenesis of inflammatory bowel disease (see below), but the best known association – between Jewish origin and Crohn's disease – deserves comment. The magnitude of the association has almost certainly been exaggerated by study methodology, but it appears real. In one representative and reasonably matched study, a relative risk fivefold (CI: 2.3–17.2-fold) higher than in non-Jewish residents was documented.[26] Carefully acquired data from Israel, however, fail to show higher incidence than in other high prevalence areas,[7] with an incidence specifically in Israeli Jews of only 2.9 per 100 000 in the 1980s.[27]

Data are scanty for within-country comparisons of other groups but there is no doubt, whatever allowance is made for poor case ascertainment and false diagnoses of intestinal tuberculosis in developing countries, that inflammatory bowel disease is much less common in Asia, Africa and South America. The rising incidence of Crohn's disease in northern Europe is paradoxically most obvious in those of an Asian background,[7] but there are very few data on the black population groups in whom it is possibly less frequent. A small study indicated an annual incidence of Crohn's disease of between 4.5 and 5.6 per 100 000 in West Indian blacks living in Derby, UK, which was less than (but not significantly so) the rate of 7.0 per 100 000 in the local Caucasian population.[28] A more recent report from Georgia (USA) on African-American children suggests annual incidences of both ulcerative colitis (5–7 per 100 000) and Crohn's disease (7–12 per 100 000) similar to those of the white population.[29]

SEASONAL VARIATION IN THE ONSET OF INFLAMMATORY BOWEL DISEASE

Patients are often convinced that new and relapsing symptoms from inflammatory bowel disease are concentrated at certain times of year; there is some clinical and epidemiological support for this. Peak times for first presentation in the autumn and early winter, and for clinical relapses in the spring and autumn, with a relative dearth of clinical events in summer months, have been suggested by several retrospective analyses,[30,31] but not all.[32] A large prospective study of incident cases[33] argues against such any such association for Crohn's disease, but is strongly indicative of a continuing cyclical incidence for ulcerative colitis, with regular peaks in winter, and troughs in late spring. Pooling data for 4 consecutive years provides December with a 1.48-fold increased risk for colitis presentation, whereas May is favoured at a relative rate of 0.76 (overall significance for departure from uniform distribution: $P = 0.028$). The obvious question as to why the month should influence presentation with colitis is unanswered but lends further credence to the hypothesis that there is an infective trigger for presentation if not necessarily one of a truly pathogenic nature (see below). Moum and colleagues speculate[33] that winter upper respiratory tract infections or the antibiotics often used in their treatment are implicated, and are inclined to dismiss the more obviously gastrointestinal pathogens which are more commonly isolated during summer months in Scandinavia. It is not clear why the peak months for incidence should appear to differ from those for relapse.

Aetiology and pathogenesis

INTRODUCTION

The aetiology and pathogenesis of the inflammatory bowel diseases have limited immediate bearing on clinical practice, but it is hoped that the following analysis will aid an understanding of the disease process and of the mechanisms by which some therapeutic agents may act. It should also help to provide comprehensible answers to some of the justifiable and increasingly frequent questions being asked by patients about the cause(s) of their disease.

It is conventional to consider separately the inherited factors, assumed to be controlled genetically, and the environmental and other influences, which predispose to inflammatory bowel disease. It is probable, however, that (in the absence of simple Mendelian inheritance) the genetic factors act predominantly as risk factors that place the predisposed individual at greater risk of sustaining inflammatory bowel disease when exposed to a subsequent environmental challenge. Pragmatism dictates that until such time as the relative apportionment of these influences is known, convention is followed: inherited and environmental aspects will therefore be considered separately.

GENETICS OF INFLAMMATORY BOWEL DISEASE

General aspects and family studies

There is a clear familial link to both major forms of inflammatory bowel disease, with supportive data from studies of twins and individual families, and from population groups.[34,35] The risk of a second first-order family member being affected lies between 1 in 15 and 1 in 10, which is in the region of 20 times the highest population prevalences seen (see above). The concordance rate for Crohn's in twin pairs is at least at the level of that seen in other conditions (such as insulin-dependent diabetes) for which a genetic link is uncontroversial. No fewer than 8 of 18 individuals with a monozygotic twin affected by Crohn's disease developed the disease themselves (compared with only 1 of 26 dizygotic twins) in Tysk's study.[34] Extended family pedigrees make it clear that

simple monogenic Mendelian-type inheritance is unlikely to be relevant, even with a complex attribution of incomplete penetrance. Although the technique of segregation analysis indicates that genetic predisposition is present in as few as 10 per cent of inflammatory bowel disease patients,[36] this is probably an underestimate, given accumulating evidence for a variety of distinct genetic sites being involved, each with low penetrance (and perhaps also dependent on additional environmental factors for disease expression).

Concordance for type of inflammatory bowel disease is generally stronger for Crohn's disease than for ulcerative colitis. There was, for example, only one pair of identical twins in whom both had ulcerative colitis of 16 pairs in whom the index twin had the disease, compared with the 8 (of 18) with Crohn's in Tysk's study.[34] An Oxford study which concentrated on affected siblings confirmed a general tendency for the nature of the disease to be concordant.[37] Thus, ulcerative colitis affected both of 29 sibling pairs, Crohn's 42 pairs, and only 12 pairs with disease were discordant.

Anticipation

Ulcerative colitis seems to occur at a younger age in familial cases in comparison with those without a family history, with a significantly different mean age at diagnosis (28.5 versus 35 years; $P < 0.02$) in one representative study.[37] Genetic anticipation may also occur. This concept has been established in other fields, and refers to the phenomenon of a genetically influenced disease presenting at an earlier age with each successive generation. Anticipation was sought in studies from Baltimore and New York in families concordant for Crohn's disease.[38,39] Family members from at least two generations were included. The mean age of diagnosis was more than 12 years earlier in the younger generation (at 18.9 years versus 31.4 years in Baltimore, and 21 versus 35 in New York) – statistically significant results. These differences were also carried across three generations in the few families thus afflicted. The possible biases introduced by earlier diagnosis being prompted by an informed family milieu, or by missing late-affected offspring, are considered by the authors. It is probable that these are insufficient to explain all the differences seen (especially since in some Baltimore families the child was diagnosed before the parent). When analysis was restricted to pairs where parents had an age at diagnosis of under 28 years, significant evidence for anticipation was retained only for New York Jewish families. In non-gastrointestinal conditions for which genetic anticipation is recorded, there is an association with paternal transmission. Interestingly, in the Baltimore family series, the second-generation patient had more extensive disease in 15 of 27 parent/child pairs; in 13 of these 15, the affected parent was the father.[38] There are otherwise no other obvious phenotypic differences between familial and non-familial cases for either ulcerative colitis or Crohn's.

HLA in inflammatory bowel disease

HLA links have long been sought in ulcerative colitis, in part because of the original descriptions of a link with positivity for HLA-B27 in patients also affected by ankylosing spondylitis (see Chapter 6), and the postulates that there were autoimmune phenomena operating in colitis (see below). A variety of HLA-A and HLA-B associations were reported in the 1980s, but with marked international differences and not a little controversy. The field is not an easy one for the amateur, given continuing uncertainty and the multiple, overlapping names used for antigens and alleles. Methodological criticisms, particularly of small studies, have been invoked to explain many of the differences between past reports, and interest has increasingly converged on the class II antigens.

Meta-analysis has now been performed on Medline-listed publications using standard techniques.[40] DR2, DR9 and DRB1*0103 were positively associated with ulcerative colitis, and a negative association was found between DR4 and ulcerative colitis. Positive data for HLA linkage in Crohn's disease have been fewer than in ulcerative colitis, but meta-analysis points to a positive association with DR7, DRB3*0301 and DQ4, and a negative association with DR2 and DR3.[40] It should be recognized, however, that these associations are population-specific and do not apply similarly strongly in all geographical areas.

Many authors have tried to attribute phenotypic characteristics of inflammatory bowel disease to the underlying genotype. All of these conclusions must remain somewhat speculative as the subgroup analyses performed have rarely had adequate power, but there are strong indications that certain HLA types favour, or protect from, more extensive or more severe disease.

Cytokine gene polymorphism

The influence of altered cytokine expression as part of the inflammatory response and its contribution to the pathogenesis of inflammatory bowel disease is considered later, but there is also evidence that the cytokine milieu is significantly influenced through a series of gene polymorphisms. The genes for tumour necrosis factor alpha (TNF-α) and for the interleukin-1 receptor antagonist (IL-1RA) have attracted most attention (coding respectively for a key inflammatory mediator and for an endogenous antagonist to another).

The TNF gene is intimately associated with the HLA complex on chromosome 6 and most studies have dealt with its types 1 and 2 alleles. Targan's group found significant linkage to a particular TNF-α haplotype in 75 patients with Crohn's disease compared both to patients with ulcerative colitis and to normal controls (relative risk 4.4–7.4),[41] while the Belgian group suggest more that the type 2 allele determines a more severe disease phenotype (steroid dependence, etc.) than primarily the susceptibility to Crohn's disease *per se*.[42] Three novel TNF gene polymorphisms were positively associated with Crohn's disease in a reasonably sized Japanese study and are also claimed to influence both susceptibility to Crohn's and its phenotype.[43] Our own data, however, strongly question any linkage to specific TNF alleles in inflammatory bowel disease patients of European origin.[44]

The gene for IL-1RA, which is on chromosome 2, has a number of alleles. There is evidence that allele 2 is important in ulcerative colitis in some populations[45,46] but not others,[47] albeit at a low relative risk (no more than 1.4 times).[45,46] It does not appear to have any relevance to Crohn's disease.[46,47]

It is possible that certain alleles of the gene for IL-2 predispose to ulcerative colitis,[48] but there is no support for any link with the IL-10 gene.[48]

The inflammatory bowel disease genes

IBD1

The first paper putting forward a cogent case for an IBD gene was published in 1996,[49] and since then (in addition to the associations already described to chromosomes 2 and 6) numerous other potential loci have been proposed. The IBD1 locus was identified from a genome-wide scan of European families with multiple affected members, using markers at roughly 13 centimorgan (cM) intervals.[49] The locus, which is near to (probably between) D16S409 and D16S419, has been demonstrated in most of the subsequent studies and in most (but not all) population groups; the conventional requirements for confirmed linkage are established.[50–52] The IBD1 gene lies near to, but is distinct from, functionally pertinent genes such as the IL-4 receptor.[53] In all series, IBD1 is linked to Crohn's disease and much less,[51,54] or not at all,[50] to ulcerative colitis. The magnitude of linkage in Crohn's disease is, however, low. The relative risk to an allele-identical sibling is only 1.46.[54] This locus can only account for a proportion of the overall

increase in Crohn's risk in affected families, perhaps around 12.5 per cent. The phenomenon of epistasis, by which the influence of one susceptibility gene is made more apparent by the congruent expression of another susceptibility gene, has been explored by Cho et al., and lends support not only to IBD1 but also to a locus on chromosome 1p.[50]

IBD2

The systematic genome-wide search in the Oxford sibling pair study supported linkage to IBD1 but also provided the first evidence for IBD2 on chromosome 12,[55] with statistically significant support. This association has been widely confirmed, and in most series the association holds mainly or exclusively for ulcerative colitis.[56,57] The precise location and function of the gene, which lies near to but distinct from that for interferon-gamma (IFN-γ),[58] remain similarly ill-defined to those of IBD1. We have studied the gene for natural resistance-associated macrophage protein 2 because of its location close to the IBD2 locus, but find no clear evidence for linkage.[59]

Putative IBD3

The 150 000-strong Chaldean population in North America represents something of a human Galapagos Island; they are a devout Catholic Iraqi group living in the Detroit area who rarely marry out of their community, and who suffer a high frequency of inflammatory bowel disease. A link to chromosome 1p had been suggested in several of the early genome scans,[50,60] and has been followed using a single nucleotide polymorphism (SNP) approach in the Chaldeans. The link to 1p is confirmed and haplotype analysis has narrowed the proposed locus to around 1 cM.[61] Although technically the 1p site is 'confirmed' for inflammatory bowel disease, this association is an uncommon finding and has been absent from many of the genome scans performed.

Putative IBD4

Genome scanning in North America has identified a potential susceptibility locus on chromosome 14q (at 14q11.2).[62] As this has now been supported by data (placing a link to D14S261 and to the consecutive loci D14S:50/80/49) from two other groups,[63,64] there is some justification for awarding it recognition as *IBD4*. The link appears more particular to Crohn's disease.

Other putative IBD gene sites

Mucin genes have also been studied because of their potential functional significance (see below). Certain polymorphisms of *MUC3* (chromosome 7), which are rare in the general population, are found in the Oxford genome scan[65] positively linked to ulcerative colitis. *MUC1* is overexpressed in diseased but not normal-looking ileal mucosa, and the expression of *MUC3*, *MUC4* and *MUC5b* is more prevalent in Crohn's ileum than in normals.[66]

Evidence in favour of linkage to inflammatory bowel disease has now been suggested for all but three of the chromosomes! The nature of inflammatory bowel disease as a complex polygenic disorder is all too clear. It should also be remembered that the linkages currently described are mostly for regions of up to 40 cM, which leaves room for several hundred potential genes. Nonetheless, the replication of linkages in IBD is generally better than for other polygenic disorders, and the present elucidation of the human genome should make the next steps easier and substantially more rapid.

pANCA

Some years ago, a circulating antibody to a neutrophil cytoplasmic antigen (ANCA) was found in patients with inflammatory bowel disease. It was thought initially to be that identified in systemic vasculitic conditions such as Wegener's granulomatosis, but subsequent work has shown that it is a different antigen, the site of expression in inflammatory bowel disease having a

distinct perinuclear focus – hence pANCA. The most relevant of the several potential antigens detected has remained unclear. Although catalase, alpha-enolase, and lactoferrin are prominent, it does not appear that definition of the antigenic specificities of ANCA is clinically helpful.[67]

There is interest in whether patients with pANCA represent a clinically or biologically distinct subgroup and whether the expression of the antibody is genetically determined. There seem to be links between pANCA positivity and certain HLA subtypes, the DR3, DQ2, TNF-α2 haplotype being particularly strongly associated in the Oxford database.[68] There have been reports of pANCA in healthy first-order relatives of colitics,[69,70] but the Oxford group found no cases of pANCA positivity in family members who did not themselves have an inflammatory condition with which the antibody is associated.[71] It remains possible that expression and familial risk vary between populations, but probable that pANCA is not itself a crucial marker of increased genetic risk.

Antibodies to pANCA are very frequently found in ulcerative colitis, but rarely in patients with Crohn's disease, in whom the rates of detection are similar to those of the relevant control populations. There is a strong association between presence of antibody and concurrent primary sclerosing cholangitis (see Chapter 6). It does not seem likely that the antibody has a directly harmful effect or that neutrophils are activated by the antibody. Expression of the antibody does not seem to reflect disease activity,[72] although some authors find that antibody levels slowly diminish after colectomy. Estève *et al.* join those who predict a reduction in antibody positivity postoperatively, but base this on a comparison of postoperative patients with those who have not needed surgery, thereby neglecting the possibility that pANCA positivity (rather than diminishing because of successful surgery) is a good prognostic marker that indicates the patient who will not need resection.[73] Whether positivity for pANCA is associated with a particular inflammatory bowel disease phenotype remains controversial, apart from the strong link with sclerosing cholangitis; however, more than one group has felt that patients with Crohn's disease and pANCA have more ulcerative colitis-like features than those without. The patients with pANCA in one Crohn's study all had colitis, compared with only just over half of those without the antibody, were less likely to have a positive family history (17 versus 35 per cent), were less likely to have fistulating disease (28 versus 39 per cent), and were less likely to have intestinal obstruction (39 versus 65 per cent) or to need prolonged steroid therapy (1.8 years versus 4.2 years mean duration).[74] Clearly, these factors are not entirely independent and most do not reach statistical significance, but it does seem reasonable to consider that pANCA is a marker for some of the clinical features of Crohn's disease. It is doubtful that there is a causal link.

Intestinal permeability

Intestinal permeability is increased in both Crohn's and ulcerative colitis when the disease is active. The global changes (as measured by excretion of orally administered polyethylene glycol, simple sugars or EDTA) reflect abnormal permeability, predominantly at sites of macroscopic disease.[75] There is an identifiable defect in tight junction function, with associated abnormality of sodium transport, which is not of a secretory nature, but rather the result of profound barrier dysfunction and concurrent malabsorption.[76]

Abnormal permeability could simply reflect the results of tissue damage once inflammation is established, but there is increasing evidence that it occurs earlier and has aetiopathogenic significance. The pioneering study of Hollander and colleagues demonstrated changes not only in patients with Crohn's disease, but also in their healthy relatives,[77] results that were challenged by others in the field, with vigorous objections to the

use of the polyethylene glycol technique for assessing permeability. It is, however, probable that there is a subgroup of healthy relatives in whom permeability is increased, whilst other relatives (or other families) have normal permeability. A dynamic study by Sutherland's group tested this further.[78] Patients with Crohn's disease and their first-degree relatives were compared with controls. Permeability was measured by the widely accepted post-absorption lactulose/mannitol ratio, subjects being studied before and after the administration of two 1.3 g doses of aspirin. Permeability rose between the two study periods by 57 per cent in unrelated controls, but by 110 per cent in healthy relatives, of whom 35 per cent were considered 'hyper-responders'. The relatives were statistically distinguishable from the controls but not from those with Crohn's disease (133 per cent increase). Comparable data were found in a paediatric series, with 20 per cent of healthy relatives demonstrating an exaggerated response to non-steroidal administration.[79]

The majority of patients with Crohn's disease and a subset of their relatives with increased permeability also prove to have an associated phenotypic alteration of circulating B cells, which is absent in controls.[80] The CD45RO isoform appeared almost exclusively and specifically in those with abnormal permeability, but independently of the presence of inflammation, again indicative of a primary role for abnormal permeability. The CD45RO isoform is itself strongly related to the immune response to antigen challenge. It thus seems probable that there is an inherited increase in permeability in some families with Crohn's disease, and that this might be aetiologically relevant. These affected relatives are probably those at especial risk of Crohn's disease if exposed to necessary additional factors. In other words, the increased permeability may be legitimately considered as a genetic risk factor that predisposes to the development of inflammatory bowel disease. Sutherland's group indicate one such possible mechanism, since exposure to quantities of aspirin similar to those used in their study[78] is a common environmental challenge (and one that would not be likely to have been ascertained epidemiologically).

Abnormalities of permeability are generally evident before other manifestations of disease when sequential observation has been performed. In an illustrative study performed in Crohn's patients in remission, a high lactulose/mannitol ratio (indicative of increased permeability) predicted relapse within a year. Relapse occurred in 70 per cent of such patients compared with only 17 per cent of those with an initially normal result ($P < 0.01$).[81]

Cell adhesion molecules, growth factors and mucins

At the cellular level, in addition to information on tight junctions, there is an increasing literature based around the cell adhesion molecules. These molecules have a key role in the normal behaviour of cells in relation to their neighbours, whether of the same or distinct morphological type. Understandably, much of the early interest focused on issues of oncogenesis and metastasis,[82] but the cell adhesion molecules are also pertinent to the development of inflammation, to abnormalities of permeability and to mucosal repair in inflammatory bowel disease. They may be considered in two main groups: the vascular and the epithelial adhesion molecules. There is clear overlap with the function of a number of the growth factors and much interaction with cytokines and chemokines. It is probable that current interpretations are over-simplified.

Vascular cell adhesion molecules

Migration of circulating leucocytes into intestinal tissues is clearly an important component of the inflammatory response and leads to some of the pathological changes recognized in inflammatory bowel disease. Leucocyte immigration is preceded by 'rolling' and subsequent adhesion – both governed to a large extent by the endothelial cell adhesion molecules. Bacteria also can make use of cell adhesion molecule receptors to gain access to mammalian cells, the particular case of *Yersinia* and its postulated entry via Peyer's patches using its invasin protein to bind to integrins[83] being of interest, given the similarities between some forms of yersiniosis and Crohn's disease (see Chapter 2).

The vascular cell adhesion molecule (VCAM-1) has a role in leucocyte adherence (predominantly of monocytes) to the endothelial luminal surface, but although it is constitutively expressed in the colonic vasculature, there has been disagreement as to whether there are alterations in its expression in patients with inflammatory bowel disease relative to controls.[84,85] It is probable that it is increased, but perhaps only after the development of inflammation;[86] there appears to be a positive association with disease activity.[84]

The endothelial leucocyte adhesion molecule (ELAM-1), which is normally absent from colonic endothelium, is consistently found in the vessels of inflamed tissues in both ulcerative colitis and Crohn's disease, and within neutrophils in crypt abscesses.[83] There is a probable positive correlation with sites of free radical damage (see below).

The intercellular adhesion molecule (ICAM-1), which promotes the initial T cell–macrophage interaction, also is significantly elevated in active inflammatory bowel disease, and behaves in parallel with more traditional markers of inflammation such as C-reactive protein (CRP) and orosomucoid.[84,85] Work combining inflammatory bowel disease tissues with an endothelial cell line confirms the link with ICAM-1, and adds comparable data implicating E-selectin.[87] This study also claims a significant difference in this over-expression between Crohn's disease and ulcerative colitis, with much greater levels of the adhesion molecules in Crohn's despite apparently similar degrees of inflammation histologically.

P-selectin (also known as CD62), which, like

the other selectins, binds to carbohydrate ligands rather than to other proteins, is also over-expressed in the vessels of both forms of inflammatory bowel disease when active.[88] Perhaps more important, however, is the observation that it is also focally over-expressed in tissues from patients in remission. *In vitro* work has also suggested that these molecules may have a role in the evolution of the granuloma.[89]

Vascular endothelial growth factor is increased in serum in inflammatory bowel disease (at higher levels in Crohn's disease than ulcerative colitis),[90] and probably comes at least in part from the peripheral blood mononuclear cell at times of inflammation (but not when disease is quiescent).[91]

Epithelial cell adhesion molecules

E-cadherin, which is expressed predominantly at the adherens junction, is probably the most important of the epithelial cell adhesion molecules, in its own right and through key interactions with the catenins and related mediators such as the p120 protein. There is loss of E-cadherin, alpha-catenin and p120 expression at sites of ulceration in ulcerative colitis and in many ulcerated Crohn's disease samples.[92] These observations imply not so much a causative role but a potentially important contribution to the facilitation of cell migration once ulceration has occurred. An interesting study in which a mutated colorectal carcinoma cell line failed to express normal levels of E-cadherin and concurrently demonstrated features suggestive of a colitic phenotype raises the possibility that abnormalities of E-cadherin may also have an aetiological role.[93] Our own recent work has focused on syndecan-1 which is an epithelial adhesion molecule expressed somewhat more diffusely than E-cadherin, with an important role in adhesion not only between adjacent epithelial cells but also between the epithelium and the underlying basement membrane. Syndecan-1 is grossly deficient in reparative epithelium in

inflammatory bowel disease; whilst this may be helpful in facilitating cell motility (as suggested for E-cadherin), the trimolecular interaction between basic fibroblast growth factor, syndecan and the growth factor receptor – needed for tissue restitution – is interrupted and is likely to be defective *in vivo*.[94]

There is also an intriguing chimeric murine model in which there is a mutant N-cadherin.[95] Wild-type N-cadherin is normally present in the healthy intestine, but when mutant N-cadherin is expressed along the crypt–villus axis, a transmural inflammation, with many features common to Crohn's disease, occurs. Abnormal expression of this cadherin in the crypts was also found to be associated with abnormal proliferation and adenoma formation, suggesting a possible link between a cell adhesion defect associated with inflammation and the increased risk of neoplasia in inflammatory bowel disease (see Chapter 8).

Mucus and mucins

There are deficiencies and abnormalities of the intestinal mucus layer in ulcerative colitis[96] and associated abnormality of the mucus glycoproteins, with evidence in both colitis and Crohn's disease that there may be deranged restitution of damaged mucosa, perhaps mediated by defects in normal functioning of transforming growth factor beta (TGF-β), intestinal trefoil peptide, or transglutamase.[97] The colonocyte is known to be partially dependent on short-chain fatty acids, and it appears that there are reductions in both availability and utilization of butyrate in active ulcerative colitis, and, moreover, that butyrate exposure and mucin production are directly linked.[98] It is probable that the mucus loss in active colitis is the result of faecal mucinase activity,[99] given differences in levels in stools from patients with ulcerative colitis and from those in Crohn's disease patients and normal controls. The links between smoking and inflammatory bowel disease also implicate mucins (see below).

Neutrophil dysfunction and antibody to *Saccharomyces cerevisiae* antigen

There are at least two human conditions in which a disorder of neutrophil function coexists with some features of Crohn's disease. In chronic granulomatous disease (CGD) the classic presentation with excess infections is most often accompanied by steroid-responsive inflammatory, ulcerative or stenotic disease of various parts of the gastrointestinal tract.[100] In CGD, there is a mutation of the gene for NADPH oxidase on the X chromosome. This causes an inability of the affected individual's neutrophils and macrophages to kill phagocytosed bacteria; the consequent infective morbidity is readily understood. In glycogen storage disease type 1b, excess infections are key features of the clinical presentation, but gastrointestinal manifestations are, again, well-established corollary features, and include ileitis, colitis and perianal disease. The underlying molecular defect is responsible for impaired mobility of, and reduced absolute numbers of, neutrophils.[101] A similar defect of chemotaxis exists in Crohn's disease,[102] perhaps because of a circulating inhibitor.[103]

Antibody to *Saccharomyces cerevisiae* antigen (ASCA) is present in a majority of patients with Crohn's disease (and a minority with ulcerative colitis) and it has been suggested that it may have pathogenic significance. The epitope is probably an oligomannan (a mannose polymer) of cell walls, and may itself inhibit neutrophil function and provoke granuloma formation via the inhibition of normal bacterial killing and clearance.[104] Most of the research effort with ASCA has been devoted to its potential role as a diagnostic marker (see Chapter 2), which is a shame given this intriguing insight into its potential pathogenicity.

VASCULAR AETIOLOGIES AND PLATELETS

Speculation that Crohn's disease is of primarily vascular origin, arising via multifocal but microscopic infarction of the relevant areas of intestine, remains controversial,[105] there being equivalent data supporting a primary defect affecting the lymphatic endothelium[106] and the considerable difficulties in distinguishing vascular from lymphatic endothelium. The granulomas characteristic of Crohn's disease do at least appear associated with vascular structures. In a study of 485 granulomas from the tissues of 15 patients, 85 per cent were intimately associated with vascular injury, suggesting that abnormality of the intestinal microvasculature plays an early (if not necessarily causative) role in the pathogenesis of Crohn's disease.[107] It does not appear that any such vasculitis is mediated in an autoimmune fashion, since even when vasculitis is demonstrable histologically there is little evidence of a humoral immune response.[108]

There is also evidence for platelets having more than an incidental role.[109] There is usually a degree of thrombocytosis in active inflammatory bowel disease, with enhanced platelet aggregation and expression of platelet surface markers, including P-selectin and GP53. There is increased release of inflammatory mediators and other intracellular proteins into the plasma.[109] In an interesting peroperative study, it has been demonstrated that as blood passes from mesenteric artery to vein there is the expected loss of neutrophils into the tissues in both ulcerative colitis and Crohn's disease,[110] but that in Crohn's there is also a substantial increase in platelet aggregation as blood crosses the mesenteric capillary bed. This all suggests that platelets can contribute to microinfarction and local inflammation, and also presents the possibility that they may be a major influence on vascular events distant from the gut (see Chapter 7).

Platelet-activating factor (PAF), which is found in high concentration in mucosal biopsies in both Crohn's disease and ulcerative colitis, may be integral to these effects. It has a pro-inflammatory effect on other cells, is a potent stimulator of intestinal secretion, and is responsible for a secretory response in cultured mucosal biopsies.[111] Whether this is important in contributing to diarrhoea *in vivo* remains to be clarified, but there is good evidence that faecal PAF levels correlate well with other markers of disease activity.[112]

The marginal artery and ulcerative colitis

The striking demarcation of the upper limit of ulcerative colitis (see Chapter 2) might suggest a vascular explanation. In a small study, still not replicated in other centres, *in vitro* angiography and detailed pathological examination of colitis resection specimens indicated that the point of demarcation was coincident with the proximal extent of the marginal artery – a normally small branch of the inferior mesenteric artery.[113] The observation as it stands is impressive, but it is difficult to conceptualize why this 'additional' blood supply should predispose to colitis, and difficult to understand how initially distal colitis can spread to involve more proximal sites (see Chapter 2), given the embryological determination of the extent of the marginal artery, unless the vascular status merely defines the maximum possible extent of disease.

INFECTION AS THE CAUSE OF INFLAMMATORY BOWEL DISEASE

Introduction

For many years, and arguably for the entire history of recognized Crohn's disease, infective aetiologies have been sought, and postulated pathogenic organisms promulgated. Mycobacteria were first suspected even before the work of Crohn and his colleagues. Before considering individual organisms, however, it may be instructive to explore the epidemiological pointers. Inflammatory bowel disease remains relatively rare in the developing world (see above), even when allowance is made for underdiagnosis. An intriguing three-centre study performed in the UK[114] examined the childhood socioeconomic circumstances of patients with inflammatory bowel disease in comparison with controls matched by age, sex and general practice registration. Access to hot running water and a separate bathroom in the first 5 years of life were associated with greatly *increased* risk of Crohn's disease (relative risks after correction for social class of 5.0 and 3.3, respectively), but not of ulcerative colitis. This is presumably not a causal association but might be taken to suggest that protection from 'ordinary' environmental organisms in early childhood renders some individuals more prone to Crohn's disease in later life. Countries with a high mortality from childhood diarrhoeal illnesses consistently have a low frequency of inflammatory bowel disease. An untestable supplementary assertion may be constructed that endemic gastrointestinal infection kills those who would otherwise go on to develop inflammatory bowel disease.[115] It is hypothesized that helminth infestation is especially protective. As helminths provoke a Th2 response, this should be most pertinent to Crohn's disease, as is partially supported by data from two mouse models in which infection with *Heligmosomoides polygyrus* and *Trichuris muris* appears to ameliorate inflammation.[116] Parallel studies in the respiratory field have confirmed that atopic disease is less frequent in people heavily exposed to orofaecal and foodborne microbes. In a retrospective case–control study of 240 atopic military recruits, serological surrogate markers were used for childhood hygiene and orofaecal/foodborne transmission. There was significantly less evidence for prior infection with these organisms in the atopic group, whereas past infection with organisms thought independent of socioeconomic status was similar to that in controls.[117] The semi-sterile modern diet is implicated by a postulated influence on the gut microflora and thence on the gut-associated lymphoid tissue. The 'unhygienic' traditional diet is thought protective by providing regular daily stimulation of the mucosal immune system, or by favouring gut colonization and high turnover of commensals such as enterobacteria and *Lactobacillus*, but no data on these aspects exist at present.[117] Ulcerative colitis and atopic disease are strongly positively correlated (more than double the rates in controls),[118] and it may not be unreasonable to extrapolate directly from atopy in general to inflammatory bowel disease in particular. It does seem to be the case, nonetheless, that the prevailing gut flora is of profound importance (see below).

An interesting study from Guinea-Bissau may provide part of the explanation for the link between infection and inflammatory bowel disease.[119] The study was of adults, and hinges on documentation of measles infections during an epidemic in their childhood; it is accordingly subject to some reservations. Nevertheless, atopy (skin-prick positive) proved almost twice as common in those who had been vaccinated and avoided infection in 1979, compared with their unvaccinated compatriots who developed measles (25.6 per cent versus 12.8 per cent). The difference remained significant when corrected for such factors as breast-feeding. If childhood measles infection can in some way prevent development of atopy, then it seems very reasonable to suppose that it might have other long-term immunological effects. Equally, there is no reason that this response (or responses) should be unique to measles amongst putative pathogens. Measles is considered further below.

Independently of a true role in aetiology, infective organisms may act as triggers for relapses of inflammatory bowel disease: this is certainly many patients' experience. Particular organisms loosely associated with this phenomenon include *Clostridium difficile*, *Campylobacter* species and toxigenic *Escherichia coli*. There is no reliable evidence that what is being described is any more than a more severe clinical manifestation of an otherwise mild gastrointestinal infection in a patient with an underlying inflammatory bowel disease. Infection may aggravate an underlying mucosal barrier defect (see above), and thereby promote disease in a situation in which the normal individual would be protected. It is striking that when injury, ischaemia or severe inflammation leads to perforation of the intestinal wall, profound adverse consequences follow, with, at the very least, the formation of a circumscribed intra-abdominal abscess, if not frank peritonitis and septicaemia. These life-threatening illnesses are, however, caused by organisms that belong to the normal gut flora and which are benign or actively beneficial when in their correct location. It is not surprising that the intestinal mucosa is well equipped to *contain* such potential pathogens but it is a little remarkable that normally no inflammatory response is demonstrable.

Tolerance to the resident intestinal flora therefore exists normally, but is broken in active inflammatory bowel disease. This important phenomenon has been carefully studied by a leading German group.[120] The immune response to endogenous microflora was examined in peripheral blood, in inflamed and in non-inflamed mucosa. They demonstrated that lamina propria mononuclear cells (LPMC) from inflamed areas of intestine actively proliferated after co-culture with sonicates of bacteria from that person's gut. Peripheral blood mononuclear cells (PBMC) or LPMC from the non-inflamed gut of the same patient, and PBMC and LPMC from controls did not. This effect was apparently antigen driven (as it was inhibited by anti-MHC class 2 antibody). Proliferation could, however, be induced by using bacterial sonicates from other human subjects. In other words, there is selective tolerance to autologous intestinal flora (but not heterologous intestinal flora), and this tolerance is lost in intestinal inflammation. This provides a potential mechanism for the perpetuation of idiopathic inflammatory bowel disease.

Specific organisms in inflammatory bowel disease aetiology

There are a small number of specific organisms and a rather larger number of pathogen groups that have been seriously proposed as the cause of Crohn's disease and, to a lesser extent, of ulcerative colitis. Each has its protagonists, and it remains the area above all others that has led inflammatory bowel disease research workers to follow faith rather than science. This is unfortunate, as there are still debates based on opinion rather than fact that have conspired to delay a fuller understanding of the pathogenesis of these diseases. The evidence in favour of the specific candidate organisms is incomplete and in each case falls short of fulfilling Koch's postulates.

Mycobacterium paratuberculosis *and* Avium intracellulare *complex*

Mycobacterium paratuberculosis is causatively associated with a granulomatous disease of cattle – Johne's disease – which shares a number of features with Crohn's disease. Avium infections are well recognized in the severely immunocompromised (particularly in HIV infection). These organisms are relatively ubiquitous in the human environment, and are both present in cows' milk and prone to survive pasteurization as currently practised. There was early evidence that *M. paratuberculosis* was to be found in intestine from Crohn's disease patients, with only occasional intact bacteria but bacterial antigens or DNA present in around 65 per cent of samples studied, compared with frequencies of well under 20 per cent in control tissues (including those from ulcerative colitis patients and normals).[121] In distinction

from Johne's disease, there was usually no associated inflammatory response at the sites of these antigens. Immediately, concerns were expressed that polymerase chain reaction (PCR) assay techniques had been responsible for some false positives. No series has been able to demonstrate anything near to a 100 per cent association in well-documented Crohn's disease, and there was a maximum frequency of detection of DNA even at the sites of granulomata of under 15 per cent in one positive study.[122] Although these observations have been supported by reports from several centres, careful use of more modern technology, which is both more sensitive and more specific, mostly fails to demonstrate a different prevalence of detection of the organism in Crohn's disease from that in other patient groups. The Leeds study used oligonucleotide primers to the species-specific *M. paratuberculosis* IS*900* DNA insertion element with PCR on intestinal tissue DNA extracts. The method was considered capable of detecting one to two mycobacterial genomes. Tissue from 68 patients with Crohn's, 49 with ulcerative colitis, and 26 non-inflammatory bowel disease controls was studied. In no inflammatory bowel disease case was *M. paratuberculosis* detected.[123] Several immunocytochemistry studies have now failed to find mycobacterial antigens in diseased tissues and there are four other negative PCR studies. Numerous serological studies have failed to demonstrate antibody to *M. paratuberculosis* and attempts to show cell-mediated immunity are also unrewarding. Inoculation of experimental animals with Crohn's disease tissue has failed to induce Johne's disease, and inoculation of animals with *M. paratuberculosis* fails to cause Crohn's disease (or indeed Johne's disease in most species). Only the Texas group seem still to be persuaded by a positive association with the p65 heat-shock protein and a p36 antigen.[124] Although Johne's disease is common in farm animals, and infected animals shed *M. paratuberculosis* in large numbers, no record of zoonotic transmission to man has been recorded. There is no substantial body of epidemiological evidence favouring a higher frequency of Crohn's disease in those particularly closely exposed to *M. paratuberculosis*; indeed, rather the opposite, given the lower incidence in farmers,[125] and the comparative incidence of Crohn's disease in the developed and underdeveloped world. The question of antibiotic therapy in inflammatory bowel disease is discussed further in Chapter 3, but the general failure of antimycobacterial regimens to help in Crohn's disease and the generally positive effects of corticosteroids also argue against the case for continuing infection with *M. paratuberculosis*. Two relatively recent literature reviews have concluded firmly that the evidence is insufficient to implicate mycobacteria in the causation of Crohn's disease.[126,127]

Measles

A number of human diseases have been linked to persistent infection with paramyxoviruses, of which subacute sclerosing panencephalitis is now very firmly associated with prior measles infection. Although, until the advent of immunization, acute measles infection was virtually the rule in childhood, preliminary epidemiological evidence and the observation of putative viral particles in tissues from Crohn's disease patients prompted further exploration of measles as a causative agent. Clinical support is arguably lent by the occurrence of oral aphthous ulcers (and vasculitis) in both acute measles and Crohn's disease. Measles antigens were detected in Crohn's disease tissues by an immunogold technique, supporting the view that the virus may persist in the intestine after acute infection.[128] Low levels of antigen were also found in ileocaecal tuberculosis, leaving open the possibility that persistently infected immune cells aggregate in foci of inflammation without necessarily having a causal association. It is also possible that the (immune) patient with intestinal disease who is re-exposed to measles is not able to prevent uptake of the virus into the inflamed tissues,

though obviously able to mount an immunological response sufficient to avoid a recurrence of measles. Comparable studies in other laboratories have mostly failed to lend support to a specific involvement of measles virus, however, and Haga *et al.* were unable to demonstrate any evidence of genetic material from measles, mumps, or rubella viruses in intestinal resections from patients with Crohn's or ulcerative colitis, or in controls without inflammatory bowel disease,[129] a failure now replicated by a more recent study from the Royal Free group who first described it.[130]

There are interesting epidemiological links between perinatal measles infection and the subsequent development of Crohn's disease, with infants born during epidemics being almost 1.5 times more likely to develop Crohn's disease within 30 years than those born in non-epidemic periods.[131] The four (of 25 000) pregnancies complicated by clinically diagnosed measles in Uppsala between 1940 and 1949 prove especially striking. Of the offspring of these four women, no fewer than three have required multiple resections for severe Crohn's disease.[132] Interestingly, the fourth child, without Crohn's disease, was the only one of the four to have suffered clinical measles. The dramatic reductions in clinical measles infections in developed and developing countries have not, however, been associated with a reduction in the incidence of Crohn's disease – rather the converse, a phenomenon perhaps even exaggerated by the administration of measles vaccination.[133] The proposed explanations require that the timing of exposure to measles virus or its antigens is crucial, and it is plausible that some of those who previously died of overwhelming measles infection and now survive (because of improved social circumstances or vaccination) are those who now go on to develop Crohn's disease. The UK 1970 prospective birth cohort study yields information on a number of viral and bacterial infections.[134] If measles and mumps occurred before the age of 7 and (crucially) within 1 year of each other, the risk of Crohn's disease and of ulcerative colitis was increased more than sixfold; sequential infections in the first 3 years of life predisposed to Crohn's, whereas those around the age of 6 were more likely to develop ulcerative colitis. An almost unbelievable 96 per cent of subjects for whom both infections were recorded in the same 12-month period were subsequently reported to have inflammatory bowel disease.[134] Wakefield's group suggested that the combined measles, mumps and rubella (MMR) vaccine also was strongly implicated. There are important questions still to be answered in respect of ulcerative colitis, linked to measles and rubella, but without a comparable rationalizing hypothesis, and with possible linkage between influenza epidemics and later inflammatory bowel disease. The position has not been made less controversial by the discovery that a variant form of autism in which the normally developing child regresses to an autistic state is associated with chronic enterocolitis.[135] There is little doubt that there are objective histological changes in the intestine of these children; an hypothesis that this also is causally related to the MMR vaccine is under scrutiny.

Unsurprisingly, given the implications for national immunization programmes, this topic has engendered vigorous controversy, with reviews by government-appointed panels in the UK and USA. The Working Party appointed by the UK Committee on Safety of Medicines published its conclusions in June 1999,[136] and pulled no punches in declaring the MMR vaccine to be safe. It is true that there was no clear 'step' in the incidence of inflammatory bowel disease associated with the introduction of MMR into the UK in 1988,[137] but the epidemiology is greatly confused by the 'catch-up' campaign in which children too old to have received the vaccine at the normal age (13–15 months) received it at older ages (usually 4 years). It is difficult to feel entirely comfortable about MMR vaccination in this context, and the Japanese strategy of administering each component of the vaccine separately may just be logical until we have better data, since it is very clear that there are substantial risks to the population from losing ground in immunization uptake.

Other specific organisms of possible causal association

Listeria

Listeriosis antigens are over-represented in Crohn's tissues, with expression in 75 per cent of 16 patients, particularly at sites of ulceration and inflammation, in comparison with only 13 per cent of colitics and in no controls.[138] *Listeria monocytogenes*, like *M. paratuberculosis*, is ubiquitous in the environment, is known to invade intestinal M cells and can produce an experimental ileocolitis in which it is found to be an intracellular pathogen. The fact that the very same study records similar data for *E. coli* and streptococci (57 per cent and 44 per cent positive, respectively) weakens the case for a true aetiological link, but rather confirms that the (already) abnormal intestine is excessively permeable to, or poor at eliminating, a range of microbial antigens.[139] Greater significance might be drawn from the absence of other putative pathogens such as the measles virus. Corroborative data remain absent.[140,141]

Enteropathic E. coli

Since the excitement in the late 1950s when cross-reaction between a circulating antibody and the colon was demonstrated in ulcerative colitis,[142] and the subsequent demonstration of an *E. coli* antigen that is shared by colonic mucosa,[143] there has been a quest for evidence of destructive autoimmunity. This has been relatively unproductive as these antibodies are not specific for inflammatory bowel disease, and are not themselves cytopathic. It seems probable that this is not an important mechanism. There is, however, now evidence from studies of ileal mucosa of patients with Crohn's disease that adherent and invasive (enteropathic) *E. coli* are associated with the disease. Adherent *E. coli* were found in 65 per cent of ileal resections and in all biopsies taken from sites of postoperative recurrence.[144] An abstract from the same group indicates that the bacteria found have invasive properties in a cell culture model.[145] This is yet to be supported by work from other centres which, to date, although confirming the presence of these organisms, show no evidence of an invasive or pathogenic effect in human disease.[141,146]

Helicobacter *species*

Murine *Helicobacter* species have been implicated in colitis,[147] and there is now also some evidence that the cotton-top tamarin (see below) may develop colitis in conjunction with *Helicobacter* infection.[148] These are distinct from *H. pylori* and had not been considered to cause human disease. Fox's group in particular is taking an active role in this area and it will probably soon become clear whether this is important in inflammatory bowel disease.

Cytomegalovirus

There have been suggestions that cytomegalovirus (CMV) infection is pathogenic in ulcerative colitis, but most recent data have tended to allocate it a bystander role of uncertain or no significance even when virus is demonstrable in tissue from patients with colitis. There is no doubt, however, that CMV infection can lead to exacerbation of inflammatory bowel disease, and there is now evidence that failure of its eradication may be an important contributing factor to an inability to achieve remission in some colitic patients.[149,150] It is probably also the case that CMV exposure is more likely to provoke gastrointestinal manifestations in the immunocompetent individual if there is concurrent ulcerative colitis.[151]

Helminths

Infestation with helminths has been suggested to be protective (see above) but there are also interesting Crohn's-like features in human infection with the fish parasite *Anisakis*, which is responsible for a granulomatous reaction in the ileocaecal region when it affects the intestine. In a serum-based study, 29 per cent of Spanish patients with Crohn's disease had antibodies to the parasite.[152] This was more likely to be IgA antibody, and at higher concentrations, in patients with active disease, suggesting that this is a response to rather than a cause of disease. As *Angiostrongylus* – another helminth – also causes a condition similar to Crohn's disease,[153] a closer investigation of patients with primary infestations may be fruitful.

Hydrogen sulphide-producing bacteria

Many inflammatory bowel disease patients describe offensive flatus and it is generally the case that sulphur-containing gases are responsible. It is difficult to perform objective studies of flatus for obvious reasons,[154] but data do exist, and Levine *et al.*[155] have examined gas production in sealed samples of faeces, demonstrating striking differences between control and colitic stools, the latter producing up to four times as much hydrogen sulphide (but no differences in other metabolites studied). Hydrogen sulphide is not only unpleasant, it is also toxic, with an effect on mice not dissimilar to equimolar amounts of cyanide. It is possible that excess luminal sulphide overwhelms a genetically determined capacity for mucosal detoxification, with consequent impaired butyrate oxidation and the initiation of colitis.[156] There is evidence that patients with colitis have increased serum levels of thiol methyltransferase,[157] which may represent a response to such a series of effects in the colon. However, the same group have been unable to confirm that counts or carriage rates of sulphur-reducing bacteria in patients with ulcerative colitis are different from those in controls, leaving a role for hydrogen sulphide as a casual metabolic toxin at the circumstantial level.[158]

Other pathogenic organisms

There is evidence for a humoral immune response to a number of other intestinal organisms, with significant levels of circulating antibodies to a variety of antigens. Purified subcellular bacterial components such as lipopolysaccharide and peptidoglycan polysaccharide can produce intestinal inflammation (sometimes with an associated systemic reaction). A reproducible granulomatous enterocolitis can be provoked by intramural injection of streptococcal cell wall fragments into rat intestine. This persists to give chronic inflammation and is associated with mesenteric and lymph node disease in nearly half of the challenged animals.[159]

Normal gastrointestinal flora in pathogenesis of inflammatory bowel disease

It is probable that the link between micro-organisms and Crohn's disease reflects a dysregulated host immune response to ubiquitous normal intestinal flora or to not especially damaging pathogens. A failure of normal tolerance has already been referred to, and the sites most commonly involved (terminal ileum, caecum and left colon) are also those at which concentrations of micro-organisms tend to be maximal in the normal individual. Many measures that reduce intestinal microflora (such as gut lavage, intestinal bypass, creation of ileostomy, exclusive elemental or parenteral nutrition, antibiotic regimens) may also produce therapeutic benefit (see Chapters 3 and 4). This has been explored further by D'Haens et al.[160] They studied the effect of autologous intestinal fluids instilled into surgically excluded ileum in three patients with Crohn's disease who had undergone a 'curative' ileocolonic resection with an ileocolonic anastomosis and an upstream diverting loop ileostomy. Contact with intestinal fluids for as little as 8 days induced infiltration of mononuclear cells, eosinophils and polymorphonuclear cells into the lamina propria, small vessels and epithelium in excluded neoterminal ileum

that was previously normal. Epithelial HLA-DR expression increased, and mononuclear cells expressed activation markers. There was evidence of epithelioid transformation and transendothelial lymphocyte recruitment, associated with consistent ultrastructural changes. It seems a reasonable conclusion that normal intestinal contents can trigger postoperative recurrence of Crohn's disease in the terminal ileum proximal to an ileocolonic anastomosis. This expands on the German data already referred to,[120] as here the contact with intestinal fluid (and presumably flora) precedes the existence of overt inflammation.

MODELS OF INFLAMMATORY BOWEL DISEASE

There are many models of inflammatory bowel disease, each of which has its own strengths and weaknesses. A very comprehensive review (139 references) has recently been published by Wirtz and Neurath, to which the interested reader is referred.[161]

Few animals get spontaneous inflammatory bowel disease, but an endangered monkey, the cotton-top tamarin, and a particular mouse strain (C3H/HeJBir) are exceptions. The tamarin (*Saguinus oedipus*) develops a colitis which has much in common with ulcerative colitis, including the propensity for colorectal carcinoma; the disease mainly affects animals held in captivity. The tamarin has only a single class I MHC locus, and it is thought that this predisposes both to the risk of colitis and to a high incidence of viral infections in these animals. The C3H/HeJBir mouse develops a proximal patchy colitis with a prominent Th1 response akin to Crohn's disease. The colitis appears to be dependent on exposure to normal gut flora.

There is a burgeoning family of genetically engineered models, in which a mutated or inactivated gene leads to expression of an inflammatory bowel disease phenotype. Probably best known are the IL-2 knock-out mouse, which develops a condition similar to ulcerative colitis, and the IL-10 knock-out mouse and the HLA-B27 transgenic rat which exhibit features more like Crohn's disease. There are now at least five transgenic mouse models, and a further seven knock-out mouse models, each of which is reviewed by Wirtz and Neurath.[161] In each case there are high-level demands placed on standards of animal husbandry, and in almost every example the animal will be protected wholly or partially from inflammation if raised in a germ-free environment. The only definite exception to this rule is the $G_{i\alpha}2$-deficient mouse in which there is no amelioration of the colitis in germ-free conditions. $G_{i\alpha}2$ is a G protein involved in the adenylate cyclase-regulated signal transduction of numerous cell types (including intestinal epithelia); deficient mice suffer a condition similar to ulcerative colitis and may progress to colorectal adenocarcinoma. Potentially relevant mechanisms suggested above for the human diseases are supported by the observation that genetically determined disorders of trefoil factor and cadherin function are associated with colitis in animal models. Interestingly, available models tangentially implicate infection by cytomegalovirus (the STAT-4 transgenic mouse) and herpes simplex virus (the HSV tyrosine kinase transgenic mouse) in the pathogenesis of inflammatory bowel disease. Another interesting hint comes from a case report of a patient with X-linked agammaglobulinaemia, who required ileal resection for stenosing chronic granulomatous ileitis,[162] itself associated with enterovirus infection.

Adoptive transfer models employ the selective transfer of certain cell types to an immunocompromised animal model (usually the severe combined immunodeficiency SCID mouse). They have confirmed (*inter alia*) the importance of T cells in the immune dysregulation of inflammatory bowel disease, and point to relevance of the heat-shock proteins in colitis and Crohn's. The heat-shock proteins provide a link to the mycobacterial hypothesis as these are antigens of both mycobacteria and man, in whom they are identified with autoimmune phenomena and yet occur at high level in antigen-presenting cells of the colonic mucosa.[163] Adoptive transfer experiments have also implicated TGF-α in Crohn's disease. This is, broadly speaking, an anti-inflammatory cytokine, but it also promotes fibrosis. Its expression is increased in inflammatory bowel disease lamina propria. TGF-β subtypes 1 and 3 and their receptors are upregulated in the lamina propria in Crohn's disease.[164]

The older animal models, whether chemical, hapten-based, or from physical insult, are much simpler but generally less satisfactory, as they tend to induce a short-term, self-limiting disease lacking the chronic self-perpetuating nature that defines spontaneous inflammatory bowel disease. It is striking that, even in these models, the endogenous bacterial flora is sometimes needed for the initiation of disease and always for its perpetuation.

Anastomotic recurrence as an aetiological model for Crohn's disease

Post-resection relapse in Crohn's disease affects up to 100 per cent on endoscopic criteria by 3–5 years postoperatively, with up to 40 per cent affected by symptomatic relapse over the same time period (see Chapters 2 and 4). Relapse is much rarer if a terminal ileostomy is performed (< 20 per cent), but if continuity is then restored, relapse is frequent and usually occurs at or just above the anastomosis. Recurrence typically affects the neoterminal ileum rather than the previously defunctioned bowel distal to the anastomosis, as might appear more intuitively obvious. Rutgeerts *et al.* suggested that reflux of the faecal stream was crucial to this phenomenon,[165] but their more recent work (alluded to above) indicates that antegrade contact between intestinal contents and ileum in continuity with the lower bowel is sufficient.[160]

The importance of the faecal stream was addressed in a study of patients with Crohn's disease undergoing faecal diversion or (different patients) having continuity restored, in comparison with those without Crohn's having the same procedures.[166] Faecal diversion, as expected, produced improvement in the activity of Crohn's disease. This was associated with a fall in rectal mucosal glycoprotein synthesis and maintenance of the pre-operative levels of rectal crypt cell production, and significant *deterioration* of the macroscopic and microscopic appearance of the rectum. In the control patients having faecal diversion (mostly for cancer, non-Crohn's-related fistula, or incontinence), however, rectal crypt cell production rate fell, and rectal mucosal glycoprotein synthesis was maintained postoperatively, with no deterioration in rectal appearance. Following restoration of continuity, mucosal glycoprotein synthesis and crypt cell proliferation then rose. In Crohn's disease, mucosal synthesis and proliferation rose, but not significantly so, following restoration of continuity. These observations do not explain the pattern of recurrence, but indicate that the distal defunctioned bowel continues to behave abnormally even when global evidence of inflammation is absent or quiescent. They provide important clues as to why diversion colitis (see Chapter 4) is over-represented in Crohn's disease, and further support for the view that the distal bowel is vulnerable to deprivation of luminal nutrients or trophic factors (short-chain fatty acids being particularly implicated).

Other suggestions to explain the predominance of the neoterminal site of recurrence include mechanical or neurovascular impediments imposed by the surgery itself, but why these influences should apply to the bowel in continuity and not to the arguably more pathological end-ileostomy is difficult to conceptualize. Some light may be shed in this area by a curious epidemiological observation. Meckel's diverticulum – a relic of vitelline duct embryology – is found in 0.6–3.0 per cent of Caucasian populations, depending on how the data are collected. In a study of 294 patients having their first resection for Crohn's disease, we found a 5.8 per cent prevalence of these diverticula.[167] Their presence was not associated with heterotopic, acid-secreting mucosa, and they are not obviously pathogenic in any conventional sense, but we have speculated that they may mark zones of local alteration in gastrointestinal permeability or immune reactivity, and they do, of course, lie in the high-risk area of distal ileum most affected by Crohn's disease. It is feasible that surgical re-anastomosis, as opposed to an exteriorized ileostomy, behaves in some degree like a Meckel's diverticulum and influences the expression of recurrent Crohn's disease in a comparable but exaggerated fashion.

The ileoanal pouch as a model for ulcerative colitis

The rationale for, and clinical aspects of, creation of the ileoanal pouch for patients with ulcerative colitis are discussed in Chapter 4, but its inflammatory complication – 'pouchitis' – deserves attention here as it represents a fascinating and unique disease model for ulcerative colitis itself. The pouch has, intentionally, a marked degree of luminal stasis, and consequently an altered exposure to bacterial flora, bile acids and other potential inflammatory mediators, which are relatively foreign to the small bowel from which it is formed. The pouch quite rapidly takes on a number of colonic features with colonic metaplasia of the mucosa (see Chapter 4). All these elements are common to the pouch for colitis and that performed for familial adenomatous polyposis, for which the surgical procedure is identical. Pouchitis, however, occurs at some time in around 20 per cent of patients who previously had ulcerative colitis, but hardly ever in patients having the operation for familial polyposis. The histological (and endoscopic) features of pouchitis have much in common with ulcerative colitis, and earlier thoughts that pouchitis was always the result of re-emergent (previously misdiagnosed) Crohn's disease have now been dismissed. The dispropor-tionate coexistence of extra-intestinal manifesta-tions of inflammatory bowel disease and pouchitis[168] suggests a systemic link and (as with the absence of pouchitis in polyposis patients) that the exposure of the ileum in the pouch to unfamiliar content is not an adequate explanation. It may be worth noting here the evidence for abnormalities of small intestinal permeability in a majority of patients with ulcerative colitis[169] – ulcerative colitis begins to appear a more diffuse intestinal or systemic disorder than is convention-ally accepted. Study of unselected patients after pouch creation should help to determine the factors that lead to pouchitis and perhaps those that predispose to colitis in the first place.

IMMUNOGLOBULINS IN INFLAMMATORY BOWEL DISEASE

The principal immunoglobulin in the normal intestine is IgA, but in inflammatory bowel disease there is increased production of IgG (especially IgG1). The antigens provoking this change in anti-body profile are becoming better understood, with recent evidence from the King's group suggesting, at least in Crohn's disease, that much of the exag-gerated mucosal response is directed against non-pathogenic faecal bacteria.[170] The implied breakdown in tolerance to normal commensal gut flora is readily accounted for by a prior disruption of intestinal permeability – a point not lost on these authors, who have long been interested in this field.

There is a 40 kDa colonic protein which is specifically recognized by tissue-bound IgG in samples from patients with ulcerative colitis, and circulating antibodies to this protein are found only in (a large majority of) patients with active ulcerative colitis.[171] It is suggested that an autoimmune response to this antigen leads to complement activation via IgG1 and thus to epithelial damage and continuing inflamma-tion.[172] Interestingly, the protein is also expressed in certain of the epithelial tissues of the skin, eye, synovium and biliary tract but not at other sites,[173,174] raising the question as to its possible relevance to extra-intestinal manifestations of ulcerative colitis at these sites (see Chapter 6). Although this could be important in respect of sclerosing cholangitis, which is much more often seen in ulcerative colitis, it does not so readily fit with the other extra-intestinal manifestations of inflammatory bowel disease that are seen as often in patients with Crohn's disease (see Chapter 6).

CYTOKINES, CHEMOKINES AND PATHOGENESIS

In inflammatory bowel disease, as in other inflam-matory conditions, polypeptide cytokines and chemokines are expressed by immunoreactive cells.[175–177] Increased chemokine expression has also been observed in epithelial cells, endothelial cells, and smooth muscle cells.[177] Polypeptide cytokines and chemokines play an important role in mediation of the disease process and contribute to the destructive effects on the target tissues. Most of the cytokines and chemokines can be demonstrated in tissue and in circulation at higher than normal levels in patients with inflammatory bowel disease, and there is usually a positive correlation with disease activity. It is less certain that they have a primarily aetiological role, but they are strongly influenced by traditional therapeutic agents and specifically so by the more innovative pharmacolog-ical measures (see Chapter 3). In Crohn's disease, there is an ongoing excessive response of the Th1 type, manifest (in part) by increased intramucosal levels of TNF-α and IFN-γ – both also implicated in granuloma formation – as opposed to ulcerative colitis where the profile has more in common with a Th2 response and in which IFN-γ levels are low.[175]

This is not the place for a detailed review of these mediators, but it may be helpful to recognize that they fall into broad functional groups including those with (for example) predominantly pro-inflammatory effects (e.g. IL-1, IFN-γ or TNF-α), those with a more regulatory role (e.g. IL-2 or IL-10), those which are predominantly chemokine (e.g. IL-8, MCP-1 or ENA-78), or those with more specific roles in healing and repair (e.g. TGF-β).[175–177] This has been exploited most obviously in the case of TNF-α, which is considered fully in Chapter 3. It is entirely characteristic of the interactions between the different types of mediator that we can find an important influence of elevated TNF-α on the expression of a major epithelial cell adhesion molecule.[178]

Inflammatory bowel disease is associated with an enhanced activation of T cells,[179] but the effect is more pronounced in Crohn's disease than in ulcerative colitis. This is exemplified by the different response of lymphocytes of the lamina propria to IL-2. In Crohn's disease there is enhanced cytotoxicity, whereas ulcerative colitis cells tend to be inhibited.[180] The distinct cytokine profiles of the Th1 and Th2 classes of CD4-positive T-helper cells (hence Th) may be a reflection of these differences. Th1 lymphocytes predominantly produce IFN-γ and IL-2 and are most involved with cell-mediated immunity, whereas Th2 cells, which secrete IL-4, 5, 10 and 13, are more associated with stimulation of the B cells and a brisk antibody response. This in turn suggests that differential cytokine expression may contribute to the differences in disease expression between ulcerative colitis and Crohn's disease, but it is unlikely that the distinction is of a black and white nature.

The concentration of soluble IL-2 receptor is increased in active inflammatory bowel disease to the extent that it has been suggested as a useful marker of disease activity (see Chapter 2), and the typical increases in IL-2 receptor are associated with an impairment of T-cell proliferation in Crohn's disease, which could be normalized by exogenous IL-2 despite the apparent normality of endogenous IL-2 production.[181] IL-4 tends to influence the balance of Th1 and Th2 cells in an anti-inflammatory direction. It is deficient in lamina propria lymphocytes (mRNA and protein product) from patients with Crohn's disease and ulcerative colitis.[182] As its expression is most obviously impaired in cells from actively inflamed intestine, it is likely that it is not an initiating abnormality. IL-10 is also an immunoregulatory cytokine with predominantly inhibitory effects on other T cells and on antigen presentation, with downregulation of class II histocompatibility antigens. The production and release of a variety of pro-inflammatory cytokines are suppressed by IL-10 both *in vitro* and *in vivo*.[183] Although IL-10 levels are well preserved or high in inflammatory bowel disease, there is evidence that the concentrations are inadequate to the demand and that supplementary therapeutic IL-10 may be beneficial (see Chapter 3). IFN-γ appears capable of increasing antibody-dependent cellular cytotoxicity in ulcerative colitis,[184] and may have a further role in pathogenesis in addition to its well known effects on antigen presentation: it is possible that some of the therapeutic influence of aminosalicylates is by this route.

The eosinophil/eotaxin pathway is of special interest. Intramucosal and low levels of systemic eosinophilia have long been associated with ulcerative colitis, and more recently have been described also in Crohn's disease, quite apart from the special case of eosinophilic colitis (see Chapter 2). T lymphocytes co-localize with eosinophils at sites of allergic inflammation, and in ulcerative colitis express the eotaxin receptor, CCR3, suggesting that this interaction may represent a novel mechanism of T-lymphocyte recruitment. Surface CCR3 may mark a subset of T lymphocytes that induce eosinophil mobilization and activation through local production of Th2-type cytokines.[185] The mucosal release of eosinophilic cationic protein (ECP) is substantially increased in ulcerative colitis with a degree of eosinophil activation/degranulation related to the intensity of the overall inflammatory reaction. Activated eosinophils and extracellular deposits of ECP were, in particular, seen in crypt abscesses and in areas with damaged surface epithelium. Since ECP is highly cytotoxic, its release at the site of inflammatory bowel lesions might reflect a potential pathophysiological mechanism.[186]

REACTIVE OXYGEN SPECIES, FREE RADICALS AND NITRIC OXIDE

Free radicals are responsible for tissue damage in most inflammatory conditions to some extent, including acute infective secretory diarrhoea. The diarrhoea in both Crohn's disease and ulcerative colitis has a secretory component, and it is reasonable to explore the possibility that oxygen radicals may contribute.[187] *In vitro* studies of inflammatory cells from inflammatory bowel disease patients confirm that they are able to generate reactive oxygen metabolites in excess, and it is likely that the same occurs *in vivo*.[188–190] The specific case of iron is considered below amongst environmental influences.

Nitric oxide is produced to excess in biopsies from patients with active ulcerative colitis,[191] and is liberated into the lumen at levels 100-fold greater than in controls.[192] Comparable though less dramatic changes are found in biopsies from patients with active Crohn's colitis, and revert towards normal with steroid therapy.[193] Increased expression of inducible nitric oxide synthase (iNOS) leads, concomitantly, to release of the highly injurious peroxynitrite via generation of superoxide when arginine is deficient. In this context it is intriguing to find that nitric oxide levels are higher still in patients with the more benign, non-ulcerating condition, collagenous colitis (see Chapter 2).[194] This suggests that the nitric oxide is protective, and fits with the observation that the iNOS knock-out mouse, which is

entirely deficient in mucosal nitric oxide, routinely develops a form of colitis.[194] Selective inhibition of iNOS or arginine supplementation may therefore yield therapeutic potential.

ENTERIC NEURONES AND MAST CELLS IN INFLAMMATORY BOWEL DISEASE

The enteric neurones are probably abnormal in Crohn's disease, but it is difficult to establish whether the various changes observed are primary or epiphenomena. Several lines of enquiry have suggested that there is abnormal innervation of the submucosa, muscularis mucosae and mucosa in ulcerative colitis. This is supported by immuno-histochemical staining, demonstrating increased numbers of mucosal nerve fibres, and of the expression of neuropeptide Y and tyrosine hydroxylase.[195] Evidence that Substance P, a pro-inflammatory neurotransmitter released from mast cells, is over-expressed in both Crohn's disease and ulcerative colitis[196] can be assumed to be of some significance given improvement in animal models of colitis if specific inhibitors are administered. Gastrointestinal mast cell hyperplasia is a feature of inflammatory bowel disease and, whilst Substance P fails to induce mast cell activation in histologically normal mucosa from controls, or apparently normal proximal ulcerative colitis mucosa, it invokes a brisk histamine response from mucosal specimens taken from inflamed inflammatory bowel disease tissue and from uninvolved Crohn's disease tissue.[197]

In a more global approach, Burnstock's group have explored the neurochemical composition of enteric nerve fibres and cell bodies using whole mount preparations of human ileum from normals and those with Crohn's disease. A whole series of abnormalities were confirmed including increased tyrosine hydroxylase, 5-hydroxytryptamine and neuropeptide Y immunoreactivity in the myenteric plexus, increased neurofilaments in the myenteric plexus and the nerve fibres of the circular muscle layer, and thick bundles of immunoreactive nerve fibres in the serosa. Increased vasoactive intestinal polypeptide, nitric oxide synthase, and pituitary adenylate cyclase-activating peptide immunoreactivity was seen in the myenteric plexus and nerve fibres of the circular muscle layer. In addition, there was a chaotic display of nerve fibres containing some of the neuroactive substances, with a high frequency of enlarged varicosities in the myenteric ganglia and/or nerve fibres of the circular muscle.[198] It must be reasonable to conclude that even if these findings are not of aetiological relevance, they have functional consequences.

ENVIRONMENTAL FACTORS

Non-steroidal anti-inflammatory drugs

Non-steroidal anti-inflammatory drugs (NSAIDs) are implicated in the aetiology of some cases of inflammatory bowel disease. Labelled white-cell scanning demonstrates small bowel ulceration (of a magnitude similar to that seen in Crohn's disease) in two-thirds of those receiving long-term NSAID therapy for arthritis,[199] which can persist for more than a year after the drugs are discontinued, and may be associated with frank ileal disease on contrast radiography. A number of studies examining the colon have reached similar conclusions.[200] The commoner ill-effects include watery diarrhoea and chronic blood loss with or without anaemia. These problems tend to be exaggerated in patients with inflammatory bowel disease – and prove a limiting factor in the use of NSAIDs in those with arthropathy (see Chapter 6). A case–control study of over 300 000 residents of Tayside linked hospital events and dispensed drug data between 1989 and 1993. Of 785 patients admitted with active colitis, 200 had inflammatory bowel disease. These were matched to 1198 community controls. The odds ratios (with 95 per cent confidence intervals) for current and recent exposure to NSAIDs were 1.77 (1.01–3.10) and 1.93 (1.20–3.09) respectively. Current and recent exposures to NSAIDs were also strongly associated with *de novo* incidence of inflammatory bowel disease, with odds ratios of 2.96 (1.32–6.64) and 2.51 (1.13–5.55).[201] That the study was limited to prescribed non-steroidals and to episodes of inflammatory bowel disease sufficient to warrant admission to hospital strengthens the argument, as both of these might be expected to diminish the apparent strength of association. The possibility that non-steroidals might have been used for symptoms of inflammatory bowel disease or for associated arthropathy is not excluded and requires further clinical study. Data from the Channel Islands[202] suggest that NSAIDs may be responsible for a higher proportion of apparent new cases of inflammatory bowel disease – 72 per cent of cases on NSAIDs compared to 7 per cent of hospital controls – when non-prescribed NSAIDs also are considered. The odds ratio of 33 is highly significant (CI: 17–63) and could logically be considered, on epidemiological grounds, to explain most cases of acute self-limiting colitis. There has probably been some ascertainment bias in the study, which has not been published as a full paper, but the striking preponderance of NSAID usage in patients is unlikely to be accounted for entirely on this basis.

Smoking and inflammatory bowel disease

Smoking proves one of the more intriguing environmental factors yet identified in inflammatory bowel disease, not least from the clear differences found between its frequency in Crohn's and in ulcerative colitis. Studies from many different centres around the world have confirmed and extended the original observation from the South Wales group[203] that smoking is less common in ulcerative colitis than in healthy controls, with the highest frequency of ulcerative colitis being found in ex-smokers.[204] Initial concerns that these observations might be influenced by recall bias were effectively refuted by prospective data collection.[205] It is now generally agreed that, by contrast, smokers are over-represented amongst patients with Crohn's disease.

The effects of smoking on the success or otherwise of pouch surgery (see Chapter 4) for ulcerative colitis indicate that the link with non-smoking and colitis holds good for the ileoanal pouch.[206] Amongst 72 non-smokers there were 46 episodes of pouchitis in 18 patients, compared to 14 episodes in 4 of the 12 ex-smokers, and only a single episode of pouchitis in one of 17 current smokers.

In Crohn's disease there is good evidence that smokers, as well as being over-represented, form a group with a worse prognosis,[207] and that continued smoking is associated with more frequent relapse.[208] In a French retrospective study of 400 patients followed for a mean of over 8 years, smokers constituted 55 per cent of the total.[209] The sites of intestinal involvement were similar in smokers and non-smokers, and age at diagnosis was comparable. The need for a first surgical procedure did not differ significantly, but there was a higher frequency of repeated surgery in heavy smokers (20 versus 11 per cent) which did not quite reach statistical significance. There was, however, a significantly greater cumulative use of systemic steroids and of other immunosuppressive therapy in smokers, an effect which was more pronounced in females. At 10 years' follow-up, 52 per cent of female smokers had required immunosuppression compared to only 24 per cent of non-smokers ($P < 0.001$). In this group's follow-up study, the overall relative risk of relapse adjusted for confounding factors was 1.35 (1.03–1.76) in current smokers. This risk was increased in patients with previously inactive disease and in those who had no colonic lesions, and became significant above a threshold of 15 cigarettes per day. Former smokers behaved like non-smokers. Obesity, hyperlipidaemia, and alcohol consumption had no significant effect.[210] In a German study of 346 patients,[211] there were 59 ex-smokers

(who were not considered further), 144 smokers and 143 non-smokers. There were no important demographic differences between patients at the time of diagnosis, and the distribution of disease within the bowel was similar, but there was a higher cumulative recurrence rate in smokers. Within 5 years of first surgery, 43 per cent of smokers had relapsed compared to only 26 per cent of non-smokers (RR: 3.1; CI: 1.7–5.8), independent of the initial site of disease. The adverse effects again appeared more pronounced in women, and in those of both sexes having surgery early in the course of their disease, partly answering a question of bias introduced by the higher proportion of non-smokers who had had their disease for less than 5 years at the time of study (57 versus 47 per cent). Many more surgical procedures had been required in the smokers – at least one operation in 73 per cent versus 39 per cent – and multiple episodes of surgery were 10.8 times more likely in smokers (CI: 5.3–22.1). The overall frequency of fistula and/or abscess formation also was higher, at 40 per cent compared with only 13 per cent in non-smokers. The differences between the French and German studies are of degree and emphasis only, and are readily explained by differing criteria for surgical as opposed to immunosuppressive intervention in the two countries. The French GET AID investigators also demonstrated the benefit of life-long non-smoking in a smaller but prospective study (performed to examine the value of mesalazine after surgical resection), in which endoscopic recurrence by 12 weeks was significantly less in non-smokers (odds ratio 0.2; $P < 0.002$).[212] A Spanish study yielded a small excess of smokers with Crohn's disease, and they had a less favourable clinical course. As neither feature was significant, the effect was dismissed by the authors;[213] in my view this reflected a relatively underpowered study that is, in fact, numerically consistent with the literature in general.

The mechanisms for the differential effect of smoking on the different forms of inflammatory bowel disease remain speculative, but an altered production of arachidonic acid metabolites, disruption of mucus-producing capacity, and alterations to the protective barrier function of the colon are probably important.[214] The predominant mucin in the normal colon is the glycoprotein MUC-2; this also predominates in ulcerative colitis.[215] However, there are higher levels of synthesis and secretion of MUC-2 in patients with quiescent disease than in (different) patients with active disease.[216] The relevance of the differential degree of sulphation of MUC-2 remains unclear.

The Cleveland Clinic group have examined the effect of smoking on the mucosal cytokine profile in inflammatory bowel disease. The concentration of IL-8 proved significantly higher in healthy smokers than in non-smokers, but was lower in inflammatory bowel disease patients, and was significantly lower in smokers with Crohn's than in non-smokers with Crohn's. Concentrations of IL-1β and IL-8 were significantly reduced in smokers with ulcerative colitis compared with non-smokers with ulcerative colitis.[217] Animal data suggest that neural pathways are also important,[218] but further studies are clearly warranted.

The clinical significance of the link between smoking and Crohn's disease is, in any event, substantial, especially when one considers that the differences observed for relapse-free intervals equal or exceed those attainable with current options for maintenance therapy (see Chapter 3). However, it remains unknown, and is probably untestable (a controlled trial of stopping smoking being the necessary tool) whether stopping smoking would remove the problem. It is possible that the 'smoking phenotype' marks a subgroup with poor-prognosis Crohn's and that stopping smoking would therefore be irrelevant. The evidence, though not secure, indicates that this would probably be unnecessarily nihilistic. Stopping smoking after a diagnosis of Crohn's disease is made reduces the need for surgical intervention and improves duration of remission, stopping

smoking being associated with a reduction of relapse rate by around 40 per cent at 1 year.[219] Moreover, ex-smokers, despite having an elevated frequency of ulcerative colitis, do not have a higher incidence of Crohn's disease, and are, of course, protected from the many other hazards of smoking. Patients, and especially women, with Crohn's disease who smoke should be strongly advised to stop. Sadly, evidence to date suggests that few health care professionals are adequately addressing this issue.[220]

Appendicectomy and inflammatory bowel disease

Studies from the early 1990s suggested that previous appendicectomy was under-represented in patients with ulcerative colitis, with relative risks well under 0.5.[114,221] In one such study of 174 consecutive patients with ulcerative colitis, only one (0.6 per cent) had had a previous appendicectomy compared to 25.4 per cent of those attending an orthopaedic clinic.[221] There were methodological issues with some of these studies as they were mostly not designed with this hypothesis in mind, and there was particular uncertainty in respect of a possible confounding effect from smoking. There are, however, now numerous papers which are all concordant (the great majority with statistical significance), with appendicectomy some three to five times more common in those without ulcerative colitis.[222] In a meta-analysis (currently only available in abstract form), the overall odds ratio from 13 case–control studies is 0.31 (CI: 0.25–0.38), implying that appendicectomy yields a 69 per cent reduction in the risk of subsequent presentation with ulcerative colitis.[223] This is probably independent of smoking in adults,[224] but possibly influenced by passive smoking in children.[225] Whether acute appendicitis or laparotomy for assumed appendicitis is the protective association is unclear, as the number of normal appendices removed is unknown, but that the link is with appendiceal disease appears more persuasive. It would be unreasonable to propose a direct causal relationship, but speculation that the absence of the appendix is of local immunological significance is supported by the not infrequent histological finding of inflammation in the appendix in otherwise more distal ulcerative colitis (the appendix skip lesion) (see Chapter 2). An influence on permeability also is possible (see above).

A past history of appendicectomy has a neutral or weak positive association with later development of Crohn's disease.[114,226] However, epithelioid granulomas in appendicectomy specimens are occasionally identified, with consequent concern that the patient – despite an absence of other features – has Crohn's disease. In a major epidemiopathological survey, 6 of 6051 appendicectomies performed in Copenhagen County had granulomas at contemporary histological examination.[227] Follow-up of these patients for a minimum of 9 years revealed no further gastrointestinal symptoms. Of 373 patients with an initial clinical diagnosis of Crohn's, there were three in whom the only evidence of disease was in the appendix. Follow-up of these patients to a median of 6 years revealed no recurrence and led the authors to suggest that isolated granulomatous disease of the appendix is not Crohn's disease. An earlier report[228] concluded that there was a 14 per cent recurrence rate in such patients, but the nature of the report, culling incomplete information from many other sources, makes this less secure. It is probably correct to consider isolated granulomatous disease of the appendix as a separate condition with a good prognosis (and perhaps one that incidentally protects against ulcerative colitis).

Sex steroids in the pathogenesis of inflammatory bowel disease

The combined oral contraceptive pill has been associated with an increased risk of Crohn's disease (and possibly of ulcerative colitis).[205,229] Whether this remains true for the lower hormone doses

currently in use has not been fully addressed, but a link between hormonal status and inflammatory bowel disease expression is indicated. The frequent association that women with Crohn's find between their symptoms and certain phases of the menstrual cycle, and altered behaviour of inflammatory bowel disease in pregnancy (see Chapter 5), lend clinical support to this assertion. The prothrombotic effects of the pill may also have relevance to thrombosis in inflammatory bowel disease (see Chapter 7), and there is clear evidence implicating contraceptive steroid usage in ischaemic colitis in young women.[230]

Environmental and dietary exposure to metals and inflammatory bowel disease

The observations that certain metals may be responsible for a cell-mediated granulomatous inflammation of the skin, and that granular pigment containing aluminium, silica and titanium can be found in the intestine and mesenteric nodes of those with Crohn's disease, led us to give intradermal injections of putative pathogenic metals to patients with granulomatous Crohn's and to normal controls.[231] Although foreign-body granulomas could be elicited, there was no evidence to suggest that metal sensitivity is an important contributing cause of granulomatous Crohn's disease. However, Thompson's group in London have further developed this area, with interesting results. In Crohn's disease tissues they find spheres of diameter 100–200 nm composed only of titanium and oxygen, and larger ones (up to 700 nm) containing aluminium, silicon, iron or other elements. The small particles appear to be titanium dioxide of a purity and morphology characteristic of anatase, which is used as a food and pharmaceutical additive, mainly to procure a vivid white coloration. The time course over which these additives have been used corresponds to the emergence of Crohn's disease in the developed world, and exposure is accordingly suggested to be of aetiological significance.[232]

Iron exposure in inflammatory bowel disease may be a special case, given its probable contribution to oxidative stress.[233] Exposure of the colonic mucosa to iron is probably increased in inflammatory bowel disease. Dietary iron may well be concentrated in faecal material because of limited proximal absorption, a situation potentially exacerbated by therapeutic iron and iron from mucosal bleeding. This, in combination with oxidative stress, could lead to extension and propagation of crypt abscesses, directly or via toxic intermediaries, thus leading to acute exacerbations of the disease.[233] These effects in turn may be amplified by a tendency for the inflammatory bowel disease patient to be deficient in antioxidants.[234] Interestingly, even patients with systemic iron deficiency exhibit elevated levels of iron in mucosal biopsies from sites of active colitis.[234] There is scant but supportive clinical evidence in favour of therapeutic iron as a pro-inflammatory agent in inflammatory bowel disease.[235]

Other dietary factors

The response of some patients with Crohn's to dietary therapy (see Chapter 3) has led to speculation that a 'trigger' exists at the point of contact of food/digests and the intestine wall, and that one or more dietary factors may be a contributing cause of inflammatory bowel disease. Although a question very frequently asked by patients, and again a postulated reason for the increase in prevalence of Crohn's disease during the past half century, there is remarkably little evidence on which to base a scientific reply.[236] Various problem foods have been proposed, including refined sugar, cornflakes, margarine and vitamin A. There is now a widespread feeling that carbohydrate consumption – especially of sucrose – is higher in patients with Crohn's disease, to an odds ratio in excess of 2.5, even before the first symptoms of the disease,[237–239] and that consumption of fruit and vegetables (together with potassium, magnesium and vitamin C) is lower than in controls. This

position, however, falls short of a consensus view.[240] The role of dietary amendment in Crohn's therapy is discussed later (see Chapter 3).

Milk consumption and its involvement in the postulated link between mycobacteria and Crohn's disease have already been mentioned; a positive association is not borne out by any of the studies of diet in Crohn's disease. However, there are animal data (reversed ileal loops in pigs) that suggest that lipid may be implicated in ileal inflammation.[241]

There have not been so many associations drawn between dietary factors and ulcerative colitis, but a Western-style diet in Japanese patients is positively associated with the disease,[242] as is a high consumption of cola drinks and chocolate in the Netherlands;[239] clearly, dietary elements here are not independent risk factors. An Israeli study also suggests that high sucrose and high fat intake are positively associated with ulcerative colitis, with protection from fructose.[238]

References

1 Kirsner JB. Historical origins of medical and surgical treatment of inflammatory bowel disease. *Lancet* 1998; **352**: 1303–5.

2 Dalziel TK. Chronic interstitial enteritis. *Br Med J* 1913; **2**: 1068–70.

3 Crohn BB, Ginzburg L, Oppenheimer GD. Regional ileitis, a pathologic and clinical entity. *JAMA* 1932; **99**.

4 Coombe C, Saunders W. A singular case of stricture and thickening of the ileum. *Med Trans R Coll Phys* 1813; **4**: 16–21.

5 Sonnenberg A. Geographic variation in the incidence of and mortality from inflammatory bowel disease. *Dis Colon Rectum* 1986; **29**: 854–61.

6 Ekbom A, Helmick C, Zack M, Adami HO. The epidemiology of inflammatory bowel disease: a large, population-based study in Sweden. *Gastroenterology* 1991; **100**: 350–8.

7 Shivananda S, Lennard-Jones J, Logan R, *et al.* Incidence of inflammatory bowel disease across

Europe: is there a difference between north and south? Results of the European Collaborative Study on Inflammatory Bowel Disease (EC-IBD). *Gut* 1996; **39**: 690–7.

8 Trallori G, D'Albasio G, Palli D, *et al.* Epidemiology of inflammatory bowel disease over a 10-year period in Florence (1978–1987). *Ital J Gastroenterol* 1991; **23**: 559–63.

9 Riegler G, Tartaglione M, Marmo R, *et al.* Ulcerative colitis in old age: men more frequent than women? *Gastroenterology* 1996; **110**: A1002.

10 Loftus EV Jr, Silverstein MD, Sandborn WJ, Tremaine WJ, Harmsen WS, Zinsmeister AR. Ulcerative colitis in Olmsted County, Minnesota, 1940–1993: incidence, prevalence, and survival. *Gut* 2000; **46**: 336–43.

11 Moum B, Ekbom A, Vatn MH, *et al.* Inflammatory bowel disease: re-evaluation of the diagnosis in a prospective population based study in south eastern Norway. *Gut* 1997; **40**: 328–32.

12 Bernstein CN, Blanchard JF, Rawsthorne P, Wajda A. Epidemiology of Crohn's disease and ulcerative colitis in a central Canadian province: a population-based study. *Am J Epidemiol* 1999; **149**: 916–24.

13 Logan RFA. Inflammatory bowel disease incidence: up, down or unchanged? *Gut* 1998; **42**: 309–11.

14 Srivastava ED, Mayberry JF, Morris TJ, *et al.* Incidence of ulcerative colitis in Cardiff over 20 years: 1968–87. *Gut* 1992; **33**: 256–8.

15 Ranzi T, Bodini P, Zambelli A, *et al.* Epidemiological aspects of inflammatory bowel disease in a north Italian population: a 4 year prospective study. *Eur J Gastroenterol Hepatol* 1996; **8**: 657–61.

16 Gower-Rousseau C, Salomez J-L, Dupas J-L, *et al.* Incidence of inflammatory bowel disease in northern France (1988–1990). *Gut* 1994; **35**: 1433–8.

17 Munkholm P, Langholz E, Nielsen OH, Kreiner S, Binder V. Incidence and prevalence of Crohn's disease in the county of Copenhagen, 1962–87: a six-fold increase in incidence. *Scand J Gastroenterol* 1992; **27**: 609–14.

18 Loftus EV Jr, Silverstein MD, Sandborn WJ, Tremaine WJ, Harmsen WS, Zinsmeister AR. Crohn's disease in Olmsted County, Minnesota,

1940–1993: incidence, prevalence, and survival. *Gastroenterology* 1998; **114**: 1161–8.

19 Moum B, Vatn MH, Ekbom A, *et al.* Incidence of Crohn's disease in four counties in southeastern Norway, 1990–93. A prospective population-based study. The Inflammatory Bowel South-Eastern Norway (IBSEN) Study Group of Gastroenterologists. *Scand J Gastroenterol* 1996; **31**: 355–61.

20 Lee FI, Nguyen-Van-Tam JS. Prospective study of incidence of Crohn's disease in north-west England: no increase since the late 1970s. *Eur J Gastroenterol Hepatol* 1994; **6**: 27–31.

21 Lapidus A, Bernell O, Hellers G, Persson PG, Lofberg R. Incidence of Crohn's disease in Stockholm County 1955–1989. *Gut* 1997; **41**: 480–6.

22 Fonager K, Sorensen HT, Olsen J. Change in incidence of Crohn's disease and ulcerative colitis in Denmark. A study based on the National Registry of Patients, 1981–1992. *Int J Epidemiol* 1997; **26**: 1003–8.

23 Timmer A, Breuer-Katschinski B, Goebell H. Time trends in the incidence and disease location of Crohn's disease 1980–1995: a prospective analysis in an urban population in Germany. *Inflamm Bowel Dis* 1999; **5**: 79–84.

24 Cosgrove M, Al-Atia RF, Jenkins HR. The epidemiology of paediatric inflammatory bowel disease. *Arch Dis Child* 1996; **74**: 460–1.

25 Moum B, Bentsen B, Ekbom A, *et al.* Incidence of inflammatory bowel disease in childhood. A prospective population based study of the IBSEN study group in south-eastern Norway 1990–93. *Gastroenterology* 1996; **110**: A974.

26 Mayberry JF, Judd D, Smart H, Rhodes J, Calcraft B, Morris JS. Crohn's disease in Jewish people – an epidemiological study in south-east Wales. *Digestion* 1986; **35**: 237–40.

27 Shapira M, Tamir A. Crohn's disease in the Kinneret sub-district, Israel, 1960–1990. Incidence and prevalence in different ethnic subgroups. *Eur J Epidemiol* 1994; **10**: 231–3.

28 Fellows IW, Mayberry JF, Holmes GK. Crohn's disease in West Indians. *Am J Gastroenterol* 1988; **83**: 752–5.

29 Ogunbi SO, Ransom JA, Sullivan K, Schoen BT, Gold BD. Inflammatory bowel disease in African-American children living in Georgia. *J Pediatr* 1998; **133**: 103–7.

30 Cave DR, Freedman LS. Seasonal variations in the clinical presentation of Crohn's disease and ulcerative colitis. *Int J Epidemiol* 1975; **4**: 317–20.

31 Tysk C, Järnerot G. Seasonal variation in exacerbations of ulcerative colitis. *Scand J Gastroenterol* 1993; **28**: 95–6.

32 Sonnenberg A, Jacobsen SJ, Wasserman IH. Periodicity of hospital admissions for inflammatory bowel disease. *Am J Gastroenterol* 1994; **889**: 847–51.

33 Moum B, Aadland E, Ekbom A, Vatn MH. Seasonal variations in the onset of ulcerative colitis. *Gut* 1996; **38**: 376–8.

34 Tysk C, Linberg E, Järnerot G, Flodrus-Myrhed B. Ulcerative colitis and Crohn's disease in an unselected population of monozygotic and dizygotic twins. A study of heritability and the influence of smoking. *Gut* 1988; **29**: 990–6.

35 Roth MP, Petersen GM, McElree C, *et al.* Familial empiric risk estimates of inflammatory bowel disease in Ashkenazi Jews. *Gastroenterology* 1989; **96**: 1016–20.

36 Orholm M, Iselius L, Sorensen TI, *et al.* Investigation of inheritance of chronic inflammatory bowel diseases by complex segregation analysis. *Br Med J* 1993; **306**: 20–4.

37 Satsangi J, Welsh KI, Bunce M, *et al.* Contribution of genes of the major histocompatibility complex to susceptibility and disease phenotype in inflammatory bowel disease. *Lancet* 1996; **347**: 1212–17.

38 Polito JM II, Rees RC, Childs B, Mendeloff AI, Harris ML, Bayless TM. Preliminary evidence for genetic anticipation in Crohn's disease. *Lancet* 1996; **347**: 798–800.

39 Heresbach D, Gulwani-Akolkar B, Lesser M, *et al.* Anticipation in Crohn's disease may be influenced by gender and ethnicity of the transmitting parent. *Am J Gastroenterol* 1998; **93**: 2368–72.

40 Stokkers PC, Reitsma PH, Tytgat GN, van Deventer SJ. HLA-DR and -DQ phenotypes in inflammatory bowel disease: a meta-analysis. *Gut* 1999; **45**: 395–401.

41 Plévy SE, Targan SR, Yang H, Fernandez D, Rotter JI, Toyoda H. Tumor necrosis factor microsatellites define a Crohn's disease-associated haplotype on chromosome 6. *Gastroenterology* 1996; **110**: 1053–60.

42 Louis E, Peeters M, Franchimont D, *et al.* Tumour necrosis factor (TNF) gene polymorphism in Crohn's disease (CD): influence on disease behaviour? *Clin Exp Immunol* 2000; **119**: 64–8.

43 Negoro K, Kinouchi Y, Hiwatashi N, *et al.* Crohn's disease is associated with novel polymorphisms in the 5'-flanking region of the tumor necrosis factor gene. *Gastroenterology* 1999; **117**: 1062–8.

44 Hampe J, Shaw SH, Saiz R, *et al.* Linkage of inflammatory bowel disease to human chromosome 6p. I *Am J Hum Genet* 1999; **65**: 1647–55.

45 Mansfield JC, Holden H, Tarlow JK, I Novel genetic association between ulcerative colitis and the anti-inflammatory cytokine interleukin-1 receptor antagonist. Gastroenterology 1994; **106**: 637–42.

46 Tountas NA, Casini-Raggi V, Yang H, *et al.* Functional and ethnic association of allele 2 of the interleukin-1 receptor antagonist gene in ulcerative colitis. *Gastroenterology* 1999; **117**: 806–13.

47 Stokkers PC, van Aken BE, Basoski N, Reitsma PH, Tytgat GN, van Deventer SJ. Five genetic markers in the interleukin 1 family in relation to inflammatory bowel disease. *Gut* 1998; **43**: 33–9.

48 Parkes M, Satsangi J, Jewell D. Contribution of the IL-2 and IL-10 genes to inflammatory bowel disease susceptibility. *Clin Exp Immunol* 1998; **113**: 28–32.

49 Hugot J-P, Laurent-Puig P, Gower-Rousseau C, *et al.* Mapping of a susceptibility locus for Crohn's disease on chromosome 16. *Nature* 1996; **379**: 821–3.

50 Cho JH, Nicolae DL, Gold LH, *et al.* Identification of novel susceptibility loci for inflammatory bowel disease on chromosomes 1p, 3q, and 4q: evidence for epistasis between 1p and IBD1. *Proc Natl Acad Sci U S A* 1998; **95**: 7502–7.

51 Annese V, Latiano A, Bovio P, *et al.* Genetic analysis in Italian families with inflammatory bowel

disease supports linkage to the IBD1 locus – a GISC study. *Eur J Hum Genet* 1999; 7: 567–73.

52 Brant SR, Fu Y, Fields CT, *et al.* American families with Crohn's disease have strong evidence for linkage to chromosome 16 but not chromosome 12. *Gastroenterology* 1998; **115**: 1056–61.

53 Olavesen MG, Hampe J, Mirza MM, *et al.* Analysis of single-nucleotide polymorphisms in the interleukin-4 receptor gene for association with inflammatory bowel disease. *Immunogenetics* 2000; **51**: 1–7.

54 Mirza MM, Lee J, Teare D, *et al.* Evidence of linkage of the inflammatory bowel disease susceptibility locus on chromosome 16 (IBD1) to ulcerative colitis. *J Med Genet* 1998; **35**: 218–21.

55 Satsangi J, Parkes M, Louis E, *et al.* Two stage genome-wide search in inflammatory bowel disease provides evidence for susceptibility loci on chromosomes 3, 7 and 12. *Nat Genet* 1996; **14**: 199–202.

56 Curran ME, Lau KF, Hampe J, *et al.* Genetic analysis of inflammatory bowel disease in a large European cohort supports linkage to chromosomes 12 and 16. *Gastroenterology* 1998; **115**: 1066–71.

57 Duerr RH, Varmada MM, Zhang L, *et al.* Linkage and assocaition betweeen inflammatory bowel disease and a locus on chromosome 12. *Am J Hum Genet* 1998; **63**: 95–100.

58 Hampe J, Hermann B, Bridger S, *et al.* The interferon-γ gene as a positional and functional candidate gene for inflammatory bowel disease. *Int J Colorect Dis* 1998; **13**: 260–3.

59 Mirza M, Rowley GT, Hampe J, *et al.* Analysis of single nucleotide polymorphisms in the NRAMP2 gene for association with inflammatory bowel disease. *Gastroenterology* 2000; **118**: A594–5.

60 Hampe J, Schreiber S, Shaw SH, *et al.* A genomewide analysis provides evidence for novel linkages in inflammatory bowel disease in a large European cohort. *Am J Hum Genet* 1999; **64**: 808–16.

61 Bonen DK, Ramos R, Lee S, *et al.* Characterizing IBD risk alleles on chromosome 1p36. *Gastroenterology* 2000; **118**: A708.

62 Ma Y, Ohmen JD, Li Z, *et al.* A genome-wide search identifies potential new susceptibility loci for Crohn's disease. *Inflamm Bowel Dis* 1999; **5**: 271–8.

63 Duerr RH, Barmada MM, Zhang L, Pfuetzer R, Weeks DE. A genome scan at 751 microsatellite loci reveals linkage between Crohn's disease and chromosome 14q11–12; the IBD4 locus. *Gastroenterology* 2000; **118**: A708.

64 Vermeire S, Vlietinck R, Groenen P, Peeters M, Rutgeerts P. Replication of linkage on 14q11–12 in inflammatory bowel disease. *Gastroenterology* 2000; **118**: A338.

65 Kyo K, Parkes M, Takei Y, *et al.* Association of ulcerative colitis with rare VNTR alleles of the human intestinal mucin gene MUC3. *Hum Mol Genet* 1999; **8**: 307–11.

66 Buisine M-P, Desreumaux P, Debailleul V, *et al.* Abnormalities in mucin gene expression in Crohn's disease. *Inflamm Bowel Dis* 1999; **5**: 24–32.

67 Roozendaal C, Pogany K, Horst G, *et al.* Does analysis of the antigenic specificities of antineutrophil cytoplasmic antibodies contribute to their clinical significance in the inflammatory bowel diseases? *Scand J Gastroenterol* 1999; **34**: 1123–31.

68 Satsangi J, Landers CJ, Welsh KI, Koss K, Targan S, Jewell DP. The presence of anti-neutrophil antibodies reflects clinical and genetic heterogeneity within inflammatory bowel disease. *Inflamm Bowel Dis* 1998; **4**: 18–26.

69 Shanahan F, Duerr R, Rotter JI, *et al.* Neutrophil autoantibodies in ulcerative colitis: familial aggregation and genetic heterogeneity. *Gastroenterology* 1992; **103**: 456–61.

70 Seibold F, Slametschka D, Gregor M, Weber P. Neutrophil autoantibodies: a genetic marker in primary sclerosing cholangitis and ulcerative colitis. *Gastroenterology* 1994; **107**: 532–6.

71 Bansi DS, Lo S, Chapman RW, Fleming KA. Absence of antineutrophil cytoplasmic antibodies in relatives of UK patients with primary sclerosing cholangitis and ulcerative colitis. *Eur J Gastroenterol Hepatol* 1996; **8**: 111–16.

72 Lo SK, Fleming KA, Chapman RW. Prevalence of antineutrophil antibody in primary sclerosing

cholangitis and ulcerative colitis using an alkaline phosphatase technique. *Gut* 1992; **33**: 1370–5.

73 Estève M, Mallolas J, Klaasen J, *et al.* Antineutrophil cytoplasmic antibodies in sera from colectomised ulcerative colitis patients and its relation to the presence of pouchitis. *Gut* 1996; **38**: 894–8.

74 Vasiliauskas EA, Plévy SE, Landers CJ, *et al.* Perinuclear antineutrophil cytoplasmic antibodies in patients with Crohn's disease define a clinical subgroup. *Gastroenterology* 1996; **110**: 1810–19.

75 Teahon K, Somasundaram S, Smith T, Menzies I, Bjarnason I. Assessing the site of increased intestinal permeability in coeliac and inflammatory bowel disease. *Gut* 1996; **39**: 864–9.

76 Schmitz H, Barmeyer C, Fromm M, *et al.* Altered tight junction structure contributes to the impaired epithelial barrier function in ulcerative colitis. *Gastroenterology* 1999; **116**: 301–9.

77 Hollander D, Vadheim CM, Brettholz E, Petersen GM, Delahunty T, Rotter JI. Increased intestinal permeability in patients with Crohn's disease and their relatives. *Ann Intern Med* 1986; **105**: 883–5.

78 Hilsden RJ, Meddings JB, Sutherland LR. Intestinal permeability changes in response to acetylsalicylic acid in relatives of patients with Crohn's disease. *Gastroenterology* 1996; **110**: 1395–403.

79 Zamora SA, Hilsden RJ, Meddings JB, *et al.* Intestinal permeability before and after ibuprofen in families of children with Crohn's disease. *Can J Gastroenterol* 1999; **13**: 31–5.

80 Yacyshyn BR, Meddings JB. CD45RO expression on circulating CD19+ B cells in Crohn's disease correlates with intestinal permeability. *Gastroenterology* 1995; **108**: 132–7.

81 Wyatt J, Vogelsang H, Hübl W, Waldhöer T, Lochs H. Intestinal permeability and the prediction of relapse in Crohn's disease. *Lancet* 1993; **341**: 1437–9.

82 Frenette PS, Wagner DD. Adhesion molecules – Part 1. *N Engl J Med* 1996; **334**: 1526–9.

83 Koizumi M, King N, Lobb R, Benjamin C, Podolsky DK. Expression of vascular adhesion molecules in inflammatory bowel disease. *Gastroenterology* 1992; **103**: 840–7.

84 Jones SC, Banks RE, Haidar A, *et al.* Adhesion molecules in inflammatory bowel disease. *Gut* 1995; **36**: 724–30.

85 Nielsen OH, Langholz E, Hendel J, Brynskov J. Circulating soluble intercellular adhesion molecule-1 (sICAM-1) in active inflammatory bowel disease. *Dig Dis Sci* 1994; **39**: 1918–23.

86 Binion DG, West GA, Volk EE, *et al.* Acquired increase in leucocyte binding by intestinal microvascular endothelium in inflammatory bowel disease. *Lancet* 1998; **352**: 1742–6.

87 Pooley N, Ghosh L, Sharon P. Up-regulation of E-selectin and intercellular adhesion molecule-1 differs between Crohn's disease and ulcerative colitis. *Dig Dis Sci* 1995; **40**: 219–25.

88 Schürmann GM, Bishop AE, Facer P, *et al.* Increased expression of cell adhesion molecule P-selectin in active inflammatory bowel disease. *Gut* 1995; **36**: 411–18.

89 Mishra L, Mishra BB, Harris M, Bayless TM, Muchmore AV. In vitro cell aggregation and cell adhesion molecules in Crohn's disease. *Gastroenterology* 1993; **104**: 772–9.

90 Bousvaros A, Leichetner A, Zurakowski D, *et al.* Elevated serum vascular endothelial growth factor in children and young adults with Crohn's disease. *Dig Dis Sci* 1999; **44**: 434–40.

91 Griga T, Gutzeit A, Sommerkamp C, *et al.* Increased production of vascular endothelial growth factor by peripheral blood mononuclear cells in patients with inflammatory bowel disease. *Eur J Gastroenterol Hepatol* 1999; **11**: 175–9.

92 Karayiannakis AJ, Syrigos KN, Efstathiou J, *et al.* Expression of catenins and E-cadherin during epithelial restitution in inflammatory bowel disease. *J Pathol* 1998; **185**: 413–18.

93 Perry I, Hardy R, Jones T, Jankowski J. A colorectal cell line with alterations in E-cadherin and epithelial biology may be an in vitro model of colitis. *Mol Pathol* 1999; **52**: 231–42.

94 Day R, Ilyas M, Daszak P, Talbot I, Forbes A. Expression of syndecan-1 in inflammatory bowel disease and a possible mechanism of heparin therapy. *Dig Dis Sci* 1999; **44**: 2508–15.

95 Hermiston ML, Gordon JI. Inflammatory bowel disease and adenomas in mice expressing a

dominant negative N-cadherin. *Science* 1995; **270**: 1203–7.

96 Pullan RD, Thomas GA, Rhodes M, *et al.* Thickness of adherent mucus gel on colonic mucosa in humans and its relevance to colitis. *Gut* 1994; **35**: 353–9.

97 Poulsom R, Chinery R, Sarraf C, *et al.* Trefoil peptide gene expression in small intestinal Crohn's disease and dietary adaptation. *J Clin Gastroenterol* 1993; **17**: S78–91.

98 Finnie IA, Dwarakanath AD, Taylor BA, Rhodes JM. Colonic mucin synthesis is increased by sodium butyrate. *Gut* 1995; **36**: 93–9.

99 Dwarakanath AD, Campbell BJ, Tsai HH, Sunderland D, Hart CA, Rhodes JM. Faecal mucinase activity assessed in inflammatory bowel disease using 14C threonine labelled mucin substrate. *Gut* 1995; **37**: 58–62.

100 Barton LL, Moussa SL, Villar RG, Hulett RL. Gastrointestinal complications of chronic granulomatous disease: case report and literature review. *Clin Pediatr (Phila)* 1998; **37**: 231–6.

101 Sanderson IR, Bisset WM, Milla PJ, Leonard JV. Chronic inflammatory bowel disease in glycogen storage disease type 1B. *J Inherited Metab Dis* 1991; **14**: 771–6.

102 Segal AW, Loewi G. Neutrophil dysfunction in Crohn's disease. *Lancet* 1976; **2**: 219–21.

103 Rhodes JM, Potter BJ, Brown DJ, Jewell DP. Serum inhibitors of leukocyte chemotaxis in Crohn's disease and ulcerative colitis. *Gastroenterology* 1982; **82**: 1327–34.

104 Sendid B, Colombel JF, Jacquinto PM, *et al.* Specific antibody response to oligomannoside epitopes in Crohn's disease. *Clin Diagn Lab Immunol* 1996; **3**: 219–26.

105 Wakefield AJ, Sawyerr AM, Dhillon AP, *et al.* Pathogenesis of Crohn's disease: multifocal gastrointestinal infarction. *Lancet* 1989; **2**: 1057–62.

106 Matson AP, Van Kruiningen HJ, West AB, Cartun RW, Colombel JF, Cortot A. The relationship of granulomas to blood vessels in intestinal Crohn's disease. *Mod Pathol* 1995; **8**: 680–5.

107 Wakefield AJ, Sankey EA, Dhillon AP, *et al.* Granulomatous vasculitis in Crohn's disease. *Gastroenterology* 1991; **100**: 1279–87.

108 Sawyerr M, Pottinger BE, Savage CO, *et al.* Serum immunoglobulin G reactive with endothelial cells in inflammatory bowel disease. *Dig Dis Sci* 1994; **39**: 1909–17.

109 Collins CE, Rampton DS. Review article: platelets in inflammatory bowel disease – pathogenetic role and therapeutic implications. *Aliment Pharmacol Ther* 1997; **11**: 237–47.

110 Collins CE, Rampton DS, Rogers J, Williams NS. Platelet aggregation and neutrophil sequestration in the mesenteric circulation in inflammatory bowel disease. *Eur J Gastroenterol Hepatol* 1997; **9**: 1213–17.

111 Wardle TD, Hall L, Turnberg LA. Platelet activating factor: release from colonic mucosa in patients with ulcerative colitis and its effect on colonic secretion. *Gut* 1996; **38**: 355–61.

112 Hocke M, Richter L, Bosseckert H, Eitner K. Platelet activating factor in stool from patients with ulcerative colitis and Crohn's disease. *Hepatogastroenterology* 1999; **46**: 2333–7.

113 Hamilton MI, Dick R, Crawford L, Thompson NP, Pounder RE, Wakefield AJ. Is proximal demarcation of ulcerative colitis determined by the territory of the inferior mesenteric artery? *Lancet* 1995; **345**: 688–90.

114 Gent AE, Hellier MD, Grace RH, Swarbrick ET, Coggon D. Inflammatory bowel disease and domestic hygiene in infancy. *Lancet* 1994; **343**: 766–7.

115 Montgomery S, Pounder RE, Wakefield AJ. Infant mortality and the incidence of Crohn's disease. *Lancet* 1997; **349**: 472–3.

116 Elliott DE, Crawford C, Li J, *et al.* Helminthic parasites inhibit spontaneous colitis in IL-10 deficient mice. *Gastroenterology* 2000; **118**: A863.

117 Matricardi PM, Rosmini F, Riondino S, *et al.* Exposure to foodborne and orofaecal microbes versus airborne viruses in relation to atopy and allergic asthma: epidemiological study. *Br Med J* 2000; **320**: 412–17.

118 D'Arienzo A, Manguso F, Astarita C, *et al.* Allergic diseases and the mucosal eosinophil infiltrate in ulcerative colitis. *Gut* 1999; **45**(Suppl V): A279.

119 Shaheen SO, Aaby P, Hall AJ, *et al.* Measles and atopy in Guinea-Bissau. *Lancet* 1996; **347**: 1792–6.

120 Duchmann R, Kaiser I, Hermann E, Mayet W, Ewe K, Meyer zum Büschenfelde KH. Tolerance exists towards resident intestinal flora but is broken in active inflammatory bowel disease. *Clin Exp Immunol* 1995; **102**: 448–55.

121 Sanderson JD, Moss MT, Tizard MLV, Hermon-Taylor J. *Mycobacterium paratuberculosis* DNA in Crohn's disease tissue. *Gut* 1992; **33**: 890–6.

122 Fidler HM, Thurrell W, Johnson NMcI, Rook GAW, McFadden JJ. Specific detection of *Mycobacterium paratuberculosis* DNA associated with granulomatous tissue in Crohn's disease. *Gut* 1994; **35**: 506–10.

123 Rowbotham DS, Mapstone NP, Trejdosiewicz LK, Howdle PD, Quirke P. *Mycobacterium paratuberculosis* DNA not detected in Crohn's disease tissue by fluorescent polymerase chain reaction. *Gut* 1995; **37**: 660–7.

124 El-Zaatari FA, Naser SA, Hulten K, Burch P, Graham DY. Characterization of *Mycobacterium paratuberculosis* p36 antigen and its seroreactivities in Crohn's disease. *Curr Microbiol* 1999; **39**: 115–19.

125 Sonnenberg A. Occupational mortality of inflammatory bowel disease. *Digestion* 1990; **46**: 10–18.

126 Hubbard J, Surawicz CM. Etiological role of mycobacterium in Crohn's disease: an assessment of the literature. *Dig Dis* 1999; **17**: 6–13.

127 Van Kruiningen HJ. Lack of support for a common etiology in Johne's disease of animals and Crohn's disease in humans. *Inflamm Bowel Dis* 1999; **5**: 183–91.

128 Lewin J, Dhillon AP, Sim R, Mazure G, Pounder RE, Wakefield AJ. Persistent measles virus infection of the intestine: confirmation by immunogold electron microscopy. *Gut* 1995; **36**: 564–9.

129 Haga Y, Funakoshi O, Kuroe K, *et al.* Absence of measles viral genomic sequence in intestinal tissues from Crohn's disease by nested polymerase chain reaction. *Gut* 1996; **38**: 211–15.

130 Chadwick N, Bruce IJ, Schepelmann S, Pounder RE, Wakefield AJ. Measles virus RNA is not detected in inflammatory bowel disease using hybrid capture and reverse transcription followed by the polymerase chain reaction. *J Med Virol* 1998; **55**: 305–11.

131 Ekbom A, Wakefield AJ, Zack M, Adami HO. Perinatal measles infection and subsequent Crohn's disease. *Lancet* 1994; **344**: 508–10.

132 Ekbom A, Daszak P, Kraaz W, Wakefield AJ. Crohn's disease after in-utero measles virus exposure. *Lancet* 1996; **348**: 515–17.

133 Thompson N, Montgomery S, Pounder RE, Wakefield AJ. Is measles vaccination a risk factor for Crohn's disease? *Lancet* 1995; **345**: 1071–4.

134 Montgomery SM, Morris DL, Pounder RE, Wakefield AJ. Paramyxovirus infections in childhood and subsequent inflammatory bowel disease. *Gastroenterology* 1999; **116**: 796–803.

135 Kawashima H, Mori T, Kashiwagi Y, Takekuma K, Hoshika A, Wakefield A. Detection and sequencing of measles virus from peripheral mononuclear cells from patients with inflammatory bowel disease and autism. *Dig Dis Sci* 2000; **45**: 723–9.

136 Anon. The safety of MMR vaccine. *Curr Prob Pharmacovig* 1999; **25**: 9–10.

137 Taylor B, Miller E, Farrington EP. Autism and measles, mumps, and rubella vaccine: no epidemiological evidence for a causal association. *Lancet* 1999; **353**: 2026–9.

138 Liu Y, Van Kruiningen HJ, West AB, Cartun RW, Cortot A, Colombel JF. Immunocytochemical evidence of *Listeria, Escherichia coli*, and *Streptococcus* antigens in Crohn's disease. *Gastroenterology* 1995; **108**: 1396–404.

139 Tiveljung A, Soderholm JD, Olaison G, Jonasson J, Monstein HJ. Presence of eubacteria in biopsies from Crohn's disease inflammatory lesions as determined by 16S rRNA gene-based PCR. *J Med Microbiol* 1999; **48**: 263–8.

140 Chiba M, Fukushima T, Inoue S, Horie Y, Iizuka M, Masamune O. *Listeria monocytogenes* in Crohn's disease. *Scand J Gastroenterol* 1998; **33**: 430–4.

141 Walmsley RS, Anthony A, Sim R, Pounder RE, Wakefield AJ. Absence of *Escherichia coli, Listeria monocytogenes,* and *Klebsiella pneumoniae* antigens within inflammatory bowel disease tissues. *J Clin Pathol* 1998; **51**: 657–61.

142 Broberger O, Perlmann P. Autoantibodies in human ulcerative colitis. *J Exp Med* 1959; **110**: 657–74.

143 Perlmann P, Hammarstrom S, Lagercrantz R, Gustafsson BE. Antigen from colon of germfree rats and antibodies in human ulcerative colitis. *Ann NY Acad Sci* 1965; **124**: 377–94.

144 Darfeuille-Michaud A, Neut C, Barnich N, *et al.* Presence of adherent *E. coli* strains in ileal mucosa of patients with Crohn's disease. *Gastroenterology* 98; **115**: 1405–13.

145 Boudeau J, Glasser AL, Masseret E, Desreumaux P, Colombel J-F, Darfeuille-Michaud A. Invasive ability of *Escherichia coli* associated with Crohn's disease. *Gut* 1999; **45**(Suppl V): A277.

146 Schultsz C, Moussa M, van Ketel R, Tytgat GN, Dankert J. Frequency of pathogenic and entero-adherent *Escherichia coli* in patients with inflammatory bowel disease and controls. *J Clin Pathol* 1997; **50**: 573–9.

147 Cahill RJ, Foltz CJ, Fox JG, *et al.* Inflammatory bowel disease: an immunity-mediated condition triggered by bacterial infection with *Helicobacter hepaticus*. *Infect Immun* 1997; **65**: 3126.

148 Saunders KE, Shen Z, Dewhirst FE, Paster BJ, Dangler CA, Fox JG. Novel intestinal *Helicobacter* species isolated from cotton-top tamarins (*Saguinus oedipus*) with chronic colitis. *J Clin Microbiol* 1999; **37**: 146–51.

149 Vega R, Bertran X, Menacho M, *et al.* Cytomegalovirus infection in patients with inflammatory bowel disease. *Am J Gastroenterol* 1999; **94**: 1053–6.

150 Begos DG, Rappaport R, Jain D. Cyto-megalovirus infection masquerading as an ulcerative colitis flare-up: case report and review of the literature. *Yale J Biol Med* 1996; **69**: 323–8.

151 Rachima C, Maoz E, Apter S, Thaler M, Grossman E, Rosenthal T. Cytomegalovirus infection associated with ulcerative colitis in immunocompetent individuals. *Postgrad Med J* 1998; **74**: 486–9.

152 Guillen-Bueno R, Gutierrez-Ramos R, Perteguer-Prieto MJ, *et al.* Anti-anisakis antibodies in the clinical course of Crohn's disease. *Digestion* 1999; **60**: 268–73.

153 Liacouras CA, Bell LM, Aljabi MC, Piccoli DA. *Angiostrongylus costaricensis* enterocolitis mimics Crohn's disease. *J Pediatr Gastroenterol Nutr* 1993; **16**: 203–7.

154 Grimble G. Fibre, fermentation, flora and flatus. *Gut* 1989; **30**: 6–13.

155 Levine J, Ellis CJ, Furne JK, Springfield JR, Levitt MD. Fecal hydrogen sulfide production in ulcerative colitis. *Am J Gastroenterol* 1998; **93**: 83–7.

156 Pitcher MCL, Cummings JH. Hydrogen sulphide: a bacterial toxin in ulcerative colitis? *Gut* 1996; **39**: 1–4.

157 Pitcher MC, Beatty ER, Harris RM, Waring RH, Cummings JH. Sulfur metabolism in ulcerative colitis: investigation of detoxification enzymes in peripheral blood. *Dig Dis Sci* 1998; **43**: 2080–5.

158 Pitcher MC, Beatty ER, Cummings JH. The contribution of sulphate reducing bacteria and 5-aminosalicylic acid to faecal sulphide in patients with ulcerative colitis. *Gut* 2000; **46**: 64–72.

159 Sartor RB, Cromartie WJ, Powell DW, Schwab JH. Granulomatous enterocolitis induced in rats by purified bacterial cell wall fragments. *Gastroenterology* 1985; **89**: 587–95.

160 D'Haens GR, Geboes K, Peeters M, Baert F, Penninckx F, Rutgeerts P. Early lesions of recurrent Crohn's disease caused by infusion of intestinal contents in excluded ileum. *Gastroenterology* 1998; **114**: 262–7.

161 Wirtz S, Neurath MF. Animal models of intestinal inflammation: new insights into the molecular pathogenesis and immunotherapy of inflammatory bowel disease. *Int J Colorectal Dis* 2000; **15**: 144–60.

162 Cellier C, Foray S, Hermine O. Regional enteritis associated with enterovirus in a patient with X-linked agammaglobulinemia. *N Engl J Med* 2000; **342**: 1611–12.

163 Peetermans WE, D'Haens GR, Ceuppens JL, Rutgeerts P, Geboes K. Mucosal expression by B7-positive cells of the 60-kilodalton heat-shock protein in inflammatory bowel disease. *Gastroenterology* 1995; **108**: 75–82.

164 Di Mola F, Friess H, Scheuren A, *et al.* Transforming growth factor-betas and their signalling receptors are coexpressed in Crohn's disease. *Ann Surg* 1999; **229**: 67–75.

165 Rutgeerts P, Geboes K, Peeters M, *et al.* Effect of faecal stream diversion on recurrence of Crohn's disease in the neoterminal ileum. *Lancet* 1991; **338**: 771–4.

166 Winslet MC, Allan A, Poxon V, Youngs D, Keighley MRB. Faecal diversion for Crohn's colitis: a model to study the role of the faecal stream in the inflammatory process. *Gut* 1994; **35**: 236–42.

167 Andreyev HJN, Owen RA, Thompson I, Forbes A. Association between Meckel's diverticulum and Crohn's disease: a retrospective review. *Gut* 1994; **35**: 788–90.

168 Thomas PD, Keat AC, Forbes A, Ciclitira PJ, Nicholls RJ. Extraintestinal manifestations of ulcerative colitis following restorative proctocolectomy. *Eur J Gastroenterol Hepatol* 1999; **11**: 1001–5.

169 Oriishi T, Sata M, Toyonaga A, Sasaki E, Tanikawa K. Evaluation of intestinal permeability in patients with inflammatory bowel disease using lactulose and measuring antibodies to lipid A. *Gut* 1995; **36**: 891–6.

170 MacPherson A, Khoo UY, Forgacs I, Philpott-Howard J, Bjarnason I. Mucosal antibodies in inflammatory bowel disease are directed against intestinal bacteria. *Gut* 1996; **38**: 365–75.

171 Takahasi F, Shah HS, Wise LS, Das KM. Circulating antibodies against human colonic extract enriched with a 40kDa protein in patients with ulcerative colitis. *Gut* 1990; **31**: 1016–20.

172 Halstensen TS, Das KM, Brandtzaeg P. Epithelial deposits of immunoglobulin G1 and activated complement colocalise with the M(r) 40kD putative autoantigen in ulcerative colitis. *Gut* 1993; **34**: 650–7.

173 Das KM, Vecchi M, Sakamaki S. A shared and unique epitope(s) on human colon, skin, and biliary epithelium detected by a monoclonal antibody. *Gastroenterology* 1990; **98**: 464–9.

174 Bhagat S, Das KM. A shared and unique peptide in the human colon, eye, and joint detected by a monoclonal antibody. *Gastroenterology* 1994; **107**: 103–8.

175 McDonald TT. Effector and regulatory lymphoid cells and cytokines in mucosal sites. *Curr Top Microbiol Immunol* 1998; **236**: 113–36.

176 Luster AD. Chemokines – chemotactic cytokines that mediate inflammation. *N Engl J Med* 1998; **338**: 436–45.

177 MacDermott RP. Chemokines in the inflammatory bowel diseases. *J Clin Immunol* 1999; **19**: 266–72.

178 Day R, Rowlands D, Knight S, Forbes A. Epithelial syndecan-1 expression is reduced by tumour necrosis factor alpha in vitro. *Gut* 1999; **45**(Suppl 5): A125.

179 Raedler A, Schreiber S, Weerth A, Voss A, Peters S, Greten H. Assessment of in vivo activated T cells in patients with Crohn's disease. *Hepatogastroenterology* 1990; **37**: 67–71.

180 Kusugami K, Youngman KR, West GA, Fiocchi C. Intestinal immune reactivity to interleukin 2 differs among Crohn's disease, ulcerative colitis and controls. *Gastroenterology* 1989; **97**: 1–9.

181 Roman LI, Manzano L, De la Hera A, Abreu L, Rossi I, Alvarez-Mon M. Expanded CD4+CD45RO+ phenotype and defective proliferative response in T lymphocytes from patients with Crohn's disease. *Gastroenterology* 1996; **110**: 1008–19.

182 West GA, Matsuura T, Levine AD, Klein JS, Fiocchi C. Interleukin 4 in inflammatory bowel disease and mucosal immune reactivity. *Gastroenterology* 1996; **110**: 1683–95.

183 Moore KW, O'Garra A, de Waal Malefyt R, *et al.* Interleukin-10. *Annu Rev Immunol* 1993; **11**: 165–90.

184 Hibi T, Ohara M, Watanabe M, *et al.* Interleukin 2 and interferon-gamma augment anticolon antibody dependent cellular cytotoxicity in ulcerative colitis. *Gut* 1993; **34**: 788–93.

185 Gerber BO, Zanni MP, Uguccioni M, *et al.* Functional expression of the eotaxin receptor CCR3 in T lymphocytes co-localizing with eosinophils. *Curr Biol* 1997; **7**: 836–43.

186 Raab Y, Fredens K, Gerdin B, Hallgren R. Eosinophil activation in ulcerative colitis: studies on mucosal release and localization of eosinophil granule constituents. *Dig Dis Sci* 1998; **43**: 1061–70.

187 Gaginella TS, Kachur JF, Tamai H, Keshavarzian A. Reactive oxygen and nitrogen metabolites as mediators of secretory diarrhea. *Gastroenterology* 1995; **109**: 2019–28.

188 Simmonds NJ, Allen RE, Stevens TRJ, *et al.* Chemiluminescence assay of mucosal reactive

oxygen metabolites in inflammatory bowel disease. *Gastroenterology* 1992; **103**: 186–96.

189 Keshavarzian A, Sedghi S, Kanofsky J, *et al.* Excessive production of reactive oxygen metabolites by inflamed colon: analysis by chemiluminescence probe. *Gastroenterology* 1992; **103**: 177–85.

190 Roediger WEW, Lawson MJ, Nance SH, Radcliffe BC. Detectable colonic nitrite levels in inflammatory bowel disease – mucosal or bacterial malfunction? *Digestion* 1986; **35**: 199–204.

191 Middleton SJ, Shorthouse M, Hunter JO. Increased nitric oxide synthesis in ulcerative colitis. *Lancet* 1993; **341**: 465–6.

192 Lundberg JO, Hellström, Lundberg JM, Alving K. Greatly increased luminal nitric oxide in ulcerative colitis. *Lancet* 1994; **344**: 1673–4.

193 Rachmilewitz D, Stamler JS, Bachwich D, Karmeli F, Ackerman Z, Podolsky D. Enhanced colonic nitric oxide generation and nitric oxide synthase activity in ulcerative colitis and Crohn's disease. *Gut* 1995; **36**: 718–23.

194 Perner A, Rask-Madsen J. The potential role of nitric oxide in chronic inflammatory bowel disorders. *Aliment Pharmacol Ther* 1999; **13**: 135–44.

195 Bjorck S, Dahlstrom A, Ahlman H. Topical treatment of ulcerative proctitis with lidocaine. *Scand J Gastroenterol* 1989; **24**: 1061–72.

196 Mazumdar S, Das KM. Immunocytochemical localization of vasoactive intestinal peptide and substance P in the colon from normal subjects and patients with inflammatory bowel disease. *Am J Gastroenterol* 1992; **87**: 176–81.

197 Raithel M, Schneider HT, Hahn EG. Effect of substance P on histamine secretion from gut mucosa in inflammatory bowel disease. *Scand J Gastroenterol* 1999; **34**: 496–503.

198 Belai A, Boulos PB, Robson T, Burnstock G. Neurochemical coding in the small intestine of patients with Crohn's disease. *Gut* 1997; **40**: 767–74.

199 Bjarnason I, Zanelli G, Smith T, *et al.* Nonsteroidal antiinflammatory drug-induced intestinal inflammation in humans. *Gastroenterology* 1987; **93**: 480–9.

200 Davies NM. Toxicity of nonsteroidal anti-inflammatory drugs in the large intestine. *Dis Colon Rectum* 1995; **38**: 1311–21.

201 Evans JM, McMahon AD, Murray FE, McDevitt DG, MacDonald TM. Non-steroidal anti-inflammatory drugs are associated with emergency admission to hospital for colitis due to inflammatory bowel disease. *Gut* 1997; **40**: 619–22.

202 Gleeson MH, Warren BF. Emergency admission to hospital for colitis due to inflammatory bowel disease. *Gut* 1998; **42**: 144.

203 Harries AD, Baird A, Rhodes J. Non-smoking: a feature of ulcerative colitis. *Br Med J* 1982; **284**: 706.

204 Lindberg E, Tysk C, Andersson K, Järnerot G. Smoking and inflammatory bowel disease. A case control study. *Gut* 1988; **29**: 352–7.

205 Vessey M, Jewell D, Smith A, *et al.* Chronic inflammatory bowel disease, cigarette smoking and use of oral contraceptives: findings in a large cohort study of women of childbearing age. *Br Med J* 1986; **292**: 1101–3.

206 Merrett MN, Mortensen N, Kettlewell M, Jewell DP. Smoking may prevent pouchitis in patients with restorative proctocolectomy for ulcerative colitis. *Gut* 1996; **38**: 362–4.

207 Sutherland LR, Ramcharan S, Bryant H, Fick G. Effect of cigarette smoking on recurrence of Crohn's disease. *Gastroenterology* 1990; **98**: 1123–8.

208 Holdstock G, Savage D, Harman M, Wright R. Should patients with inflammatory bowel disease smoke? *Br Med J* 1984; **288**: 362.

209 Cosnes J, Carbonnel F, Beaugerie L, Le Quintrec Y, Gendre JP. Effects of cigarette smoking on the long-term course of Crohn's disease. *Gastroenterology* 1996; **110**: 424–31.

210 Cosnes J, Carbonnel F, Carrat F, Beaugerie L, Cattan S, Gendre J. Effects of current and former cigarette smoking on the clinical course of Crohn's disease. *Aliment Pharmacol Ther* 1999; **13**: 1403–11.

211 Breuer-Katschinski BD, Hollander N, Goebell H. Effect of smoking on the course of Crohn's disease. *Eur J Gastroenterol Hepatol* 1996; **8**: 225–8.

212 Florent C, Cortot A, Quandale P, *et al.* Placebo-controlled clinical trial of mesalazine in the prevention of early endoscopic recurrences after

resection for Crohn's disease. *Eur J Gastroenterol Hepatol* 1996; **8**: 229–33.

213 Fraga XF, Vergara M, Medina C, Casellas F, Bermejo B, Malagelada JR. Effects of smoking on the presentation and clinical course of inflammatory bowel disease. *Eur J Gastroenterol Hepatol* 1997; **9**: 683–7.

214 Cope G, Heatley R. Cigarette smoking and intestinal defences. *Gut* 1992; **32**: 721–3.

215 Tytgat KMAJ, Opddam FJM, Einerhand AWC, Büller HA, Dekker J. MUC2 is the prominent colonic mucin expressed in ulcerative colitis. *Gut* 1996; **38**: 554–63.

216 Van Klinken BJ, Van der Wal JW, Einerhand AW, Buller HA, Dekker J. Sulphation and secretion of the predominant secretory human colonic mucin MUC2 in ulcerative colitis. *Gut* 1999; **44**: 387–93.

217 Sher ME, Bank S, Greenberg R, *et al.* The influence of cigarette smoking on cytokine levels in patients with inflammatory bowel disease. *Inflamm Bowel Dis* 1999; **5**: 73–8.

218 Galeazzi F, Qui BS, O'Byrne PM, Collins SM. The adverse effect of cigaratte smoke on experimental colitis in the rat is mediated by a neural pathway. *Gut* 1999; **45**(Suppl V): A78.

219 Duffy LC, Zielezny MA, Marshall JR, *et al.* Cigarette smoking and risk of clinical relapse in patients with Crohn's disease. *Am J Prev Med* 1990; **6**: 161–6.

220 Shields PL, Low-Beer TS. Patients' awareness of adverse relation between Crohn's disease and their smoking: questionnaire survey. *Br Med J* 1996; **313**: 265–6.

221 Rutgeerts P, D'Haens G, Hiele M, Geboes K, Vantrappen G. Appendectomy protects against ulcerative colitis. *Gastroenterology* 1994; **106**: 1251–3.

222 Sandler RS. Appendicectomy and ulcerative colitis. *Lancet* 1998; **352**: 1797–8.

223 Koutroubakis IE, Vlachonikolis IG. Appendectomy and the development of ulcerative colitis a causal relationship. Results of a meta-analysis of published case-control studies. *Gut* 1999; **45**(Suppl V): A174.

224 Dijkstra B, Bagshaw PF, Frizelle FA. Protective effect of appendectomy on the development of ulcerative colitis. *Dis Colon Rectum* 1999; **42**: 334–6.

225 Montgomery SM, Pounder RE, Wakefield AJ. Smoking in adults and passive smoking in children are associated with acute appendicitis. *Lancet* 1999; **353**: 379.

226 Koutroubakis IE, Vlachonikolis IG, Kapsoritakis AS, *et al.* Appendectomy, tonsillectomy and risk of inflammatory bowel disease. *Dis Colon Rectum* 1999; **42**: 225–30.

227 Wettergren A, Munkholm P, Larsen LG, *et al.* Granulomas of the appendix: is it Crohn's disease? *Scand J Gastroenterol* 1991; **26**: 961–4.

228 Timmcke AE. Granulomatous appendicitis: is it Crohn's disease? Report of a case and review of the literature. *Am J Gastroenterol* 1986; **81**: 283–7.

229 Lesko SM, Kaufman DW, Rosenberg L, *et al.* Evidence for an increased risk of Crohn's disease in oral contraceptive users. *Gastroenterology* 1985; **89**: 1046–9.

230 Biaggi AM, Potet F. La colite ischemique du sujet jeune. *Ann Pathol* 1995; **15**: 45–9.

231 Lee JCW, Halpern S, Lowe DG, Forbes A, Lennard-Jones JE. Absence of skin sensitivity to oxides of aluminium, silicon, titanium or zirconium in patients with Crohn's disease. *Gut* 1996; **39**: 231–3.

232 Powell JJ, Ainley CC, Harvey RS, *et al.* Characterisation of inorganic microparticles in pigment cells of human gut associated lymphoid tissue. *Gut* 1996; **38**: 390–5.

233 Babbs CF. Oxygen radicals in ulcerative colitis. *Free Radic Biol Med* 1992; **13**: 169–81.

234 Sturniolo GC, Mestriner C, Lecis PE, *et al.* Altered plasma and mucosal concentrations of trace elements and antioxidants in active ulcerative colitis. *Scand J Gastroenterol* 1998; **33**: 644–9.

235 Kawai M, Sumimoto S, Kasajima Y, Hamamoto T. A case of ulcerative colitis induced by oral ferrous sulfate. *Acta Paediatr Jpn* 1992; **34**: 476–8.

236 Persson PG, Ahlbom A, Hellers G. Crohn's disease and ulcerative colitis. A review of dietary studies with emphasis on methodological aspects. *Scand J Gastroenterol* 1987; **22**: 385–9.

237 Tragnone A, Valpiani D, Miglio F, *et al.* Dietary habits as risk factors for inflammatory bowel

disease. *Eur J Gastroenterol Hepatol* 1995; 7: 47–51.

238 Reif S, Klein I, Lubin F, Farbstein M, Hallak A, Gilat T. Pre-illness dietary factors in inflammatory bowel disease. *Gut* 1997; **40**: 754–60.

239 Russel MG, Engels LG, Muris JW, *et al.* Modern life in the epidemiology of inflammatory bowel disease: a case-control study with special emphasis on nutritional factors. *Eur J Gastroenterol Hepatol* 1998; **10**: 243–9.

240 Riordan AM, Ruxton CH, Hunter JO. A review of associations between Crohn's disease and consumption of sugars. *Eur J Clin Nutr* 1998; **52**: 229–38.

241 Nagel E, Schattenfroh S, Buhner S, *et al.* Animal experiment studies of ultrastructural changes in the lamina propria of the ileum caused by dietary fats and comparison with cytopathology in Crohn disease. *Z Gastroenterol* 1993; **31**: 727–34.

242 Epidemiology Group of the Research Committee of Inflammatory Bowel Disease in Japan. Dietary and other risk factors of ulcerative colitis. A case-control study in Japan. *J Clin Gastroenterol* 1994; **19**: 166–71.

Clinical presentation

Inflammatory bowel disease is usually responsible for diarrhoea and, when the colon is involved, the rectal passage of blood. Depending on severity and the particular site(s) affected, there may also be weight loss, anorexia and fatigue, or other systemic features such as tachycardia and pyrexia. Features that point towards Crohn's disease or ulcerative colitis (Table 2.1) reflect, on the one hand, the relative frequency of rectosigmoid involvement, and, on the other, the malabsorptive effects of small bowel involvement in Crohn's disease. The history alone will occasionally remove any significant differential diagnosis. A young adult Caucasian patient presenting with several months'

Table 2.1 Clinical features which help to distinguish Crohn's disease from ulcerative colitis

	Crohn's disease	Ulcerative colitis
General		
Diarrhoea	+++	+++
Abdominal pain	+++	+
Pyrexia	++	+
Oral ulcers	+++	+
Reflecting rectosigmoid site of disease		
Rectal bleeding	+	+++
Mucus/pus with stools	+	++
Tenesmus	+	++
Reflecting small bowel involvement and malabsorption		
Weight loss	+++	+
Growth retardation	+++	+
Reflecting penetrating tissue damage		
Abdominal mass	++	–
Perianal disease	+++	+
Fistula	++	–

Key: +++, very common; ++, frequent; +, seen but relatively uncommon; –, most unusual.

diarrhoea, weight loss and right iliac fossa pain might well be considered to have Crohn's disease until proved otherwise. Equally, gastrointestinal infection must always be considered and especially so when the history is short. We still have a long way to go given the continuing reports of prolonged delay between first symptom and a definitive diagnosis; in a large multicentre European study, ulcerative colitis patients had symptoms for a mean of over 9 years whilst Crohn's patients waited over 13 years![1]

Examination and clinical investigation

EXAMINATION

The general examination will often contribute little, beyond confirming aspects of the history, but evidence of perianal disease is much more typical of Crohn's disease – affecting upwards of 15 per cent of patients – than of ulcerative colitis. One study put the frequency of perianal fistula in Crohn's as high as 33 per cent, but was probably biased towards those with more severe disease, as all had been in-patients for at least a month at some point.[2] It would, however, be a mistake to consider that perianal disease is pathognomonic of Crohn's disease, since around 10 per cent of all perianal disease associated with inflammatory bowel disease is in patients with ulcerative colitis. Severe perianal disease is nonetheless mainly confined to patients with Crohn's.

The various extra-intestinal features of inflammatory bowel disease (considered fully in Chapter 6) are sometimes said to be more or less common in ulcerative colitis than in Crohn's disease. Reliable data are few, but there is a strong association between involvement of the colon and extra-intestinal manifestations, and patients with Crohn's disease rarely have these features if their disease is confined to the small bowel.

Up to a third of patients with predominantly distal colitis may, despite a clear history of diarrhoea, prove to be constipated to abdominal palpation; this is less common in Crohn's disease. One study has suggested that this proximal stasis is actually the cause of acute relapse in up to 10 per cent of cases.[3]

Bleeding is generally a feature of ulcerative colitis and distal Crohn's disease, but catastrophic bleeding from Crohn's disease does rarely occur – at a lifetime frequency of under 1 per cent. Unsurprisingly, most of the information is in the form of case reports, but the 34 patients collected from a single Belgian centre allow some generalizations to be drawn.[4] Most of the patients had an established diagnosis of Crohn's disease (mean > 5 years) but in only a third did the bleeding occur during a time of active diseases. No less than 95 per cent of the patients had a causative ulcer, the left colon being the most frequent site. This is consistent with impressions from the literature and from collections available only in abstract form.

Distinction from functional bowel disorders may be obvious in inflammatory bowel disease patients with bleeding, but in more subtle cases, weight loss or the presence of night-time symptoms sufficient to wake the patient from sleep may be strong pointers to an organic aetiology. There may also be differences in underlying personality type between the two principal forms of inflammatory bowel disease. Patients with Crohn's disease were found in one study to be more extrovert and with a greater psychoticism score than those with ulcerative colitis, but with no differences in respect of neuroticism.[5] A degree of caution is needed in interpreting these data as prevalent cases were studied; the possibility that the course of the disease may have affected the prevailing personality state remains open (also, relatively small numbers were studied, including only 27 with ulcerative colitis).

PROCTOSCOPY

At proctosigmoidoscopy, the confluent erythema and ulceration of ulcerative colitis are, when typically exhibited, distinguishable from more characteristic aphthoid ulceration, serpiginous ulcers, and generally patchy distribution of Crohn's disease. In a patient with a history suggestive of inflammatory bowel disease and in whom the rectum appears normal, a Crohn's diagnosis is thereby supported. It is most unusual for ulcerative colitis to present with a normal-appearing rectum (and still less with a histologically normal rectum) unless topical therapy has already been utilized, but most authorities allow that this scenario very rarely occurs. Confluent proctitis is, of course, also seen in Crohn's disease.

LABORATORY INVESTIGATIONS

Investigation will typically commence with the relatively routine laboratory tests such as full blood count and serum biochemistry. These will rarely contribute to the diagnostic process in patients with a typical history and examination, but may be helpful in cases where these are atypical, and in the differential from functional disorders, which are effectively excluded by an elevated platelet count, a low haemoglobin, or a low albumin, for example. Different blood tests to assess the magnitude of inflammation are favoured by different laboratories, for logistic and other reasons, as indicated below in the section on assessment of disease activity. Correlation between the various options is incomplete and there will inevitably be different false positives and false negatives depending on which tests are selected. None of the inflammatory markers is reliable as a specific indicator of an inflammatory bowel disease diagnosis.

The potential aetiological relevance of anti-neutrophil and anti-*Saccharomyces* antibodies is addressed in Chapter 1, and their relative expression can also be of value in the distinction between ulcerative colitis and Crohn's disease. The sensitivity and specificity of pANCA positivity for a final diagnosis of ulcerative colitis are in the region of 65 per cent and 85 per cent, respectively, and positive antibody to *Saccharomyces cerevisiae* antigen (ASCA) has sensitivity and specificity for Crohn's disease of around 60 per cent and 85 per cent. If the two tests are combined, sensitivity is sacrificed (down to about 50 per cent), but specificity and positive predictive value are improved in each case to well over 90 per cent: for ulcerative colitis if there is a positive pANCA with negative ASCA; for Crohn's disease if positive ASCA with negative pANCA.[6] Unfortunately, the diagnostic yield is probably least in indeterminate colitis when help is most needed.[7] The prevailing pANCA/ASCA pattern does, however, appear to predict part of the inflammatory bowel disease phenotype. It is possible that pANCA-positive colitics have a generally worse course, that ASCA-positive Crohn's disease patients have more tendency to fistulation and need for surgery, whilst those with pANCA and without ASCA behave more like patients with ulcerative colitis than the average Crohn's disease sufferer.[7]

DIFFERENTIAL DIAGNOSIS

The differential diagnosis of inflammatory bowel disease presenting with an acute colitis includes infection, non-steroidal drug-related, and acute, self-limiting colitis (which may itself be infective). The most likely organisms – *Shigella*, *Campylobacter*, *Escherichia coli* O157, *Entamoeba* and, to a lesser extent as bleeding is less frequent, *Salmonella*, *Aeromonas*, *Yersinia* and rotavirus – are all fairly readily identified (or excluded) by conventional laboratory microbiological examination of the stools. More rigorous microbiological attention is required if the patient is immunodeficient. Pseudomembranous colitis from *Clostridium difficile* infection should be sought, by culture and by examination for its cytotoxin, especially if the patient has recently been exposed to antibiotics. It will be remembered also that the patient with inflammatory bowel disease may present acutely because of a secondary gastrointestinal infection. In the patient presenting for the first time, but in the absence of acute dysenteric symptoms, the differential diagnosis is rather wider and includes colorectal carcinoma, ischaemic colitis and radiation enteritis if there is rectal bleeding, and intestinal tuberculosis, irritable bowel syndrome and a variety of malabsorptive and other gastrointestinal conditions, if diarrhoea is unaccompanied by bleeding. When the history does not provide obvious pointers, it is then reasonable to proceed with investigation as for inflammatory bowel disease.

Imaging of inflammatory bowel disease

The traditional radiological methods of imaging the bowel have been increasingly challenged by newer modalities. Few would now argue that even the most carefully conducted double-contrast barium enema is superior to competent colonoscopy, but they remain complementary investigations[8] (see below). The alternatives to barium-based examination of the small intestine are less established. The principal competition now comes from magnetic resonance imaging (MRI), but enteroscopy and white-cell scanning have important roles. Use of reconstructive three-dimensional computerized tomography (CT), better known as virtual endoscopy, and of newer methods of more specific isotopic imaging have not yet been exploited to the full in inflammatory bowel disease. Angiography, however, is rarely relevant in this context.

PLAIN ABDOMINAL RADIOGRAPH

The plain abdominal radiograph is an under-valued and underutilized resource in many institutions caring for patients with inflammatory bowel disease. It will often be obvious from the supine film that the patient has faecal loading in the proximal colon, which effectively excludes a diagnosis of total colitis. On the contrary, total colitis becomes an important possibility when there appears to be no faecal residue at any site (see also Chapter 4).

ABDOMINAL ULTRASONOGRAPHY

The modest abdominal ultrasonographic scan has also been underutilized in inflammatory bowel disease. Quite apart from its role in detection and assessment of abscesses (see Chapter 7), it will often identify a loop of thickened, inflamed bowel with proximal distension and fluid retention, and not infrequently make possible a strong case for a diagnosis of Crohn's disease in the newly presenting patient with abdominal pain.

Modern ultrasound technology permits ready evaluation of the intestine at most sites in the abdomen, and radiologists and gastroenterologists are become more skilled at interpreting the findings. Using a very simple single criterion to determine postoperative recurrence – namely the presence of a bowel wall thickness of greater than 5 mm – ultrasonography proved nearly as reliable as full ileocolonoscopy in a blinded study of over 40 patients, and was possible in all patients, unlike endoscopy, which was prevented by disease or its location in 13 per cent.[9] With this criterion alone there was a sensitivity of 81 per cent and a positive predictive value of 96 per cent; full ileocolonoscopy can legitimately be reserved for those with negative or uncertain results given the negative predictive value of 57 per cent.

Formal, ultrasound-based scoring systems are yet to be generally accepted, but one Japanese group has proposed a complex activity index which takes into account the thickness of the bowel wall and the ease with which the normal stratification of the intestine is discerned (i.e. mucosa versus submucosa versus muscularis).[10] It is repeated for eight segments of the intestine. A good correlation with results of other imaging techniques is seen, but the absence of a correlation with C-reactive protein (CRP) levels or clinical activity scores indicates that it is a topographical rather than an activity index. Given its complexity, despite the advantage of non-invasiveness, it is unlikely that it will gain general acceptance.

Endoscopic ultrasound has not yet been widely adopted in inflammatory bowel disease, but it offers potentially useful information in assessment of complications such as pelvic fistulae, and may provide information additive to that of colonoscopy in (for example) a questioned neoplastic region in extensive colitis.[11] It is also proposed as a route to estimation of penetration and therefore of expected histology in inflammatory bowel disease in general.[12,13] It remains to be seen if this will prove of general clinical value.

Doppler flow measurements in the mesenteric vessels of patients with inflammatory bowel disease have been reported to be of value. There is also evidence that flow in the rectal vessels is reduced in ulcerative colitis, whether or not the disease is active,[14] but without changes in patients with Crohn's disease affecting the rectum.[15] Peroperative study indicates that there is normally a flow rate gradient along the length of the intestine, higher values being recorded in the proximal than the distal small bowel,[16] but that in addition to this there is a reduction in local flow rates associated with increasing severity of involvement by Crohn's disease.[16] This finding is difficult to reconcile with our own findings[17] and those of an Italian group,[18] which show a clear *positive* correlation between flow in the superior mesenteric artery and the presence of Crohn's disease, albeit differing on whether there is a correlation between disease activity or not. As these latter two studies were done in the free-living patient rather than under anaesthetic at laparotomy, it is possible that the earlier Japanese data are of less general relevance, but it is clear that we still have much to learn in this area.

BARIUM RADIOLOGY

Contrast radiology is the longest-established imaging modality for diagnosis of inflammatory bowel disease. Barium sulphate is appropriately radiodense, is essentially inert, and is not normally absorbed from the gut. However, extraluminal barium creates a vigorous and potentially fatal inflammatory reaction in the peritoneum with a high risk of subsequent devastating fibrosis. It behoves the clinician and radiologist to avoid barium where free perforation is a possibility, and to use instead a water-soluble contrast agent. Inferior definition is then to be expected, not least because many water-soluble media have a potent osmotic effect and tend to be diluted by resultant intestinal secretions.

The classical appearances of ulcerative colitis and Crohn's disease are well documented, and reference texts and atlases such as those of Margulis and Burhenne[19] and Misiewicz *et al.*[20] allow perusal of the variation in extent and severity and the more subtle aspects of radiological diagnosis. The key colonic and small bowel abnormalities may, however, be summarized (Table 2.2).

Barium enema

Although controlled comparisons of colonoscopy and barium enema favour colonoscopy, which of course offers the advantage of permitting histological sampling, there remains a case for barium radiology. The potential value of the unprepared or 'instant' enema is discussed in the section on fulminant colitis (see Chapter 4), and it retains a role in the early assessment of a new patient with colitic symptoms in whom the extent of the disease will have an immediate influence on management.

The radiological distinction between ulcerative colitis and Crohn's colitis is based on the distribution, depth and presence/absence of complications, just as in the overall distinction of the two conditions. It is usually possible to draw

Table 2.2 Barium enema in diagnosis of inflammatory bowel disease

Feature	Crohn's disease	Ulcerative colitis	Other
Distal disease	+/–	++	+/–
Continuity	+/–	++	+/–
Asymmetry	++	–	+/–
Skip lesions	++	–	+/–
Deep perforating ulcers	+	–	+/–
Fistula	++	–	+/–

Key: ++, frequent; +, seen but relatively uncommon; –, most unusual.

Figure 2.1 Barium follow-through in an early phase of Crohn's disease. The terminal ileum is seen in the centre of the image and bears several shallow aphthoid ulcers.

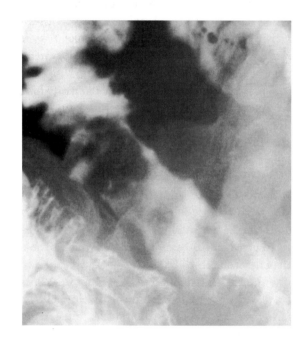

a confident interpretation from the combination of the radiological signs and the clinical features. The double-contrast enema using both air and barium has superseded the single-contrast examination (except for the 'instant' enema described above). In early/mild colitis there may be only a granularity of the mucosa, which, in ulcerative colitis, will almost always be continuous from the rectum upwards. At a relatively early stage the space between the rectum and the sacrum (the retrorectal space) becomes enlarged. It is probable that this reflects both thickening of the rectal wall and the beginnings of rectal shortening as the bowel becomes fibrotic. The so-called hosepipe colon is now infrequently seen (perhaps the result of better medical therapy or earlier surgery), but when present is strongly supportive of a diagnosis of chronic fibrotic ulcerative colitis.

Crohn's colitis may mimic ulcerative colitis but usually declares itself from deeper ulceration (the rose-thorn ulcer), and a more patchy or asymmetrical distribution (with a strong tendency to affect the mesenteric border preferentially). In mild disease the halo appearance of aphthoid ulcers is characteristic (Figure 2.1). The presence of fistulous connections with other structures makes for a sure distinction from ulcerative colitis.

When polyps are demonstrated, the radiologist may be confident that 'bridging' seen between polyps (also referred to as filiform polyposis) is the result of past inflammation, but will usually choose to defer to colonoscopic/histological assessment, since it is not possible to make a clear distinction between the inflammatory polyp (common in inflammatory bowel disease and essentially harmless) and the adenoma (which should be removed). Despite its limitations, the barium enema still provides information that cannot be obtained by other means in every centre. The proximal colon of a patient with a tight stricture can often be assessed adequately and, perhaps more importantly, radiological recognition of abnormal distensibility and contour of the bowel may be the earliest sign of malignant transformation in the long-standing colitic (see Chapter 8).

The radiological differential diagnosis for conditions other than inflammatory bowel disease includes ischaemia, which is patchy like Crohn's disease, but usually affects the vascular watershed zones such as at the splenic flexure. Infective colitides may be confused with inflammatory bowel disease (usually when the history is deficient), and there is a steady flow of accounts of mismanagement of acute amoebic colitis in which steroids have been given to treat an assumed diagnosis of inflammatory bowel disease. The classic cone-shaped caecum of chronic amoebiasis is rarely seen in Western centres, and tends to yield a differential diagnosis of neoplasia rather than of inflammatory

bowel disease when it does appear. Pseudomembranous colitis poses more of a challenge as it may complicate underlying inflammatory bowel disease, but the radiological features of plaque formation and proximal distension may be helpful if there has not already been clinical or endoscopic suspicion. All of the remaining roles of barium enema in inflammatory bowel disease are likely soon to be overtaken by developments in virtual colonoscopy, which is less invasive and which should be at least as informative as the best conventional enema.

Barium studies of the small bowel

Barium studies of the small bowel are currently more secure, clinical experience continuing to support their use in the investigation of patients with symptoms potentially attributable to the small bowel,[21] even when a centre has special expertise in colonoscopic ileoscopy.[22] There is still some debate in radiological circles as to the relative place of the traditional follow-through and the small bowel enema or enteroclysis in which the barium is instilled through a nasal tube placed into the jejunum. My colleagues prefer the former for the reason that it tends to give relatively better visualization of the lower small bowel (very often the area of greater interest in inflammatory bowel disease) and because it generally remains possible to compress the contrast-filled bowel, which in turn helps to permit separation of superimposed intestinal loops.[23] The more distended bowel created in the adequately filled bowel at enteroclysis may be more difficult or painful to compress. The decision should rightly be that of the radiologist responsible for the examination, but the speedier completion of enteroclysis may be outweighed in the patient's eyes by the added discomfort of intubation. It may also be helpful to use pharmacological manipulation with anticholinergics (such as hyoscine or atropine) not only for their influence on intestinal motility but also because patients often find that the examination is then appreciably less uncomfortable.[24]. A follow-through examination can be performed as an adjunct to assessment of the more proximal gastrointestinal tract (the meal and follow-through), but this is almost always second best for both parts of the examination as the ideal density and quantity of barium differ for the different purposes: it is not recommended and clinicians should not seek this.

It may be helpful, especially for comprehensive visualization of the terminal ileum, to introduce air into the colon (or to use an oral effervescent agent) to obtain partially double-contrast views. This is distinct from the retrograde examination of the small bowel obtained at barium enema when the ileocaecal valve is incompetent or absent, and which is not the investigation of choice if the ileum is the area of interest. Retrograde examinations are nevertheless valuable in patients with an ileostomy, and especially so when there is proximal stenosis or when the patient is unwilling or unable to retain oral barium.

The radiological features of small bowel Crohn's reflect its pathological nature and distribution. The early changes include granularity, aphthous ulcers, and fold thickening, progressing with increasing severity to nodularity, frank focal ulceration, fissuring and stenosis. The asymmetry, typical of all aspects of Crohn's disease, is usually manifest as a disproportionate involvement of the mesenteric border of the gut. The classical 'string' sign (Figure 2.2), in which lengths of bowel appear narrowed and irregular, is as much the result of inflammation as of fibrous stricturing, and the separation of adjacent loops indicates that one is dealing with thickening of the bowel. In a dynamic examination it should be possible to make a distinction between motile but severely inflamed loops and those in which there is fixed stenotic scarring. This has clear therapeutic implications. 'Cobblestones' reflect the presence of deep and intersecting transverse and longitudinal ulcers and are rarely seen in other conditions. The presence of spontaneous fistulae either between intestinal loops or from intestine to other structures is

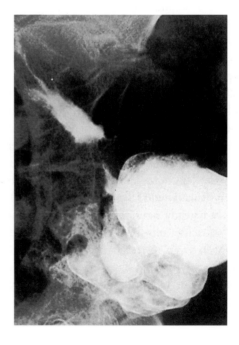

Figure 2.2 Barium follow-through in the same patient as in Figure 2.1, 12 months later when, despite 5-aminosalicylate (5-ASA) therapy, the disease has progressed, leading to stenosis of the terminal ileum, which now almost exhibits the string sign; obstructive symptoms led to a surgical intervention.

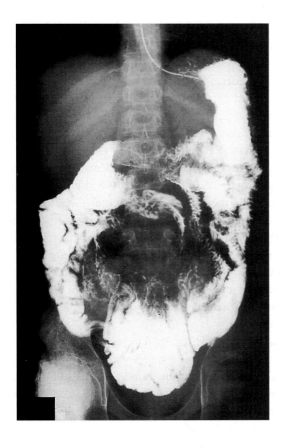

Figure 2.3 Barium follow-through in an adolescent with extreme small bowel Crohn's disease. The central loops of bowel are narrowed and their separation is indicative of their considerable thickening. The ulceration of the intestine is evident at several sites, as is the degree of distal stenosis, itself responsible for intestinal dilatation (most obvious in the left iliac fossa). The nasogastric tube was being used for primary nutritional therapy.

almost pathognomonic of Crohn's disease in developed countries.

Although involvement of the terminal ileum is characteristic, it is by no means inevitable in small bowel Crohn's disease: in a recent survey 9 of 71 patients with small bowel disease had a normal terminal ileum.[22] Patients with extensive Crohn's disease may also exhibit the characteristic malabsorption pattern of barium dilution and flocculation; a modest diffuse dilatation of the intestine (Figure 2.3) may be seen. There tends to be a loss of the intestinal fold pattern in the proximal jejunum (and sometimes an increase more distally, although this is more a feature of non-Crohn's malabsorption). The special relevance of barium studies to short bowel syndrome is considered further in Chapter 7.

Differential diagnosis for small bowel barium studies

Intestinal tuberculosis poses special problems in the differential diagnosis at centres in developed countries because its relative rarity tends to lead to its neglect. The converse problem for patients with Crohn's disease in populations in which tuberculosis is more endemic is arguably less worrying given the therapeutic implications of a wrong diagnosis in one direction rather than the other. The radiologist may help by distinguishing the characteristic multiple transverse ulcers, the classic funnelled caecum, gross thickening of the intestinal wall and fixity of the terminal ileum, or from other manifestations of tuberculosis, not least of these being the chest radiograph – although this is abnormal in only about 50 per cent of those with intestinal tuberculosis and may not be helpful.[25] A continued high index of suspicion in all population groups is needed if early infection is to be identified and late complications avoided. The differential diagnosis for terminal ileitis is often otherwise brief, but previous irradiation, Behçet's disease and yersinial infection deserve consideration. Intestinal lymphoid hyperplasia (idiopathic or related to a variety of acute and chronic infections) may be over-interpreted as Crohn's in young patients with gastrointestinal symptoms, but the experienced radiologist will usually be confident of the correct interpretation when associated ulceration is absent. At the opposite end of the age range, contrast examinations are increasingly performed in patients with intestinal ischaemia. Focal and segmental ischaemia can be difficult to distinguish from active Crohn's.

The clinician should regard a radiological verdict of Crohn's disease not as a diagnosis, but as a critical component to the formation of a global assessment. In practice, disagreement with a confident conclusion arising from a small bowel series is unusual (Table 2.3).

FISTULOGRAPHY

Fistulae are poorly demonstrated by endoscopic techniques, and the degree of filling at intraluminal contrast studies is often inadequate for their full anatomy to be discerned. CT scanning may be of some limited help in the assessment of the patient with enterocutaneous fistulae (see below and Chapter 7), but until MR methodology is a little more mature it is unlikely that the traditional 'fistulogram' will be superseded. Introduction of water-soluble contrast directly into the cutaneous opening will usually permit adequate demonstration of the fistula track and the site of its origin from the bowel. The tendency of the contrast to spill back can be overcome by its introduction through a balloon-tipped catheter, which seals the skin opening. As relatively high pressures may be required, the caution of an experienced operator is advised to avoid damage and maintain the reputation of fistulography as a safe technique.

CT SCANNING

CT scanning has mostly been used in the evaluation and management of complications of inflammatory bowel disease rather than in its initial diagnosis, but more modern scanners with helical/spiral image capturing permit detailed assessment of the entire alimentary tract. In Crohn's disease, the thickening of the bowel loops and

Table 2.3 Small bowel series in diagnosis of inflammatory bowel disease

Feature	Crohn's disease	Tuberculosis	Other infection	Ischaemia
Terminal ileal disease	++	+	+	+/−
Enteric fistula	++	+	−	−
Strictures	++	++	+/−	++
Patchy distribution	++	+	−	++
Wall thickening	++	+++	+	+
Aphthous ulcers	++	+/−	+/−	−
Asymmetry	++	+	−	++
Cobblestones	++	−	−	−

Key: +++, very common; ++, frequent; +, seen but relatively uncommon; −, most unusual.

their approximate location are easily identified, and further information in respect of significant stenoses and fistulous connections is now beginning to be of comparable reliability to that of barium follow-through. CT appearances will reliably differentiate between ulcerative colitis and Crohn's colitis in most cases, and may occasionally avoid colonoscopy.[26] The analysis of small bowel abnormalities can often differentiate causes other than Crohn's disease such as ischaemia and Behçet's.[27] The so-called 'comb' sign, which results from vascular dilatation and tortuosity, and a wider spacing of the vasa recta is proposed as a specific indicator of Crohn's disease.[28] The need for samples for histology remains, nonetheless. Enhanced CT scans are a good means to evaluate the retroperitoneum and iliopsoas region in patients with suspected abdominal sepsis, these areas often proving inaccessible to ultrasonography. Abscesses appear as relatively low-density spaces with enhancing walls, and can often be shown to contain gas (or previously administered contrast material).

Virtual colonoscopy utilizes reconstructive techniques that permit the creation of images that apparently equate to the three-dimensional intraluminal view of the colon at colonoscopy. This is beginning to take on a service role in the assessment of the colon for neoplasia in the pioneer centres,[29] but the resolution and pseudo-colour are still substantially inferior to colonoscopy. It is not yet clear that there will be a major place in inflammatory bowel disease work, but the speed at which improvements are emerging indicates that this may be just a question of time. There is no conceptual reason why the same approach should not be used to perform pseudo-endoscopy of the upper gastrointestinal tract or small intestine. It is unlikely, however, that therapeutic roles or means of obtaining biopsies will arise so as to render the comparable endoscopic routes obsolete. All forms of CT expose the patient to high radiation dose, and it is more likely that CT virtual endoscopy will itself be vanquished by equivalent reconstructions using MRI (see below).

MAGNETIC RESONANCE IMAGING

MR scanning permits non-invasive three-dimensional imaging of the abdomen and pelvis, and the speedier image acquisition of modern equipment reduces earlier difficulties associated with artefact from intestinal movement. As long ago as 1994 MR outperformed the visual diagnosis made at colonoscopy in a small controlled study.[30] MR images are particularly helpful in the pelvis – a difficult area for most other forms of imaging – where unenhanced spin-echo sequences can be invaluable in identifying and distinguishing inflammation/sepsis from surrounding normal tissues. Its application to patients with Crohn's disease has not been overlooked, but constraints of finance and availability have precluded gastroenterologists in many centres from developing adequate degrees of familiarity with its strengths and weaknesses.

MR enhanced by gadolinium (i.v.) and barium (orally) has been compared blindly with similarly enhanced, state-of the-art CT scanning in 26 patients with Crohn's disease[31] with the subsequent knowledge of all other investigations to provide a gold standard. Depiction of mural thickening was superior on the MR images, which showed over 80 per cent of 65 abnormal bowel segments, compared to helical CT, which showed only 63 per cent ($P < 0.05$). Most of this gain was in the better recognition by MR of mildly diseased segments.

In the general context of pelvic sepsis and anorectal fistulae, anal endosonography has proved the best modality, a primacy that is retained in Crohn's disease in which it outperformed MRI to a sensitivity of 89 per cent versus only 48 per cent for the MRI.[32] However, MR technology has already moved on to some extent and it is possible that the deficit has by now been largely eliminated, and with less dependence on a specially skilled operator than for the sonographic technique. See also Chapter 7.

MR scanning may prove to be of value in sequential imaging in Crohn's disease, a small blinded study having demonstrated good correlation between gadolinium-enhanced MR and a 'gold standard' derived from a composite of conventional radiography, endoscopy and/or surgery.[33] Increased bowel wall thickness and increased signal intensity on T1-weighted and on T2-weighted images were seen (only) in affected parts of the small and large intestine. All three parameters improved significantly with successful steroid treatment.

There has been less use of axial imaging in the monitoring of ulcerative colitis but this may be about to change if early data from the use of a new negative superparamagnetic oral contrast agent (ferumoxsil) are substantiated by other centres. D'Arienzo *et al.* achieved identical diagnostic information from ferumoxsil-enhanced MR scanning to that achieved from colonoscopy, with useful information about extent and severity of disease in each colonic segment.[34] An initial need for histological confirmation nonetheless remains.

It is clear that as MR scanning becomes faster (and less noisy?) and with a wider selection of contrast agents, it will replace many, if not all, CT scans and barium examinations currently performed for inflammatory bowel disease.

WHITE-CELL SCANNING, SPECT AND E-SELECTIN SCANNING

Radiolabelled white-cell scanning identifies areas of inflammation and has the potential to yield quantitative assessments. When autologous leucocytes are returned to the host circulation they migrate preferentially to areas of inflammation or, in the absence of inflammation, mainly to the bone marrow and spleen. Labelled neutrophils

re-injected into patients with inflammatory bowel disease tend to localize to areas of bowel currently involved in the disease. Initial work with indium-111 permitted a distinction between patients with active and inactive disease, and the radioactivity of timed faecal collections gave an 'excretion index' score. Indium has been superseded in most centres by labelling with technetium-99[m], which is cheaper, more readily available, has a shorter half-life, lower expected radiation exposure, and gives images more quickly and of better resolution. The usual carrier, hexamethyl propylene amine oxime (HMPAO) is lipophilic and easily able to enter white cells for labelling, but then becomes converted intracellularly to a hydrophilic form which cannot escape, leaving it and its associated technetium fixed within the cell. Crohn's disease activity and its predominant site(s) can be reliably documented.[35] It is possible to quantify disease activity (not by stool collections as there is a degree of colonic excretion of the isotope in normals), but there is difficulty in judging the accuracy and sensitivity of HMPAO scanning.

The distinction between currently active Crohn's disease, amenable to steroid therapy or other non-surgical methods, and fibrostenotic disease that can only be expected to respond to surgical resection or repair is an important one. The radiologist may be able to make an informed judgement from barium images but will often acknowledge that a trial of therapy is a better indication of the predominant problem. White-cell scanning has a logical role in this context – a normal scan in a symptomatic patient with known radiological abnormalities ought to constitute a strong indication for surgery. Unfortunately, although this is true at a statistical level, it appears not to hold good for the individual patient in whom a therapeutic decision is required,[36] and a barium image is often still needed alongside the scan to obtain the full picture.

White-cell scanning can be refined further by its combination with software developed for CT to allow creation of single photon emission CT (SPECT) images, in which a three-dimensional reconstruction becomes possible.[37] All of the variants of white-cell scanning expose the patient to a great deal less ionizing radiation than barium imaging and x-ray CT, with typical doses in the region of that of a standard chest radiograph (but more than from MRI!). Many inflammatory bowel disease centres do not use a great deal of HMPAO scanning, a stance challenged by the St George's group in London on the bases (*inter alia*) of quantitative reproducibility and low invasiveness,[38] but I am not entirely persuaded. It is especially disappointing, given the aim of minimizing irradiation, that scintigraphy was found to be unreliable in Birmingham children.[39]

E-selectin scanning has emerged from experiences with labelled white-cell scintigraphy. The selectin is overexpressed in endothelial cells at sites of inflammation and can be detected following the intravenous administration of a radiolabelled anti-E-selectin antibody. It has the theoretical advantages of studying a more fixed entity that (unlike white cells) will not be shed into the bowel lumen, and is applicable in the neutropenic patient. Preliminary data indicate an accuracy comparable to that of HMPAO scanning;[40] if indium as radiolabel can be switched to the more user-friendly technetium, it could prove to have a clinical role.

ENDOSCOPY

Colonoscopy and ileoscopy

Endoscopic assessment of the intestine is most helpful in inflammatory bowel disease, but full colonoscopy is not always required: the high proportion of the required information that can be obtained from simple sigmoidoscopy and biopsy is sometimes now underestimated. The characteristic appearances of confluent inflammation will permit the experienced endoscopist to diagnose ulcerative colitis with some confidence. Needless to say, this is substantially less reliable than the equivalent

information from the pathologist and no firm conclusion should be drawn without histological support. Colonoscopy comes into its own in ulcerative colitis (Plates 1 and 2) in determining the proximal extent of disease and in surveillance for neoplasia (see Chapter 8). The upper limit of disease at colonoscopy tends to be somewhat more proximal than predicted by concurrent barium enema, and is often very well defined.

A curious exception to the confluence of ulcerative colitis exists, however, in respect of the caecum. For years colonoscopists have worried about the significance of minor areas of inflammation around the caecal pole in patients who otherwise seemed to have ulcerative colitis, and it is probable that some patients have been labelled as having Crohn's disease on this criterion alone. In a prospective study of 20 patients with established 'left-sided ulcerative colitis', Rutgeerts' group has clarified and reassured.[41] The upper margin of inflammation was sharply demarcated in 6 patients and gradual in 14, but there was then proximal segmental inflammation, separated from the distal inflamed segment by apparently uninvolved mucosa, in no less than 75 per cent, which always included the area around the appendiceal orifice. There were no other reasons to doubt the prior diagnosis of ulcerative colitis, and the histology from all sites was concordant. The caecal patch or skip lesion may thus be considered a normal feature of distal ulcerative colitis; there are no good grounds for considering that this warrants the appellation of extensive colitis being bestowed on these patients.

In surveillance, the endoscopist will be alert to focal areas of more abnormal mucosa and to mass lesions. The oddly termed 'dysplasia-associated lesion or mass' (DALM) has especial prognostic significance, but in the main the examination serves to permit the collection of a series of biopsies from around the colon (at least 10 biopsies for a reasonable chance of representative sampling; see Chapter 8).

Sigmoidoscopy is less helpful in Crohn's disease but it is always worth taking a mucosal biopsy even of normal-looking mucosa when the differential diagnosis includes Crohn's, as a single characteristic granuloma can lend substantial weight to the diagnostic process. Full colonoscopy (Plate 3) is proportionately more valuable in diagnosis than in ulcerative colitis, given the potential for patchy disease expression and also because of the possibility of examining (and biopsying) the terminal ileum (Plate 4) in a majority of cases.

A number of centres have become interested in extending the sensitivity of colonoscopy by including optical coherence tomography (OCT). OCT can permit high-resolution, cross-sectional imaging of the microstructure of biological tissues. It is somewhat analogous to ultrasound, but instead of measuring the intensity of back-reflected sound waves it utilizes infrared light. OCT could in theory be performed through a conventional endoscope and can already provide two- and three-dimensional images of tissues *in situ*. The image resolution approaches the cellular level, and is to a depth similar to a conventional biopsy. There are preliminary clinical data suggesting that apparent rigidity and dilatation of terminal capillaries as detected by the technique are a feature peculiar to ulcerative colitis, but there are no fully published series as yet. Pitris *et al.* have, nonetheless, provided important data confirming its value in distinguishing colitis from both normal and neoplastic tissue in an *ex vivo* context.[42] If this can be replicated *in vivo*, it may prove an important addition to surveillance methodology (see Chapter 8).

Laser-induced fluorescence is another technique with a strong laboratory pedigree that is now being assessed clinically. An argon laser is used to provoke fluorescence and yields a range of fluorescence patterns with almost complete correlation, in stained tissue sections, with histological presence or absence of dysplasia.[43] It is not yet clear whether this could be of sufficient sensitivity for the distinction of dysplasia from inflammation *in vivo*.

Other endoscopy

Upper gastrointestinal endoscopy is helpful in patients with proximal symptomatology (see below), and enteroscopy has the potential to assist in the diagnostic work-up of patients in whom more standard investigations are inconclusive or contradictory. As long ago as 1993, one group was finding routine peroperative enteroscopy valuable in the full assessment of their patients with Crohn's disease,[44] and the non-operative use of push enteroscopy (with the inherent advantage over sonde enteroscopy of being able to take biopsies) in difficult Crohn's is now relatively routine in some centres.[45]

Pathology

The macroscopic pathology of inflammatory bowel disease correlates closely with the clinical, radiological and endoscopic appearances, and simple examination of resected bowel rarely presents surprises. The different topographical distributions of Crohn's and ulcerative colitis are no less key to the pathological diagnosis. In Crohn's disease, there is characteristic 'fat wrapping' around stiff, immobile, thickened bowel loops, and there may be unexpected fistulous connections or widespread adherence of the bowel to adjacent structures. While the serosal surface of the colon in ulcerative colitis often appears normal, it is not unusual for the colon of the fulminant colitic to exhibit full-thickness involvement, probably reflecting secondary ischaemia (see also Chapter 4). In all forms of aggressive disease, the bowel may be alarmingly friable.

Once the bowel is opened, the proximal limit of ulcerative colitis is often found to be very strictly demarcated (hence the proposal that the extent of disease is determined by the underlying

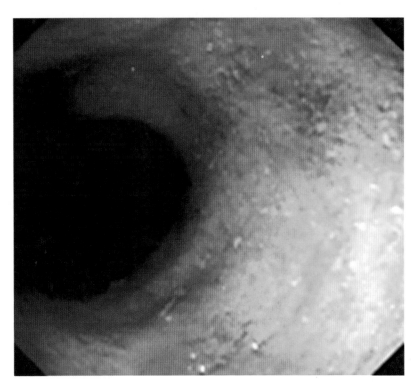

Plate 1 Colonoscopic view of the descending colon in relatively inactive ulcerative colitis – the disease is confluent with a generalized granular appearance.

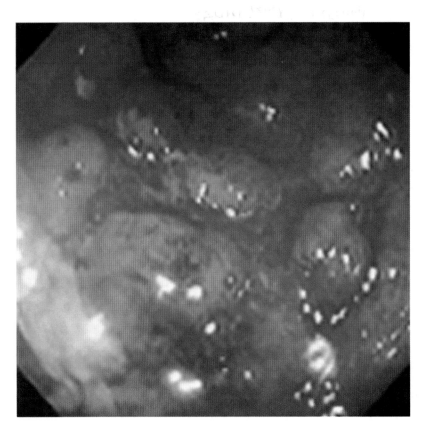

Plate 2 Post-inflammatory polyposis in a patient with a current exacerbation of ulcerative colitis – biopsies from the raised areas showed non-specific inflammation.

Plate 3 Relatively deep linear ulcer typical of Crohn's disease as seen at colonoscopy.

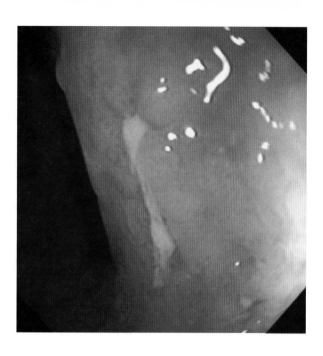

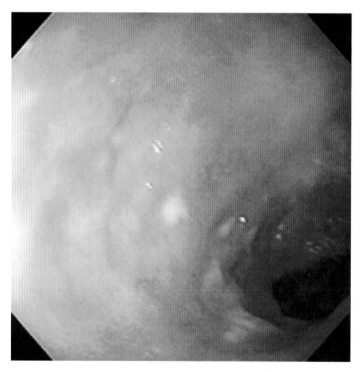

Plate 4 Multiple aphthous ulcers in the terminal ileum as visualized at ileocolonoscopy in a patient with Crohn's disease.

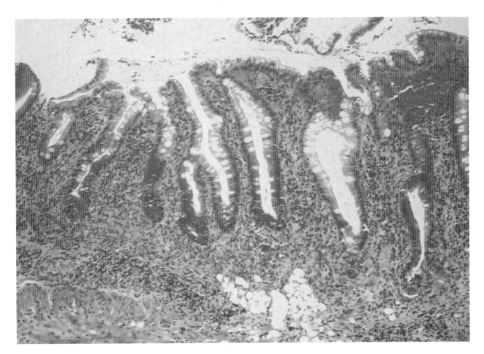

Plate 5 Histology of a rectal biopsy in ulcerative colitis. Note the loss of the normal architectural organization, the relative depletion of goblet cells and the beginnings of crypt abscess formation.

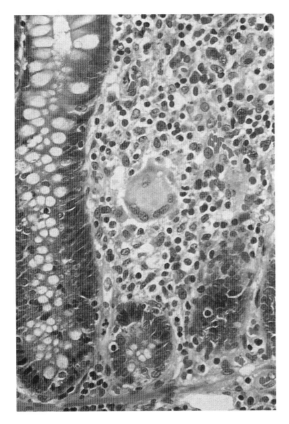

Plate 6 Colonic histology in Crohn's disease. The presence of giant cell granulomas, together with better preserved goblet cell content and overall mucosal architecture, are almost pathognomonic of Crohn's.

Plate 7 Histological appearance of collagenous colitis. The overall mucosal architecture and the mild inflammatory infiltrate are typical but the diagnosis is clinched by the thick band of collagen immediately beneath the epithelium. (Courtesy Professor A. B. Price.)

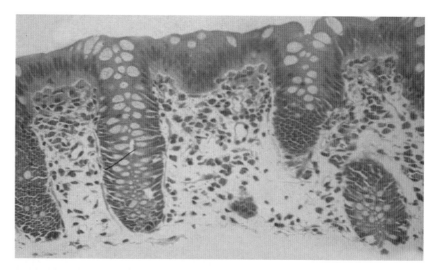

Plate 8 Histology of the normal ileoanal pouch. The ileal mucosa has taken on many colonic features, most obvious of which is the loss of villi; there is a minimal inflammatory infiltrate. (Courtesy of Professor I. C. Talbot.)

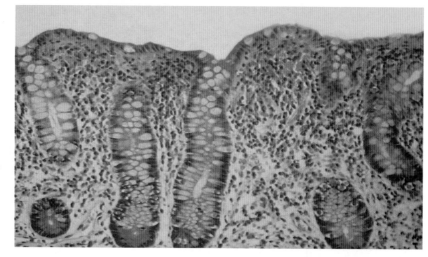

Plate 9 Histology of the ileoanal pouch with pouchitis. The colonified mucosa now exhibits destruction of the normal glandular structure and a marked inflammatory infiltrate. (Courtesy Professor I. C. Talbot.)

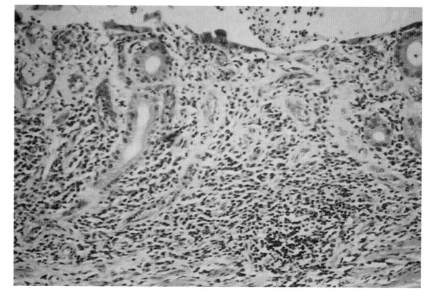

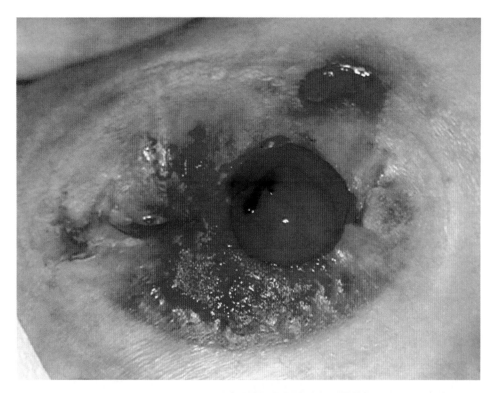

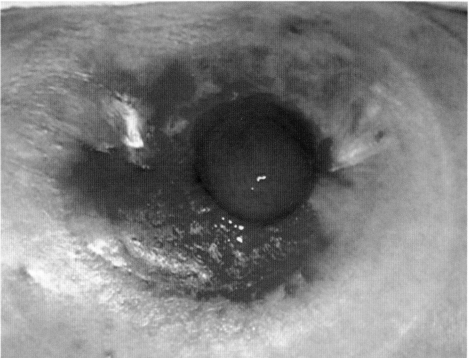

Plate 10 The appearance of the peristomal area in a Crohn's patient with multiple enterocutaneous fistulae (a) before and (b) 6 weeks after two infusions of infliximab. By the time of the second image the superior ulcer had healed and all three of the fistulae had stopped draining.

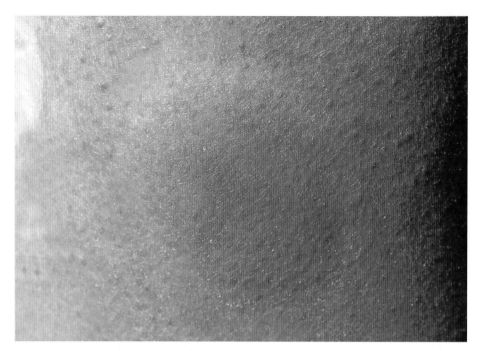

Plate 11 Characteristic appearance of erythema nodosum, which in this case was on the shin of a patient with ulcerative colitis and measured 3 cm in diameter.

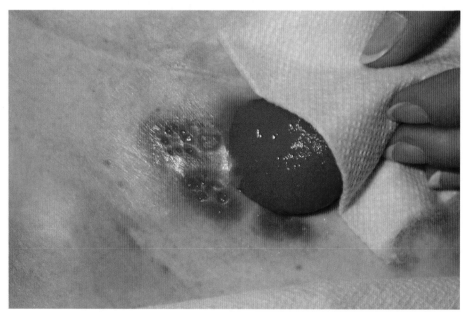

Plate 12 Pyoderma gangrenosum may occur at any site but is over-represented at sites of previous trauma (pathergy). In this case it developed shortly after the creation of an ileostomy in a patient with extensive Crohn's disease.

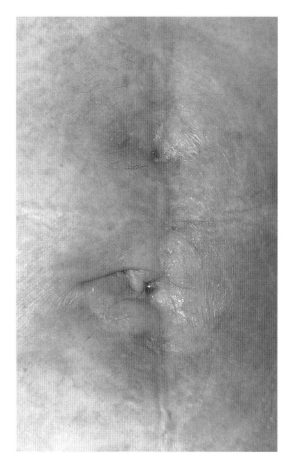

Plate 13 Small postoperative fistula in the scar of a patient with Crohn's disease. Resolution with conservative therapy might reasonably be expected.

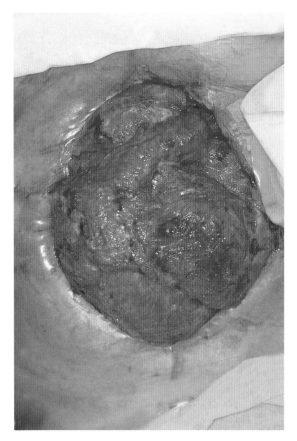

Plate 14 Catastrophic fistulation in a patient with Crohn's disease in whom surgical resection was complicated by dehiscence of the abdominal wound and by numerous enteric fistulae. At the time of this photograph, meticulous wound care and exclusive parenteral nutrition have led to the covering of the initial virtual laparostomy by clean, healthy granulation tissue, despite the continuing presence of at least four fistulous openings. Further surgery was required later.

vasculature – see Chapter 1); whatever the origin, the phenomenon itself remains striking. The colonic surface may be studded with inflammatory polyps or with pseudopolyps. There is considerable confusion in the use of these terms. The inflammatory polyp is a true polyp in the sense that it protrudes from the mucosal surface into the lumen on a stalk of variable breadth and length. These polyps occur at sites of past inflammation, and may be the only markers of extensive colitis in patients in prolonged remission. Amazing architectural formations may develop with long, interlinked polyps and bridging. Pseudopolyps, on the other hand, are truly not polyps; they may be described macroscopically, endoscopically and (particularly) in radiological reports. They represent islands of normal or regenerative mucosa, which appear elevated because of the loss of the surrounding sloughed mucosa. Their presence will always coincide with active inflammation at the site implicated.

HISTOLOGY

In ulcerative colitis the histological changes are predominantly confined to the mucosa and submucosa. In active disease there will typically be an acute inflammatory reaction with a neutrophil infiltrate, crypt abscesses, and goblet cells depleted of mucus (Plate 5); there may also be generalized oedema and vascular congestion. None of these features is pathognomonic of ulcerative colitis, although their occurrence together will be highly suggestive. With chronicity, architectural changes develop. There are then abnormal, irregular and excessively branched atrophic crypts. Typically the crypts become shortened and, unlike normal crypts, no longer reach at least two-thirds of the distance from the luminal surface to the muscularis mucosae. These changes are relatively specific to ulcerative colitis, and help greatly in the pathological distinction from acute infective colitis and acute self-limited colitis.[46]

Transmural involvement is the norm in established Crohn's disease, and there will usually be a predominantly lymphocytic infiltrate.[47] Lymphoid aggregates are especially helpful in identifying Crohn's disease as they do not normally occur in ulcerative colitis. Crypt abscesses and neutrophil infiltrates occur in acute disease, but are much less prominent features than in ulcerative colitis. Goblet cells are less often drained of mucus, and the mucosal architecture is generally better preserved than in ulcerative colitis. The most helpful specific feature in Crohn's disease is the granuloma, which, when present, occurs mainly in the submucosa, and is non-caseating (Plate 6). The differential diagnosis for granulomatous colitis/ileitis includes not only tuberculosis, yersiniosis and sarcoid, but also the foreign body reaction which may confuse if typical inclusions are absent on polarized light microscopy.

Pericryptal granulomas have been considered of lesser significance, however, and most pathologists consider them evidence of crypt damage and therefore of non-specific nature. Fourteen patients with these lesions and with no other features (clinical or pathological) of Crohn's disease were followed for between 2 and 17 years, in comparison with eight patients with pericryptal inflammation and no granulomas.[48] Unequivocal evidence of Crohn's disease became apparent with follow-up in 10 of those with granulomas, but in only one without. Although controversial, it appears that true granulomas at any site should be considered important, if not inevitable, predictors of a final Crohn's diagnosis.

The aphthoid ulcers of early Crohn's typically occur over intestinal Peyer's patches and lymphoid aggregates, but whether they are necessarily the origin of the larger, deep ulcers seen in more advanced disease is uncertain. Oral aphthous ulcers are definitely not peculiar to Crohn's disease, but those elsewhere in the gut, while not pathognomonic for inflammatory bowel disease, are sufficiently associated to make exploration of their pathogenesis of interest. It now seems probable, from a careful pathological study of lesions at various stages of their evolution, that (in the colon at least) aphthi originate in the follicle-associated epithelium in conjunction with an over-expression of HLA-DR antigens, and may reflect a role of this specialized epithelium as a portal for entry of potentially pathogenic agents.[49]

INDETERMINATE COLITIS

Because of the absence of the differentiating markers of chronicity, the histopathologist is least likely to be able to make a firm distinction between ulcerative and Crohn's colitis in the colon removed at first presentation for fulminant disease. The term indeterminate colitis is applied to this group, and to any patient in whom there is chronic colitis in the absence of features – clinical, or from imaging as well as from histology – that amount to a diagnosis of ulcerative colitis or Crohn's disease. It can be seen, therefore, that the pathologist may record indeterminate colitis in a patient where there is no ileal histology but the barium follow-through shows obvious Crohn's disease. A diagnosis of indeterminate colitis, then, to be meaningful, must carry with it the corollary that this is based on histology alone (in which case the clinician may be able to make a more or less certain assessment of whether it is Crohn's or ulcerative colitis), or that it is indeterminate colitis when all relevant disciplines have completed their deliberations, in which case the diagnosis stands until new information becomes available (which in many cases it does not). Price has helpfully reviewed this area from the perspective of the histopathologist.[50]

The difficulties of indeterminate colitis extend to the evaluation of the retained, defunctioned rectum prior to consideration of pouch surgery (see Chapter 4). Unfortunately, the histological characteristics of diversion colitis/proctitis share many of the features of Crohn's disease, and the pathologist may be unable to advise confidently as to whether the underlying diagnosis is ulcerative colitis, and that a pouch can sensibly be considered, or whether the clinician should be more wary.

Most patients categorized as having indeterminate colitis probably have ulcerative colitis, given that they will almost inevitably have continuous distal colorectal disease and disease limited to the mucosa, or have presented with fulminant colitis. Accordingly, most of them retain this semi-diagnosis in the long term, as it is unusual for a feature so characteristic of ulcerative colitis to emerge that it outweighs the earlier uncertainty. A proportion (well under 25 per cent) will nevertheless subsequently express features – especially gastric or small bowel involvement or obvious granulomas – that lead to a firm diagnosis of Crohn's disease. With this proviso, most patients with indeterminate colitis are clinically much more like those with ulcerative colitis and should probably be managed accordingly.[51] From 46 patients in whom examination of a resected colon led the pathologist to call the colitis indeterminate, clinical features pointed to probable Crohn's disease in 19 and ulcerative colitis in 11. At a median of 10 years of follow-up, only five working diagnoses had been changed. One patient thought to have Crohn's was reclassified as ulcerative colitis, three with indeterminate colitis were subsequently considered more definitely ulcerative colitis, and only one patient with a single granuloma moved from the indeterminate to the Crohn's disease group (12 remained 'indeterminate' with no small bowel features). Similar conclusions come from a more recent but otherwise comparable Italian study,[52] in which the importance of the patient with self-limiting disease is also highlighted. When follow-up investigations show no abnormality in a patient with prior acute indeterminate colitis, there need not be a lifetime label of idiopathic inflammatory bowel disease.

Clinical variants of inflammatory bowel disease, disease activity and prognosis

ORAL AND FACIAL CROHN'S DISEASE

Oral aphthous ulcers are common in the general population but are over-represented in groups of patients with inflammatory bowel disease – especially those with Crohn's disease.[49] They are, however, not the only manifestations of inflammatory bowel disease in the mouth, focal oedema and polypoid papulous hyperplasia also being frequently identifiable.[53] Oral disease may be the first evidence of Crohn's disease, particularly so in the paediatric age range. Disfiguring lip involvement can be especially distressing for adolescents, but fortunately tends to resolve spontaneously and completely with time.

Topical steroid therapy (e.g. with hydrocortisone pellets) will lead to complete remission in at least 50 per cent of cases but when this fails, intralesional injection of steroids, systemic steroids or immunosuppression are reasonable options in response to facial distortion, disabling pain and inability to eat, even in the absence of disease activity at other sites. It is not unheard of for admission to be required for the administration of parenteral opiates for severe oral ulceration. Thalidomide may also have a role for these ulcers (see Chapter 3). Orofacial granulomatosis is strongly linked with and possibly the result of Crohn's disease, and particularly affects the lips and gums. Topical laser therapy can be effective for some of these patients.[54] It is unclear whether the Melkersson–Rosenthal orofacial granulomatosis syndrome, in which chronically swollen lips and tongue populated with numerous granulomas are combined with facial palsy, is a separate condition or a variant of orofacial Crohn's.[55] A distinction from orofacial sarcoid is usually discernible from the presence of other gastrointestinal signs and the absence of pulmonary features in the patient with Crohn's.

GASTRODUODENAL CROHN'S AND *HELICOBACTER* INFECTION

Gastroduodenal Crohn's was once thought to be unusual, and frequencies of less than 2 per cent are recorded in the older literature. This perhaps reflects its tendency to affect patients who also have advanced disease at other sites, thereby deflecting attention from upper gastrointestinal symptoms. The frequency in adults is probably nearer 10 per cent.[56] Most patients with Crohn's disease coming to upper gastrointestinal endoscopy have macroscopic changes in the stomach, and this does not appear to be a result of selection bias. Data from paediatric and adolescent series indicate a very high frequency of upper gastrointestinal involvement in unselected cases.[57,58] In a study of 62 consecutive patients with ileocolic Crohn's disease, no less than 42 per cent had histologically confirmed chronic gastritis.[58] This was only associated with *Helicobacter pylori* in 9.7 per cent, and with gastric granulomas in only 6.5 per cent. The inflammatory changes were initially thought similar to those of Crohn's disease at other gastrointestinal sites, with a positive correlation between the severity of intestinal disease and the presence of gastritis. In a subsequent large adult series, the seroprevalence of *H. pylori* was less in inflammatory bowel disease patients than in age-matched controls (48 versus 59 per cent; $P < 0.05$), almost entirely accounted for by the Crohn's disease patients, of whom 15 per cent had *H. pylori*-negative chronic gastritis.

It is possible that the histology of the stomach and duodenum in Crohn's disease is characteristic of the disease. More than half of biopsied patients in one series had acute inflammation, only a fifth of whom had *H. pylori*. Focal acute inflammation in the stomach and deep, acute inflammation with surface intraepithelial neutrophils in the duodenum were sufficiently more common in *H. pylori*-negative Crohn's patients for it to be suggested that this is a characteristic of the condition (and independent of granulomas, which were present in only 9 per cent).[59] It is probable that Crohn's disease is now the commonest cause of *H. pylori*-negative chronic gastritis in the patient who is not on non-steroidal anti-inflammatory drugs (NSAIDs).

FUNCTIONAL SYMPTOMS IN INFLAMMATORY BOWEL DISEASE

It is not unusual for patients with well established inflammatory bowel disease to present with a symptom or group of symptoms – especially pain – that sounds more functional, and in whom investigations seeking evidence of current inflammation (such as raised platelet count or CRP and endoscopic assessment) are normal. Symptomatic proximal constipation in those with distal colitis (see above) might also be included within this context. There is remarkably little in the literature on this important clinical conundrum, and a disconcerting tendency for promising meeting abstracts to disappear rather than proceed to publication.

The possible impact of functional disorder should be remembered in patients with inflammatory bowel disease, and perhaps particularly so in Crohn's disease in which active disease is less easily confirmed or refuted endoscopically. There are logical reasons for considering that such patients have superimposed irritable bowel syndrome, but in this context this should be very much a diagnosis of exclusion. Management can then reasonably be along functional lines, with avoidance of the more toxic options for therapy of inflammatory bowel disease.

PSYCHOLOGICAL PROBLEMS AND PSYCHIATRIC DISEASE IN INFLAMMATORY BOWEL DISEASE

The patient with inflammatory bowel disease has a chronic and often debilitating disease that can only (in the case of ulcerative colitis) be cured by radical surgery that itself leaves variable long-term sequelae. The symptoms of the disease are unpleasant, and are not considered ones for 'polite conversation'. It is inevitable therefore that psychological morbidity runs alongside the organic physical disease. No-one now would seriously maintain that the inflammatory bowel diseases are caused by psychological disease, but there can be little doubt that psychological factors can be very important, and presumably contribute to the functional symptoms described above. The unpredictability of inflammatory bowel disease is itself a major cause of anxiety and stress, especially when faecal incontinence is or has ever been a problem. Many patients limit their social lives dramatically, and (to the physician's eyes) disproportionately, because of these fears. Lay support groups have played an important role in reducing the social stigma of diarrhoea and urgency but the problem remains.

There is some evidence for excess neuroticism and obsessiveness in inflammatory bowel disease, but it is very difficult to distinguish elements that were present before the onset of the disease, and which could have a partial causal role, from those that are in reaction to the illness. The same difficulty applies to the analysis of more formal psychological disorders such as depression and anxiety. Fully prospective studies are only just beginning to emerge, and all forms of objective quantifiable data are thin on the ground, but in a partly prospective and (incompletely) blinded study of ulcerative colitis, the level of reported stress over the previous 2 years was higher in 11 with active proctitis than in 35 with endoscopic remission ($P = 0.004$). Symptomatic patients were more likely to recall major life events in the previous 6 months ($P = 0.02$).[60] Again, it is difficult to know whether this is a cause or effect relationship, and there are obvious concerns over recall bias, but a true link between psychological factors and colitis activity is strongly suggested. A prospective study cross-relating disease activity and degree of psychological distress has concluded that almost all of the latter is the result of disease activity.[61] It is also clear that psychological factors make a major impact on the overall quality of life reported by patients with inflammatory bowel disease – indeed, of comparable impact to factors indicative of physical health.[62] The virtual absence of colitis in free-living tamarin monkeys compared to its high frequency in animals in captivity has also been taken to reflect a response to environmental stress.[63]

Given time and a sympathetic ear, patients are remarkably candid about the influence of stress and emotional issues on their intestinal symptoms, and often appear to find such discussion therapeutically valuable in its own right. They may also be greatly helped by 'permission' to use moderately potent constipating agents such as loperamide to help them through times of predictable stress. This use of opioids is more prevalent among European than North American gastroenterologists for reasons that are unclear. There does not seem to be any risk attached to such a strategy so long as the patient knows to discontinue the drug if true constipation develops or if abdominal discomfort or pain indicative of developing obstruction begins.

In a tertiary referral practice, many inflammatory bowel disease patients have major psychological and emotional problems, and especially those who have been ill during adolescence and whose ability to manage their transition from childhood to adulthood has been seriously impaired by the illness (despite the best efforts of health care workers and the best intentions of their parents). In this context the close involvement of counsellor, psychologist and psychiatrist is essential for comprehensive care, but even in the most straightforward case these issues should be addressed actively by the clinician. Faecal soiling and frank incontinence are rarely admitted to but frequently experienced, and anxiety that they may be experienced is almost universal in the patient with diarrhoea. The impact of this on (female) sexuality is alluded to elsewhere (see below and Chapter 5).

Patients with inflammatory bowel disease are not immune from other psychiatric diagnoses but these do not seem over-represented or under-represented relative to control populations, and their management can normally be conducted in a conventional fashion. Occasionally extensive small bowel Crohn's disease can lead to problems with absorption of psychoactive drugs, but in most respects therapy will be unaltered.

CHRONIC PAIN IN INFLAMMATORY BOWEL DISEASE

The acute pain associated with a specific complication or during a major relapse of inflammatory bowel disease rarely presents a management problem, but a substantial minority of patients with chronically active Crohn's disease have continual abdominal pain, which can prove intractable. In a German postoperative follow-up study of over 200 patients, chronic pain was the symptom of most concern to patients with continuing or recurrent morbidity, and was closely linked to need for therapy (including repeated surgical episodes).[64] There is some evidence that inflammation within the intestinal mucosa can result in sensitization of visceral afferent pathways, but this is not borne out by rectal balloon distension studies in Crohn's patients (with ileal but not rectal disease), which yielded significantly *higher* thresholds for discomfort and pain than in controls,[65] perhaps because the chronic inflammation leads to inhibitory descending bulbospinal influences on sacral dorsal horn neurones.

The clinician's first role is, as far as possible, to confirm or refute the presence of a remediable physical cause of pain, but when pain remains idiopathic or is hugely out of proportion to the objective findings, management becomes a problem. There is a surprising paucity of reports in the literature on this difficult topic, but the appropriate readiness of gastrointestinal physicians and nurses to resort to opiates (especially pethidine) in dealing with acute pain is probably a significant contributing cause to the emergence of opiate addiction in a high proportion of those who develop a chronic pain syndrome. One unit suggests that 5 per cent of its entire inflammatory bowel disease population is drug dependent (excluding alcohol).[66] This figure is clearly influenced by the prevalence of drug abuse in the general population to which patients belong, and informal data suggest a considerably lower figure in London at least. The problem is nevertheless real and probably reflects the gastroenterologist's management uncertainties and the reluctance of affected patients to accept help from pain clinics or drug-dependency centres. A high index of suspicion should be maintained and long-term use of opiates for pain control avoided whenever possible. Antidepressants may be valuable even in the absence of overt depression, as may alternatives such as carbamazepine, or strategies based on hypnotherapy or acupuncture. There are, however, no controlled data in respect of any of these in the context of inflammatory bowel disease. The early involvement of clinicians with skills complementary to those of the gastrointestinal team is always to be encouraged.

INFLAMMATORY BOWEL DISEASE THAT IS NOT ULCERATIVE COLITIS OR CROHN'S DISEASE

Behçet's disease
Aphthous ulcers in the mouth in conjunction with arthropathy, uveitis or a variety of dermatological or neurological features will lead rapidly to a clinical diagnosis of the idiopathic condition Behçet's disease if aphthous ulcers are also found on the genitalia.[67] When there are no urogenital ulcers, the differential diagnosis will usually include Crohn's disease, not least since around 50 per cent of patients with Behçet's have gastrointestinal symptoms such as diarrhoea, vomiting and abdominal pain.[68] There are still no definitive tests for the diagnosis. The condition is very much commoner in middle-eastern and Asian populations.[69] Up to 1 in 1000 of the Japanese population may be affected, compared with less than 1 in 500 000 in North America.

Radiologically, the typical features of Behçet's are aphthous and geographical ulcers, with a patchy distribution not dissimilar from that of Crohn's disease.[70] The ulcers may be deep and punched out, but do not often perforate or lead to fistulae formation. Intestinal lesions tend to be concentrated in the ileocaecal region and may be responsible for distortion and mass effects. The CT features, by emphasizing these differences, may help in the distinction from Crohn's disease.[27] Clinical remission is associated with parallel improvement in radiological signs. Histologically there is a non-specific chronic inflammatory process associated with the areas of ulceration. Treatment has usually included topical or systemic steroids, but a variety of alternative immunosuppressants have also been thought helpful. Controlled trial data showing useful responses to thalidomide[71] have acted as a trigger to the closer evaluation of this agent in Crohn's disease (see Chapter 3).

Ulcerative jejunitis
Ulcerative jejunitis (or chronic non-granulomatous jejunitis) usually affects patients with coeliac disease who lose or fail to achieve a response to gluten withdrawal.[72] Worsening malabsorptive symptoms, often associated with abdominal pain, lead to further investigation. The condition may

also be present at the first presentation in some older patients in whom the differential diagnosis will usually be Crohn's disease. In either case, villous atrophy in combination with proximal small bowel ulceration is demonstrable. Radiological findings include prominence of the intestinal folds but the dilatation typical of untreated coeliac disease is not a feature.[73] It is probable that ulcerative jejunitis is a preneoplastic condition with a definite association with intestinal T-cell lymphoma, of which it may be a *forme fruste*; aberrant monoclonal T cells can be identified in intestinal lesions and in some apparently normal mucosa.[74] If very careful histological assessment reveals no malignancy, then the management will normally include a strict gluten-free diet and avoidance of potentially ulcerogenic drugs such as NSAIDs. This will sometimes suffice, but progression to frank lymphoma is nevertheless still seen. There are no prospective studies of therapy. Jejunitis may also be a feature of ischaemia associated with volvulus or with microangiopathy, but there will usually be other pointers to coexistent pathology.

Lymphocytic and collagenous colitis

Definition of the microscopic colitides is problematic and there is consequent confusion clinically and in the literature. There should be first a distinction between the microscopic forms of ulcerative colitis and Crohn's disease where the endoscopist reports normal-looking mucosa but the histologist is able to give a firm or suggestive report of one of these two main forms of inflammatory bowel disease (usually ulcerative colitis). This is most obviously the case in proximal biopsies from colitics with macroscopically distal disease. These patients have 'microscopic' colitis in the sense that they have no macroscopic evidence of disease at a given site, but clearly belong to the class of patients with ulcerative colitis or Crohn's. If all patients with persistent but undiagnosed diarrhoea are subjected to colonoscopy and biopsy, other conditions emerge, some of which

may also be detected by rectal biopsy alone. There are three relatively well-defined forms of 'specific' microscopic colitis: collagenous, lymphocytic and eosinophilic. Eosinophilic cases probably have a different aetiology and pathogenesis and are considered separately. There is, however, more overlap between lymphocytic and collagenous colitis (for example at different sites in the colon or at different times).[75] A case report illustrated this point particularly vividly: there were unequivocal features of collagenous colitis only 2 weeks before colectomy (itself a most unusual requirement), but the operative specimen exhibited features only of lymphocytic colitis.[76] There is also a small group of patients with definite and persistent histological abnormalities which fall short of satisfying criteria laid down for collagenous or lymphocytic colitis, who might be considered to have non-specific microscopic colitis.[77] Experienced endoscopists reporting a colonoscopy as 'not quite normal' will often receive a histological report of a (virtually) microscopic colitis.

Collagenous colitis is the easiest to define, as it may be diagnosed from a subepithelial collagen band of 10 μm or more in thickness (Plate 7), usually but not always with an associated chronic inflammatory infiltrate. There is great variation in reported prevalence, but this may be a problem of ascertainment since it is often necessary to have a histological assessment on multiple biopsies from a full colonoscopy to obtain positive samples. As many as 95 per cent[78] or as few as 57 per cent[79] of cases are identifiable from rectal biopsy alone. It should now be standard practice to obtain multiple colonoscopic biopsies in all patients with chronic diarrhoea in whom a diagnosis is otherwise lacking.

It has been estimated that the annual incidence of collagenous colitis is as high as 1.1 per 100 000 in Spain,[79] but, as only about 4 of every 100 patients investigated at the reporting centre for chronic diarrhoea and who had a normal-looking colonoscopy proved to have the diagnosis, I am suspicious of this high population figure. All series agree, however, that collagenous colitis is much commoner in women (typically at a female to male ratio of around 4:1), usually arises in the sixth and seventh decades, and generally presents with chronic, almost watery, diarrhoea without bleeding.[75] It is associated with coeliac disease, rheumatoid arthritis, seronegative arthritis and a range of autoimmune and connective tissue diseases.[80] An autoimmune link is further supported by high levels of circulating IgM, autoantibodies to nuclear antigens, and linkage to specific HLA-DQ genotypes.[75,81] Laboratory abnormalities are otherwise scarce, and reflect mild inflammatory activity.

Treatment remains a problem and there are no controlled trials to guide us. Most patients will be exposed to 5-aminosalicylate (5-ASA) compounds, steroids, metronidazole and/or mepacrine, each of which has its protagonists. There are insufficient data to recommend one regimen over another. The collected experience of 26 cases seen in New York, still only presented in abstract form,[82] suggests that steroids and antibiotics are mostly unhelpful, but that a combination of 5-ASA and an anti-diarrhoeal is effective in about half, with up to a quarter achieving a sustained complete remission. Bismuth-based regimens also have their supporters.[83]

Lymphocytic colitis is diagnosed from biopsies in which there is an excess of intraepithelial lymphocytes, goblet cell depletion, sometimes with an increase in eosinophils, and an absence of the characteristic architectural abnormalities of conventional inflammatory bowel disease. These features have been reproducibly recorded, with only modest inter-observer variation.[84] The almost exclusive intraepithelial inflammation is analogous to that of coeliac disease, and has attracted attention to the strong association between lymphocytic colitis and coeliac disease. The rectal gluten challenge test for coeliac disease produces changes that would otherwise point to a diagnosis of lymphocytic colitis,[85] and there is evidence of abnormal small bowel morphology or permeability, together with antigliadin antibodies in a minority of lymphocytic colitis patients in whom there is no other evidence of coeliac disease.[86]

Lymphocytic colitis, too, may be proximal or patchy in distribution, and reliable detection necessitates colonoscopy with multiple biopsies. Whilst it is clear that, in general, there is substantial under-detection, the annual incidence of 3.1 per 100 000 of the Spanish epidemiology study[75] seems remarkably high. The condition typically affects those in the sixth and seventh decades, but with a more equal sex distribution than collagenous colitis (females exceeding males to a ratio of between 1.5 and 2.7).[79,87] Associations with diseases other than coeliac are less conspicuous than but similar to those of collagenous colitis.[80] Therapeutic options are again of unproven value and a regimen of withdrawal of NSAIDs, 5-ASA drugs and/or steroids is used pragmatically.

The natural or treated history of these 'lesser' forms of inflammatory bowel disease is incompletely recorded, and the retrospective reports that do exist are presumably heavily biased to the more severe cases referred to tertiary centres. There is a general impression that the prognosis is good and that many patients may be asymptomatic, or nearly so, within a few years from the time of diagnosis. Surgery is very rarely required. A group in Zurich has published an account of 35 patients with lymphocytic colitis, 27 of whom were followed in detail for a mean of more than 3 years.[87] No fewer than 25 achieved full clinical remission, and histology reverted to normal in 22. In this context, the value, if any, of the various therapies promulgated must be seriously in question. Controlled trials involving multiple centres to recruit adequate numbers are needed.

Eosinophilic enteritis and colitis

Eosinophilic enteritis usually affects the upper gastrointestinal tract, but can be responsible for both ileal and, more rarely, colitic disease.[88] There is an association with other atopic conditions in at least a third of cases, and less often with a global hypereosinophilia syndrome (Churg–Strauss disease), most patients with gastrointestinal disease lacking a dramatic excess of eosinophils in the blood. The overall incidence is uncertain, the literature comprising mainly case reports. The clinical differential diagnosis is, depending on the principal site involved, often Crohn's disease. All ages can be affected. There may be non-specific thickening and ulceration visible at upper gastrointestinal endoscopy or colonoscopy, and the intestinal wall may be sufficiently thickened for this to be apparent radiologically as fold thickening or frank stenosis.[89] The diagnosis will usually be made from the characteristic eosinophilic infiltrate at histological assessment. There is nevertheless an overlap, with excess eosinophils in many biopsies from, and a suggestion that eotaxin chemotaxis may be aetiologically important in, patients with ulcerative colitis (see Chapter 1). It is evident that parasitic infestation should be excluded before a diagnosis of eosinophilic enteritis is accepted and, as exposure to certain drugs may also lead to eosinophilic infiltrates, a careful drug history is also required. The particular case of the sulphasalazine- or mesalazine-induced pulmonary eosinophilic infiltrate is rare but pertinent because of potential therapeutic strategies.[90]

Eosinophilic enteritis at any site often proves to be steroid responsive but there are no controlled data to support this, or reliable information in respect of the various other drugs that have been advocated. In those patients with generalized hypereosinophilia, the gastrointestinal involvement is rarely the most pressing clinical issue, and management is appropriately devolved to others.

Inflammatory bowel disease of the HIV-infected patient

The special case of inflammatory bowel disease in patients infected with the HIV virus was highlighted by James, with the apparent remission of Crohn's disease on progression of HIV disease to fully established immunosuppression,[91] but this scenario is absent as often as it is present in case reports. Sharpstone *et al.* reviewed eight cases with both diagnoses,[92] including two patients with Crohn's disease and six with ulcerative colitis. The degree of inflammatory bowel disease activity did not appear to influence the gravity of immunosuppression, but there was some improvement in CD4 count after colectomy in four patients who needed surgery. Progressive immunosuppression as the viral disease advanced was associated neither with improvement nor deterioration of the inflammatory bowel disease. The most pertinent point may be that the inflamed colitic rectum places the patient at higher risk for contracting HIV infection, thus accounting for the relatively large number of patients with both diagnoses.

HIV enteritis exists but it is still unclear whether it is responsible for symptoms. It seems probable that in some patients it is the principal cause of malabsorption, but that this is relatively mild, and that the severely symptomatic patient will almost always have a second infecting organism such as a *Cryptosporidium* or *Microsporidium*, or a degree of bile salt malabsorption. Cello's group has suggested that there is also a non-specific colitis of HIV disease, which they identified in 15 of a group of 79 HIV-infected patients with diarrhoea, in whom no infecting organism (or other diagnosis) could be elicited.[93] The condition was associated with relatively modest immunosuppression and was responsive to 5-ASA therapy. Is this, in fact, a *forme fruste* of idiopathic inflammatory bowel disease?

Diverticulosis, obstructive colitis and inflammatory bowel disease

Diverticulosis and inflammatory bowel disease are both relatively common, and as diverticulum formation increases with age it is not surprising that the conditions are seen together in the elderly. This seems more common in Crohn's disease than would be expected by chance alone, however, and Shepherd[94] suggests that there may be a subtype of Crohn's disease that is associated with diverticula or indeed a new diagnosis, of diverticular colitis, indicating that the blind-ended diverticula may predispose to the adverse (bacterial?) effects of stasis. He analyses the difficulties in making a certain distinction between the two conditions, recognizing that some features considered typical (but never pathognomonic) of Crohn's may also occur in complicated diverticulosis in the absence of inflammatory bowel disease. I remain sceptical of this proposal, but agree that it deserves consideration, not least because of the link between appendicectomy and protection from ulcerative colitis (see Chapter 1). There is also a potential correlation here with the condition of obstructive colitis in which inflammation (which may proceed to ulceration and frank necrosis) occurs proximal to a stenosing lesion.[95] Obstructive colitis is more obviously the result of ischaemia, with impairment of blood supply secondary to a combination of elevation of the intraluminal pressure, distension of the colonic wall and probably other factors that impair adequate perfusion. It probably occurs to a clinically overt degree in around 4 per cent of patients with colonic obstruction but can give rise to confusion with concurrent inflammatory bowel disease if not actively considered.

Vascular and ischaemic enterocolitis, radiation enteritis and gastrointestinal endometriosis

The recognition of ischaemic colitis is often obvious from the clinical context. Most patients have other evidence of vasculopathy (ischaemic heart disease and/or peripheral vascular disease) and the colitis is concentrated at vascular watershed zones, particularly the splenic flexure and the distal sigmoid. The colonoscopic features are often considerably more prominent than the histological findings. There is no specific treatment and most patients recover spontaneously. Surgical resection is only rarely required. More proximal mesenteric ischaemia is more difficult to diagnose, as the symptoms are non-specific and standard investigations of the small intestine will often be normal. The differential diagnosis will include Crohn's disease, and Doppler sonography may be the key to a correct attribution of disease to the major vessels given the correct degree of suspicion. Vascular dilatation or reconstruction may be possible in advance of a major ischaemic loss leading to short bowel syndrome (see Chapter 7).

Acute radiation enteritis commonly results from therapeutic irradiation in cancer therapy; it presents within a few days of exposure and may be responsible for bloody diarrhoea for some weeks but usually settles spontaneously. In up to 5 per cent of patients receiving appropriate radiation dosage there is progression to the more intractable chronic radiation damage; the underlying pathogenesis is predominantly via focal ischaemia, with cell loss, fibrosis and obliterative vascular injury. Unfortunately, the condition may prove progressive; there is no established specific therapy.[96]

Endometriosis affecting the intestine can also prove a vascular cause of apparent inflammatory bowel disease. Depending on diagnostic criteria the prevalence of endometriosis may be as high as 10 per cent in women of reproductive age, and the bowel is involved in more than 10 per cent of these women.[97] Various symptoms including dysmenorrhoea, dyspareunia, chronic pelvic pain, diarrhoea, constipation, cyclic rectal bleeding, and colicky abdominal pain characterize the condition. Involvement of the distal ileum may lead to fibrosis and stricture formation that can be confused with Crohn's disease; intestinal obstruction may also occur.[98] An appropriate index of suspicion and a low threshold for diagnostic laparoscopy will usually lead to the correct diagnosis. Most patients respond to hormonal manipulation, but surgery may be required.

Clinical course and natural history of inflammatory bowel disease

The clinical course of inflammatory bowel disease is not easily predicted. With the proviso that concordance (for ulcerative colitis or Crohn's disease) is not complete, the disease does, however, tend to behave similarly in different members of an afflicted family (with an element of anticipation with succeeding generations – see Chapter 1).[99] There do not appear to be particular races or population groups in whom notably mild or severe disease can be expected. Ashkenazi Jews may be an exception to this general rule, as they seem to have a predilection for unusually aggressive Crohn's disease. A recent questionnaire study confirms a general tendency for Crohn's patients from poorer communities to fare less well, but with no independent effect from race.[100]

In ulcerative colitis, the initial extent of colonic involvement remains a good but fallible guide to its future course (as well as to the risk of neoplastic transformation – see Chapter 8), but curiously the severity of individual severe acute relapses does not itself have an adverse impact on the frequency or severity of further relapses, or on the need for surgery. If surgery is avoided despite systemic features such as fever and weight loss, the chance of remission over the subsequent 5 years is somewhat better than average. In an analysis of 1161 patients with ulcerative colitis, Langholz *et al.* provide additional detailed actuarial data for probability of relapse and remission.[101] At presentation, 44 per cent had no macroscopic disease proximal to the sigmoid. At any one time, about 50 per cent of patients were in full remission, but 90 per cent remained prone to intermittent relapses. Chronic disease activity in the first 2 years after diagnosis predicted continuing activity over the next 5 years to a high level of significance. Disease activity in a given year predicted a 70–80 per cent risk of activity in the following year. The cumulative risk of colectomy in this (surgically orientated) centre was 24 per cent at 10 years and 32 per cent at 25 years. The rate of colectomy was 9 per cent in the first year of diagnosis, 3 per cent in each of the following 4 years and about 1 per cent per year thereafter. One quarter of those coming to surgery had disease limited to the rectum and sigmoid at the time of initial presentation, but their cumulative risk at 5 years was only 9 per cent compared with 35 per cent in those with pan-colitis at diagnosis. More than 90 per cent of patients with colitis retained full working capacity at 10 years. Remarkably similar data have resulted from the British three-centre cohort study of new colitics presenting between 1977 and 1986.[102] Nearly half the patients had only a single episode of disease, and the others had a mean of 1.8 relapses in the 8 years of follow-up. Just over 9 per cent were hospitalized in any given year, and the colectomy rate rose gradually to 15 per cent at 15 years. In general, the likelihood that surgery will be necessary for non-fulminant ulcerative colitis is predicted by systemic signs, poor general condition, low serum albumin, mucopus in stools and more problematic diarrhoea.[103]

There appear to be distinct subtypes of Crohn's disease, with, for example, some patients in whom perforating, fistulating disease is the norm, and others who never suffer these potentially very disabling complications. Working on the premise that differential cytokine expression (or sensitivity) could account for the differences seen, Gilberts *et al.*[104] studied mRNA levels for a range of cytokine and related species. A bimodal distribution was found (only) for interleukin (IL-1β) and IL-1 receptor antagonist, with much higher levels of both of these in tissues from patients with non-perforating disease. These were not, perhaps, the expected results, given that levels of the mediators for fibrosis included did not distinguish between the two groups, but nevertheless support the hypothesis that underlying (genetic) differences play a significant role in determining the clinical manifestations of Crohn's disease.

Transforming growth factor beta (TGF-β) ought logically to be closely implicated in the net tendency to fibrosis or fistulation in Crohn's disease,[105] but this proved not to be the case in a clinical series in which TGF-β behaved as a disease activity marker not dissimilar to the platelet count.[106]

We should not lose sight of the considerable rarity with which Crohn's heals entirely. Long-term review of 465 patients recruited in Rome from 1978 indicates that complete remission with full endoscopic and histological resolution may be expected in 2.5 per cent without any obvious link to clinical phenotype or to treatment given.[107]

The Mayo Clinic group have applied Markov modelling to prospectively recorded data from 174 community Crohn's disease patients followed for up to 25 years.[108] They demonstrate that the average patient presented at the age of 28.1 and over the next 11 years had, on average, 4 years in spontaneous remission, 3.3 years in postoperative remission and 1 month in full remission on drug treatment. Less encouragingly they also had 2.5 months of active uncontrolled disease, 2 months in the immediate perioperative period, with 2.7 years of mild disease and 5 months of drug (usually steroid) dependency.

Increasing age is probably linked to a diminishing severity and frequency of relapses of inflammatory bowel disease, but firm data are lacking. There was, however, definite ($P = 0.01$) advantage from increasing patient age in one dose-ranging study of a 5-ASA, 27 per cent of the over-50s relapsing by 48 weeks compared with 53 per cent of otherwise matched patients under 35.[109]

Frequency and significance of proximal extension of distal colitis

Ulcerative colitis is well established as a distal disease, the inflammation of which extends proximally, in continuity, but to a variable extent. The proportion of the colon involved is clinically relevant because it has a bearing on both the severity

of disease and on the long-term risk of colitis-related colonic carcinoma (see Chapter 8). Intensity and frequency of hospital follow-up are, accordingly, greatly influenced by the extent documented. However, the extent of the colitis may advance proximally after the initial diagnostic evaluation. The clinical importance of this is exemplified by no fewer than 12 colitis-related carcinomas recorded at St Mark's Hospital, in patients who had documented distal disease and who were not therefore under special supervision, but who were found to have extensive colitis at the time of cancer surgery.[110] Proximal progression of colitis (and of ulcerative proctitis) is increasingly recognized. A number of studies have reported extension up to the next colonic 'segment' (rectum to sigmoid; sigmoid to descending, etc.) in around 10 per cent after 5 years. The Birmingham group has reviewed the literature and their own experience.[111] From 145 cases, followed for a median of more than 10 years, disease extended proximal to the sigmoid in 36 per cent (at a median of 6 years). In 29 per cent the progression was sufficient to justify a new diagnosis of macroscopic extensive colitis. Comparison between those with progression and those without presented no predictive cues. Derivative actuarial analysis predicts progression proximal to the sigmoid in about 16 per cent at 5 years (95 per cent CI: 11–24 per cent) and in 31 per cent at 10 years (CI: 23–40 per cent). The frequency of progression to involve more proximal colon seems to be somewhat higher in those with disease initially confined to the rectum than in those with initial proctosigmoiditis.

The mammoth Copenhagen study[103] included 1628 patients with ulcerative colitis and, *inter alia*, examined disease progression in the subset of those with proctosigmoiditis. Similar methodology to that employed in Birmingham was used, but a probability of progression of no less than 53 per cent at 25 years was recorded. In this series, abdominal pain and continuing diarrhoea were associated independently with a greater tendency to disease progression. There was also evidence for regression of initially extensive colitis after 25 years.

As progression of initially distal disease does not necessarily seem to lead to more frequent or severe relapses, which would draw attention to the change, and yet places the patient at higher risk of colorectal carcinoma, it is logical to re-evaluate the extent of colitis at intervals in patients with distal disease (see Chapter 8).

There are fewer data relating to the equivalent questions in Crohn's disease, but one major study indicates a very high rate of progression indeed.[112] Amongst 323 patients presenting with Crohn's affecting the colon, followed up for a mean of 9.8 years, the probability of having pan-colitis was 77.1 per cent after 15 years (higher in patients with initially left-sided or segmental colitis than in those with initially right-sided colitis). The chance of developing rectal involvement by 15 years was 78.8 per cent and of perianal fistulation, 43.3 per cent. Sixty-two per cent of patients had undergone some degree of colonic resection by 15 years, and the cumulative risk of total colectomy was 18.2 per cent. The 15-year probabilities of proctectomy (12 per cent) and of having a defunctioning stoma (21 per cent) were influenced mainly by perianal fistulation.

The constancy of the nature of disease at initial presentation and at subsequent relapse in Crohn's has been closely examined. It is intriguing that there is such great similarity between the original disease and its later relapse. Not only does the general behaviour of the disease (fibro-stenotic/fistulating) tend to run true, but so does the actual extent of bowel involved.[113] Remarkably, this implies that a patient from whom 20 cm of diseased terminal ileum is resected tends to re-present with 20 cm of disease in the neoterminal ileum. This almost implausible scenario fits the experience at other centres but is unexplained.

GUIDES TO DISEASE ACTIVITY

Crohn's disease

The most widely used and most frequently criticized scale of Crohn's disease activity is the Crohn's Disease Activity Index (CDAI) (see Appendix A).[114] This index is based on a series of self-reported symptoms during the week prior to its determination, coupled with additional scores for a number of clinical signs and complications. The most objective measures included are weight change and haematocrit. It is precisely because of the subjectivity of the score that the CDAI is so lambasted, given that it would be frequent for patients with irritable bowel syndrome to appear to have active Crohn's disease (CDAI > 150) on the basis of a perceived severe illness. The same objection is raised to the Harvey–Bradshaw scale,[115] although this is easier to compute and appears to give comparable information (see Appendix A). Most authorities in the field have tried to improve this situation, whether by including additional laboratory markers (such as the platelet count, or CRP), or by devising entirely independent measures of disease activity. Some of the more helpful of these will be discussed but it is important to recognize that we lack a gold standard either for diagnosis of Crohn's disease or its degree of activity. Comparisons of the different methods tend to be made against a global assessment made for all available information or against the CDAI.

Use of individual laboratory markers is not without value, but few biochemical tests have a positive or negative predictive value in excess of 80 per cent. Most of the data are relatively elderly, but four studies performed within the last 10 years which, between them, compared a wide range of biochemical parameters with global clinical scoring tools are representative.[116–119] IL-6 and serum amyloid A (SAA) proved the most sensitive markers, both being elevated in > 90 per cent of patients with active Crohn's disease,[119]

SAA correlating better with CDAI and global scores ($r > 0.8$), and both correlating closely with the CRP which they outperformed. Similar but less accurate conclusions were possible when the tests were applied to patients with ulcerative colitis.[119] Circulating IL-2 receptor levels are reasonably informative, but they are no more specific.[117] Other cytokines, orosomucoid, alpha-1-antitrypsin, fibrinogen, platelet count and sedimentation rate were not informative in Crohn's disease, although all but fibrinogen tend to be elevated in active ulcerative colitis.[116,118] There may be some value from measurement of alpha-1 acid glycoprotein and haptoglobin in Crohn's disease.[118] More novel options include estimation of the granulocyte marker calprotectin in faecal samples.[120]

There are no compelling arguments for a single choice, but the CRP is a less complex phenomenon than the sedimentation rate and has been shown to have a close correlation with overall disease activity, whilst the sedimentation rate often correlates only with colonic disease.[121] As things stand, unless IL-6 or SAA assays become routinely available, I will continue to use the CRP, recognizing that about 20 per cent of patients with active disease will have normal levels.

Best known of the more objective composite indices is the Dutch or Van Hees Index (see Appendix A).[122] Unsurprisingly, it correlates well with other laboratory-based assessments and relatively poorly with clinical impressions or with the CDAI. However, the scale is based on nine parameters, each of which requires multiplication by a constant, before they are summed and a further constant subtracted; it is not a tool for the busy clinician!

One suggested solution to this problem is the use of a lavage method of measuring, *inter alia*, intestinal protein loss, considered a very objective assessment of Crohn's disease activity.[123] Commentators have been less convinced and question the acceptability of the lavage technique to both patients and investigators. The Edinburgh investigators explored the degree of protein-losing enteropathy, in conjunction with the CDAI and a global clinical assessment. Importantly, they included some subjects in whom active Crohn's disease was unlikely, some thought to have only (non-inflamed) fibrous strictures, and some in whom Crohn's was subsequently excluded. Patients in whom the clinical global judgement indicated active Crohn's disease (or ulcerative colitis for which the CDAI was, somewhat unconventionally, also used) had abnormal gut lavage protein levels (particularly IgG), but those with a high CDAI thought falsely high because of prominent fibrous stricturing or predominant psychological symptoms had normal gut lavage results. One can conclude that the lavage technique (in the hands of its protagonists) provides highly plausible results, but it is neither non-invasive nor especially quick and cannot be a routine out-patient test.

Permeability testing is also suggested as a means of determining disease activity, but although one paediatric centre is confident that inactive disease is associated with normal permeability,[124] this flies in the face of data from other centres and, indeed, the presence of abnormal permeability in healthy relatives (see Chapter 1).

Altered blood flow in Crohn's disease is of potential value as a marker of disease activity but there is still too much disagreement between workers in the field for this yet to be considered a fruitful means of assessing disease activity (see above).

Ulcerative colitis

Comparable scoring systems for defining the activity of ulcerative colitis have proved less controversial as the presence (or absence) of rectal bleeding and the closer association between bowel frequency and inflammatory activity lead them to be more objective. Unfortunately, the widely quoted St Mark's or Powell-Tuck score[125] has proved too easy to misuse, given the possibility of fragmenting the score, and because of the different numbering scale used for the proctoscopic appearance score compared to the numbers utilized in the paper by Baron *et al.*,[126] on which this part of the St Mark's score is based. I increasingly favour the more recent, adequately reproducible, and very simple, Walmsley score.[127] These and other examples, together with suggested scoring systems for histological assessment are given in Appendix A.

QUALITY OF LIFE WITH INFLAMMATORY BOWEL DISEASE

It is obvious that inflammatory bowel disease has an adverse impact on the patient's quality of life, but the medical profession's attention and interest have focused historically on aspects that cause major morbidity and may prove life-threatening. The creation (and considerable success) of patient support groups (such as the National Association for Colitis and Crohn's Disease in Britain, or AMICI in Italy) has been partly in response to this perceived lack of attention. Many useful information leaflets and practical aids such as the 'Can't Wait' card (aiding urgent access to toilet facilities when away from home) have been produced, in addition to counselling services and more informal support.

Efforts made to improve patient awareness and education are prima facie a good thing, but it is pleasing to be able to record scientific support for their value. The Manchester group have devised a patient information booklet on ulcerative colitis which incorporates a synopsis of symptoms, investigations and treatments (including surgery) from a patient-based perspective. There are a few minor errors of fact and a number of unusual opinions but the overall balance is good. The authors are to be congratulated on subjecting their work to a controlled trial in 239 patients randomized to receive the booklet or to standard information alone.[128] At 9 months, knowledge and confidence in self-management were assessed by questionnaire, with a clear advantage to those with the booklet (knowledge scores, quality of life scores and general satisfaction all increased, the two former with statistical support).

Patient-led groups have also taken steps to offset discrimination in the workplace and in respect of health and life insurance. Fortunately, the profession has reacted positively, and Mayberry's group[129] in particular has taken these and related issues in hand. Despite time lost from full-time education, young patients with Crohn's disease reach comparable[129] or higher[130,131] levels of academic success relative to their unaffected peers. Sadly, this is not sufficient to preclude a somewhat higher frequency of subsequent unemployment and a desire of up to a third of these patients to wish to conceal their condition from actual or prospective employers,[129] or, indeed, an inability to carry out the activities necessary for normal employment in about 20 per cent.[130,131] The similar proportion of women with Crohn's disease achieving marriage (81 per cent versus 76 per cent of age-matched controls) is probably also an acceptable surrogate for a marker of reasonable social functioning,[132] but more women who wish to work have to stop because of irritable bowel disease (23 per cent versus 16 per cent of men).[131] Personal finance arrangements and loans (such as for mortgages) were more difficult to secure for younger and female patients than for their older, male counterparts; over 8 per cent of all patients had special terms imposed on mortgage arrangements.[131]

Internationally, the lead in the quantification of this area has been taken by Irvine and her colleagues, who devised and validated a disease-specific quality of life instrument – the Inflammatory Bowel Disease Questionnaire (IBDQ).[133] The IBDQ score ranges from a minimum of 32 to 'perfect' health at 224, patients with inflammatory bowel disease returning scores of about 180 when well and around 120 when in severe relapse; a change of more than 16 points is considered clinically significant. The IBDQ is complementary to so-called generic measures which are also applicable to the general population and to those with other diseases, such as the extensively evaluated SF36 questionnaire, a 36-item health status scale.[134] Copyright issues prevent the duplication here of these two scales, but both are readily available. It is not practicable to apply these instruments in routine practice, but recognition that the quantification of quality of life is critical to a comprehensive assessment of therapeutic endeavours has led to their now nearly universal inclusion in responsible trial protocols. Another well-validated, generic, quality of life scale is, however, sufficiently simple that it has the potential to be adopted in even a busy clinic. The EuroQol tool requires answers to only five Likert-graded questions and a single linear analogue scale point[135] (see Appendix A).

THE COST OF CARE OF INFLAMMATORY BOWEL DISEASE

It is difficult to estimate the cost of management of a chronic relapsing disease that is rarely fatal. North American and Swedish attempts have been made nonetheless.

First to publish usefully in this area were Hay and Hay[136] who estimated an average annual cost for Crohn's disease of US$6561, 81 per cent of which was accounted for by surgery and associated in-patient costs, and for ulcerative colitis of US$1488 per year. Extrapolation to the US population yields a financial demand of US$1.0–1.2 billion for Crohn's disease. They estimate that 80 per cent of all Crohn's disease costs are generated by 20 per cent of Crohn's disease patients, and that 2 per cent of the patients account for 28.9 per cent of all costs. If 5–10 per cent of all those affected don't work as a result, then Hay and Hay attribute an estimated additional US$0.4–0.8 billion per year in indirect costs. On these figures some US$200 million would be saved in the USA each

year if the number of days missed from work were reduced by 20 per cent.[136] Silverstein *et al.* produced an average lifetime figure for the cost of Crohn's disease of US$125 404 (albeit with a median of US$39 906);[108] almost half the median was on direct surgical costs, and included an estimate of US$6000 per patient per year for costs to the referral centre and US$3000 as direct community health costs. Hanauer reasons that 10 per cent of all costs are on drugs, and a little over 50 per cent on surgery.[137] Feagon *et al.* have tried to analyse this issue from the perspective of the health care purchaser.[138] They split Crohn's disease patients between: those that had ever been admitted for the disease; those on steroids or immunosuppression but not admitted for Crohn's; and the remainder. The first group cost a mean of US$37 000 per patient per year of which US$28 000 was for in-patient care, the second group cost about US$10 000, and the third about US$6000 per year with an average for all patients of US$12 417 per patient-year.

Although the Hays make an effort to reckon the indirect costs of inflammatory bowel disease, this has been measured in the Swedish study of Blomqvist and Ekbom.[139] Again, admission accounted for 68 per cent of direct costs, and in their analysis 25 per cent of patients accounted for 48 per cent of all direct costs. The estimated overall direct cost was US$690 per patient-year, this being an average figure for inflammatory bowel disease, Crohn's disease patients costing about three times as much as ulcerative colitics. For Sweden this is US$27.5m per annum. In addition to this, indirect costs of US$58.4m per year were also identified. This is from sick leave and early retirement approximately equally – few people take early retirement but when they do it is very expensive. Average sick leave is about 6 weeks a year (more for Crohn's than for ulcerative colitis) and inflammatory bowel disease accounts for 0.4 per cent of all sick leave in Sweden.

The cost-effectiveness of care of inflammatory bowel disease

We cannot and should not try to avoid stringent audit of our efforts in inflammatory bowel disease therapy, but should ensure that clinical cost-effectiveness is assessed rather than a simple counting of the financial cost of new drugs, procedures and personnel support. Fortunately, despite the inherent difficulties of study of chronic relapsing conditions, there is an increased acceptance of cost-effectiveness as linked to quality of life measures. The much quoted QALY (quality-adjusted life year) deserves a little explanation. It is based on 'utility' as a quality measure where a utility of 1 is equivalent to perfect health and 0 to death. If by intervention we can improve utility from 0.5 to 0.7 for 3 years this is a gain in QALYs of 0.6, and the cost per QALY can be calculated. Western society is usually prepared to pay for things that cost less than £30 000 per QALY gained (with exceptions). The utility measure is based on the 'standard gamble' where the subject chooses one of two options until 'utility', which is the point of equipoise where a decision between the two becomes impossible/equivalent.[140] As an example, an hypothetical patient with bad Crohn's disease offered surgical cure from an operation with no complications, but a 1 per cent risk of sudden death, would most likely choose the former, but if the figures were 90 per cent versus 10 per cent or 70 per cent and 30 per cent, the choice somewhere reaches equipoise. Interestingly, real patients with Crohn's disease in remission (defined by doctors on the basis of CDAI scores) are obviously some way from true remission as they gamble at the 20 per cent level.[140] This value comes from a decision between choice A, which is stay how you are now, or choice B, which is to take a gamble where there are the two possible outcomes – sudden painless death or cure. The patients' choice of a 20 per cent risk of death as acceptable translates to a utility score of 0.8 (which is worse than class 3–4 angina but not as bad as having an abdominoperineal excision and stoma for colorectal carcinoma). Patients with active inflammatory bowel disease prove to have utility scores of around 0.7.

Example use of the QALY has been made for the 'cost' of 5-ASA therapy in Crohn's disease maintenance (see Chapter 3). The resultant figure of US$5000 for each QALY[141] illustrates potential problems of these exercises, as this came not from actual data but from estimates from the literature and opinion, and with the costings made retrospectively!

SEXUALITY

The relatively normal fertility of patients with inflammatory bowel disease is considered in Chapter 5, but fertility is, of course, only one component of sexual life. Great morbidity can result from what may seem to be relatively minor defects in actual or perceived sexual functioning. Much has been written about the stigma of the gastrointestinal stoma, and all practitioners will aim to avoid stoma creation in the young patient if possible;[142] this has especial significance in Asian communities where it is not unusual for a young woman to be considered unmarriageable as a result of a stoma. Less attention has been focused on the concern that faecal incontinence will occur during intercourse; this is much more often a worry than an actuality, but the anxiety of the patient (particularly female) may be of such overwhelming intensity as to prevent the formation of any potentially sexual relationship. It is typical of the whole area of sexual functioning that this major concern of patients is one which is not conveyed to their medical attendants: the doctor should recognize this and introduce its discussion at an appropriate point in the consulting process. Fear of incontinence led to complete sexual abstinence in 14 per cent of women with Crohn's disease in one study.[143] Achieving secure continence is more difficult, but pre-coital loperamide may suffice and will often provide the reassurance that is needed. Dyspareunia is likewise a problem that is often not mentioned in the inflammatory bowel disease clinic, but should be enquired after in potentially sexually active women. Questionnaire data indicate a prevalence of dyspareunia as high as 38 per cent compared with 18 per cent in controls.[144] Painful intercourse in women with Crohn's disease is often the result of active inflammation and, when gynaecological causes are excluded, may itself be an indication for intestinal surgery if more intensive medical therapy is insufficient.

It is encouraging that reported frequency and enjoyment of sexual activity in inflammatory bowel disease patients seemed similar to those in controls. However, complacency should be tempered by the relatively low reply rates and the wide range of responses in both groups,[144] especially since the same authors report six times the frequency of sexual abstinence in women with Crohn's compared with controls, when interviewed face to face (24 per cent versus 4 per cent).[143]

CAUSES OF DEATH IN INFLAMMATORY BOWEL DISEASE

Those aspects of morbidity and mortality specific to colorectal carcinoma are considered in Chapter 8, but in other respects the major inflammatory bowel diseases have generally been felt to have little effect on mortality. This may reflect a tendency for subjects from relatively advantaged social classes to be affected by the diseases, and this is a major argument put forward by life assurance institutions when challenged as to why premiums for life cover are adversely loaded for inflammatory bowel disease patients. Their argument is that, whatever the mortality data for ulcerative colitis or Crohn's disease relative to standard mortality data for the population, the company must quote on the basis of its average customer, who is from the upper echelons of society. Since it cannot be denied that inflammatory bowel disease sometimes kills, a financial consequence to the patient becomes inevitable. See also above.

There is surprisingly little in the literature on all-cause mortality from inflammatory bowel disease, or whether this is changing with time; past data have been somewhat contradictory. It is therefore helpful to analyse a population study of nearly 3000 inflammatory bowel disease patients seen between 1955 and 1984.[145] The criteria for case ascertainment and diagnosis would satisfy most clinical trials, and it is unlikely that better epidemiological data will emerge for this time period. It is probable that the great majority of cases of both ulcerative colitis and Crohn's disease to occur in the Stockholm area have been identified and included. Mortality data ($n = 429$) come from the National Death Register up to 1990, with causes of death codified according to the death certificate. In only 2.5 per cent of patients was life-or-death follow-up to 1990 not available. Mortality from all causes and from specific causes was analysed by conventional relative survival statistics in comparison with the age- and sex-adjusted standard mortality data for Sweden. The relative survival for Crohn's disease was 93.7 per cent at 15 years (95 per cent CI: 91.8–95.7) with no significant differences according to the site of the bowel involved. The standardized mortality ratio (SMR) was 1.51. There was a slight worsening in prognosis in those diagnosed after 1970 (1.2 per cent worse at 15 years) but this, too, failed to reach significance. In ulcerative colitis, there was also a reduced life expectancy to the extent of 94.2 per cent at 15 years (CI: 92.4–96.1), which was most marked for those with extensive colitis (92.9 per cent), but yet again this was not statistically different even from those with proctitis alone (96.4 per cent). The SMR was 1.37. As in Crohn's disease, the prognosis was less good in those diagnosed after 1970, which was attributed to an ageing population of new colitics (albeit with the mean age at diagnosis rising only from 30.8 to 36.4 across the study period). The cause-specific mortality obviously includes patients dying from their inflammatory bowel disease (74 of the 429 deaths). When these are excluded, the SMRs remain elevated for both ulcerative colitis and Crohn's disease (1.20 and 1.14, respectively). The majority of these excesses occur within the purview of the gastroenterologist, as in addition to the three-fold increase in colorectal carcinoma deaths in ulcerative colitis, there were increases in deaths from non-alcoholic liver disease in ulcerative colitis (SMR 4.8) (presumably from sclerosing cholangitis – see Chapter 6) and from other gastrointestinal disorders in both ulcerative colitis and Crohn's (SMRs 2.4–4.0). UK data are less complete but 6 of 58 deaths documented by 1993 in the 454 patients recruited between 1977 and 1986 to the three-centre ulcerative colitis cohort were considered colitis related.[102]

There were also excess deaths in Sweden from asthma, especially in ulcerative colitis (SMR 6.21; CI: 2.50–12.8) with increased deaths from other respiratory causes also (SMRs 1.6–2.1), which was obviously not the result of a higher frequency of smokers (under-represented amongst colitics).[145] In Crohn's disease, there were very similar results, albeit with a more modestly increased SMR of 2.76 in asthmatics. The other major study of specified all-cause mortality (from Uppsala, also in Sweden)[146] also demonstrated increased mortality from respiratory causes, admittedly at a lower level (SMR 1.5; CI: 1.1–2.2); this should, accordingly, now be accepted as a true association – the explanation remains less certain.

Crohn's patients in Stockholm appeared relatively protected from death from colorectal carcinoma (SMR 0.30; CI: 0.01–1.66), and those from Uppsala were less likely to die from cerebrovascular disease (SMR 0.7; CI: 0.5–1.0).[145,146] For no other major diagnostic grouping was substantially or statistically decreased risk found. There may be a tendency in each study for over-recording of inflammatory bowel disease as the cause of death, but this would have the effect of diminishing the likelihood of seeing excesses of other causes rather than the opposite observation as found.

The reasons for the worse prognosis with time in Stockholm are not fully explained and appear to conflict with published data for follow-up data on patients in Uppsala and in other tertiary referral centres. An increased mortality in more recently diagnosed Crohn's patients was found, however, in Leicestershire.[147] Amongst 1000 patients hospitalized in New York for Crohn's disease between 1972 and 1987, 25 had died by 1994.[148] In 18 individuals, the death was considered clearly related to Crohn's disease – in seven cases because of postoperative sepsis, and in six because of gastrointestinal neoplasia. It is possible that the modest recent improvements in management are currently outweighed by an older affected population. As the statistics are not robust from a comparative point of view, these data should be considered mainly as interesting observations, and not be permitted to influence clinical or health economic planning at this stage.

References

1 Moum B, Ekbom A, Vatn MH, et al. Inflammatory bowel disease: re-evaluation of the diagnosis in a prospective population based study in south eastern Norway. Gut 1997; 40: 328–32.

2 Maeda K, Okada M, Yao T, et al. Intestinal and extra-intestinal complications of Crohn's disease: predictors and cumulative probability of complications. J Gastroenterol 1994; 29: 577–82.

3 Allison MC, Vallance R. Prevalence of proximal faecal stasis in active ulcerative colitis. Gut 1991; 32: 179–82.

4 Belaiche J, Louis E, D'Haens G, et al. Acute lower gastrointestinal bleeding in Crohn's disease: characteristics of a unique series of 34 patients. Belgian IBD Research Group. Am J Gastroenterol 1999; 94: 2177–81.

5 Barrett SML, Standen PJ, Lee AS, Hawkey CJ, Logan RFA. Personality, smoking and inflammatory

bowel disease. *Eur J Gastroenterol Hepatol* 1996; **8**: 651–5.

6 Quinton JF, Sendid B, Reumaux D, *et al.* Anti-*Saccharomyces cerevisiae* mannan antibodies combined with antineutrophil cytoplasmic autoantibodies in inflammatory bowel disease: prevalence and diagnostic role. *Gut* 1998; **42**: 788–91.

7 Targan SR. The utility of ANCA and ASCA in inflammatory bowel disease. *Inflamm Bowel Dis* 1999; **5**: 61–3.

8 Dijkstra J, Reeders JW, Tytgat GN. Idiopathic inflammatory bowel disease: endoscopic–radiologic correlation. *Radiology* 1995; **197**: 369–75.

9 Andreoli A, Cerro P, Falasco G, Giglio LA, Prantera C. Role of ultrasonography in the diagnosis of postsurgical recurrence of Crohn's disease. *Am J Gastroenterol* 1998; **93**: 1117–21.

10 Futagami Y, Haruma K, Hata J, *et al.* Development and validation of an ultrasonographic activity index of Crohn's disease. *Eur J Gastroenterol Hepatol* 1999; **11**: 1007–12.

11 Tio TL, Kallimanis GE. Endoscopic ultrasonography of perianorectal fistulas and abscesses. *Endoscopy* 1994; **26**: 813–15.

12 Shimizu S, Tada M, Kawai K. Endoscopic ultrasonography in inflammatory bowel diseases. *Gastrointest Endosc Clin North Am* 1995; **5**: 851–9.

13 Tsuga K, Haruma K, Fujimura J, *et al.* Evaluation of the colorectal wall in normal subjects and patients with ulcerative colitis using an ultrasonic catheter probe. *Gastrointest Endosc* 1998; **48**: 477–84.

14 Guslandi M, Polli D, Sorghi M, Tittobello A. Rectal blood flow in ulcerative colitis. *Am J Gastroenterol* 1995; **90**: 579–80.

15 Guslandi M, Sorghi S, Polli D, Tittobello A. Measurement of rectal blood flow by laser Doppler flowmetry in inflammatory bowel disease. *Hepatogastroenterology* 1998; **45**: 445–6.

16 Tateishi S, Arima S, Futami K. Assessment of blood flow in the small intestine by laser Doppler flowmetry: comparison of healthy small intestine and small intestine in Crohn's disease. *J Gastroenterol* 1997; **32**: 457–63.

17 Hare C, Bartram CI, Halligan S, Harvey R, Forbes A. Doppler ultrasound of the superior mesenteric artery to assess Crohn's disease. *Tech Coloproctol* 1997; **1**: 61–3.

18 Maconi G, Parente F, Bollani S, *et al.* Factors affecting splanchnic haemodynamics in Crohn's disease: a prospective controlled study using Doppler ultrasound. *Gut* 1998; **43**: 645–50.

19 Margulis AR, Burhenne HJ. *Practical Alimentary Tract Radiology*. St Louis: Mosby, 1993.

20 Misiewicz JJ, Forbes A, Price AB, Shorvon PJ, Triger DR, Tytgat GNJ (eds). *Atlas of Clinical Gastroenterology*, 2nd edn. London: Mosby, 1994.

21 Chernish SM, Maglinte DD, O'Connor K. Evaluation of the small intestine by enteroclysis for Crohn's disease. *Am J Gastroenterol* 1992; **87**: 696–701.

22 Halligan S, Saunders B, Williams C, Bartram C. Adult Crohn disease: can ileoscopy replace small bowel radiology? *Abdom Imaging* 1998; **23**: 117–21.

23 Bartram CI. Barium radiology. *Scand J Gastroenterol* 1994; **203**(Suppl): 20–3.

24 Halligan MS, Jobling JC, Bartram CI. Benefit of intravenous muscle relaxants during barium follow-through. *Clin Radiol* 1994; **49**: 179–82.

25 Palmer KR, Patil DH, Basran GS, Riordan JF, Silk DB. Abdominal tuberculosis in urban Britain – a common disease. *Gut* 1985; **26**: 1296–305.

26 Philpotts LE, Heiken JP, Westcott MA, Gore RM. Colitis: use of CT findings in differential diagnosis. *Radiology* 1994; **190**: 445–9.

27 Horton KM, Corl FM, Fishman EK. CT of nonneoplastic diseases of the small bowel: spectrum of disease. *J Comput Assist Tomogr* 1999; **23**: 417–28.

28 Meyers MA, McGuire PV. Spiral CT demonstration of hypervascularity in Crohn disease: 'vascular jejunization of the ileum' or the 'comb' sign. *Abdom Imaging* 1995; **20**: 327–32.

29 Kay CL, Kulling D, Hawes RH, Young JW, Cotton PB. Virtual endoscopy – comparison with colonoscopy in the detection of space-occupying lesions of the colon. *Endoscopy* 2000; **32**: 226–32.

30 Shoenut JP, Semelka RC, Magro CM, Silverman R, Yaffe CS, Micflikier AB. Comparison of magnetic resonance imaging and endoscopy in

distinguishing the type and severity of inflammatory bowel disease. *J Clin Gastroenterol* 1994; **19**: 31–5.

31 Low RN, Francis IR, Politoske D, Bennett M. Crohn's disease evaluation: comparison of contrast-enhanced MR imaging and single-phase helical CT scanning. *J Magn Reson Imaging* 2000; **11**: 127–35.

32 Orsoni P, Barthet M, Portier F, Panuel M, Desjeux A, Grimaud JC. Prospective comparison of endosonography, magnetic resonance imaging and surgical findings in anorectal fistula and abscess complicating Crohn's disease. *Br J Surg* 1999; **86**: 360–4.

33 Madsen SM, Thomsen HS, Schlichting P, Dorph S, Munkholm P. Evaluation of treatment response in active Crohn's disease by low-field magnetic resonance imaging. *Abdom Imaging* 1999; **24**: 232–9.

34 D'Arienzo A, Scaglione G, Vicinanza G, *et al.* Magnetic resonance imaging with ferumoxil, a negative superparamagnetic oral contrast agent, in the evaluation of ulcerative colitis. *Am J Gastroenterol* 2000; **95**: 720–4.

35 Lantto E, Jarvi K, Krekala I, *et al.* Technetium-99m hexamethyl propylene amine oxime leukocytes in the assessment of disease activity in inflammatory bowel disease. *Eur J Nucl Med* 1992; **19**: 14–18.

36 McCarthy M, Dutton J, Hirst J, Rottenberg G, Sanderson J. Can technetium white cell scintigraphy predict response to medical therapy in stricturing ileal Crohn's disease? *Gut* 1999; **45**(Suppl V): A129.

37 Bicik I, Bauerfeind P, Breitbach T, Von Schulthess GK, Fried M. Inflammatory bowel disease activity measured by positron-emission tomography. *Lancet* 1997; **350**: 262.

38 Weldon MJ, Lowe C, Joseph AEA, Maxwell JD. Review article: quantitative leucocyte scanning in the assessment of inflammatory bowel disease activity and its response to therapy. *Aliment Pharmacol Ther* 1996; **10**: 123–32.

39 Murphy MS, Grahnquist L, Romani P, Chapman S. Tc-HMPAO scintigraphy in paediatric IBD: a systematic comparison with barium follow-through, upper GI endoscopy and colonoscopy. *Gut* 1999; **45**(Suppl V): A129.

40 Bhatti M, Chapman P, Peters M, Haskard D, Hodgson HJ. Visualising E-selectin in the detection and evaluation of inflammatory bowel disease. *Gut* 1998; **43**: 40–7.

41 D'Haens G, Geboes K, Peeters M, Baert F, Ectors N, Rutgeerts P. Patchy cecal inflammation associated with distal ulcerative colitis: a prospective endoscopic study. *Am J Gastroenterol* 1997; **92**: 1275–9.

42 Pitris C, Jesser C, Boppart SA, Stamper D, Brezinski ME, Fujimoto JG. Feasibility of optical coherence tomography for high-resolution imaging of human gastrointestinal tract malignancies. *J Gastroenterol* 2000; **35**: 87–92.

43 Romer TJ, Fitzmaurice M, Cothren RM, *et al.* Laser-induced fluorescence microscopy of normal colon and dysplasia in colonic adenomas: implications for spectroscopic diagnosis. *Am J Gastroenterol* 1995; **90**: 81–7.

44 Smedh K, Olaison G, Nyström PO, Sjödahl R. Intraoperative enteroscopy in Crohn's disease. *Br J Surg* 1993; **80**: 897–900.

45 Perez-Cuadrado E, Macenlle R, Iglesias J, Fabra R, Lamas D. Usefulness of oral video push enteroscopy in Crohn's disease. *Endoscopy* 1997; **29**: 745–7.

46 Surawicz MC, Belic L. Rectal biopsy helps to distinguish acute self-limited colitis from idiopathic inflammatory bowel disease. *Gut* 1994; **24**: 519–24.

47 Price AB, Morson BC. Inflammatory bowel disease: the surgical pathology of Crohn's disease and ulcerative colitis. *Hum Pathol* 1975; **6**: 7–29.

48 Lee FD, Maguire C, Obeidat W, Russell RI. Importance of cryptolytic lesions and pericryptal granulomas in inflammatory bowel disease. *J Clin Pathol* 1997; **50**: 148–52.

49 Fujimura Y, Kamoi R, Iida M. Pathogenesis of aphthoid ulcers in Crohn's disease: correlative findings by magnifying colonoscopy, electron microscopy, and immunohistochemistry. *Gut* 1996; **38**: 724–32.

50 Price AB. Overlap in the spectrum of non-specific inflammatory bowel disease – colitis indeterminate. *J Clin Pathol* 1978; **31**: 567–77.

51 Wells AD, McMillan I, Price AB, Ritchie JK, Nicholls RJ. Natural history of indeterminate colitis. *Br J Surg* 1991; **78**: 179–81.

52 Meucci G, Bortoli A, Riccioli FA, *et al.* Frequency and clinical evolution of indeterminate colitis: a retrospective multi-centre study in northern Italy. *Eur J Gastroenterol Hepatol* 1999; **11**: 909–13.

53 Plauth M, Jenss H, Meyle J. Oral manifestations of Crohn's disease. An analysis of 79 cases. *J Clin Gastroenterol* 1991; **13**: 29–37.

54 Giller JP, Vinciguerra M, Heller A, Kunken FR, Kahn E. Treatment of gingival Crohn's disease with laser therapy. *N Y State Dent J* 1997; **63**: 32–5.

55 Lloyd DA, Payton KB, Guenther L, Frydman W. Melkersson–Rosenthal syndrome and Crohn's disease: one disease or two? Report of a case and discussion of the literature. *J Clin Gastroenterol* 1994; **18**: 213–17.

56 Parente F, Molteni P, Bollani S, *et al.* Prevalence of *Helicobacter pylori* infection and related upper gastrointestinal lesions in patients with inflammatory bowel diseases. A cross-sectional study with matching. *Scand J Gastroenterol* 1997; **32**: 1140–6.

57 Mashako MNL, Cezard JP, Navarro J, *et al.* Crohn's disease lesions in the upper gastrointestinal tract: correlation between clinical, radiological, endoscopic and histological features in adolescents and children. *J Pediatr Gastroenterol Nutr* 1989; **8**: 442–6.

58 Halme L, Kärkkäinen P, Rautelin H, Kosunen TU, Sipponen P. High frequency of *Helicobacter* negative gastritis in patients with Crohn's disease. *Gut* 1996; **38**: 379–83.

59 Wright CL, Riddell RH. Histology of the stomach and duodenum in Crohn's disease. *Am J Surg Pathol* 1998; **22**: 383–90.

60 Levenstein S, Prantera C, Varvo V, *et al.* Psychological stress and disease activity in ulcerative colitis: a multidimensional cross-sectional study. *Am J Gastroenterol* 1994; **89**: 1219–25.

61 Porcelli P, Leoci C, Guerra V. A prospective study of the relationship between disease activity and psychological distress in patients with inflammatory bowel disease. *Scand J Gastroenterol* 1996; **31**: 792–6.

62 Turnbull GK, Vallis TM. Quality of life in inflammatory bowel disease: the interaction of disease activity with psychosocial function. *Am J Gastroenterol* 1995; **90**: 1450–4.

63 Wood JD, Peck OC, Tefend KS, *et al.* Evidence that colitis is initiated by environmental stress and sustained by fecal factors in the cotton-top tamarin (*Saguinus oedipus*). *Dig Dis Sci* 2000; **45**: 385–93.

64 Post S, Kunhardt M, Herfarth C. Subjektive Einschatzung von Lebensqualitat, Schmerzen und Operationserfolg nach Laparotomien wegen Morbus Crohn. *Chirurg* 1995; **66**: 800–6.

65 Bernstein CN, Niazi N, Robert M, *et al.* Rectal afferent function in patients with inflammatory and functional intestinal disorders. *Pain* 1996; **66**: 151–61.

66 Kaplan MA, Korelitz BL. Narcotic dependence in inflammatory bowel disease. *J Clin Gastroenterol* 1988; **10**: 275–8.

67 Wechsler B, Davatchi F, Mizushima Y, *et al.* Criteria for diagnosis of Behçet's disease. *Lancet* 1990; **335**: 1078–80.

68 Kasahara Y, Tanaka S, Nishino M, *et al.* Intestinal involvement in Behçet's disease. Review of 136 surgical cases in the Japanese literature. *Dis Colon Rectum* 1981; **24**: 103–6.

69 Jorizzo JL. Behçet's disease: an update based on the 1985 international conference in London. *Arch Dermatol* 1986; **122**: 556–8.

70 Kim JH, Choi BI, Han JK, Choo SW, Han MC. Colitis in Behçet's disease: characteristics on double-contrast barium enema examination in 20 patients. *Abdom Imaging* 1994; **19**: 132–6.

71 Hamuryudan V, Mat C, Saip S, *et al.* Thalidomide in the treatment of the mucocutaneous lesions of the Behçet syndrome. A randomized, double-blind, placebo-controlled trial. *Ann Intern Med* 1998; **128**: 443–50.

72 Robertson DAF, Dixon MF, Scott BB, *et al.* Small intestinal ulceration: diagnostic difficulties in relation to coeliac disease. *Gut* 1983; **24**: 565–8.

73 Lamont CM, Adams FG, Mills PR. Radiology in idiopathic chronic ulcerative enteritis. *Clin Radiol* 1982; **33**: 283–6.

74 Ashton-Key M, Diss TC, Pan L, Du MQ, Isaacson PG. Molecular analysis of T-cell clonality

in ulcerative jejunitis and enteropathy-associated T-cell lymphoma. *Am J Pathol* 1997; **151**: 493–8.

75 Schiller LR. Microscopic colitis syndrome: lymphocytic colitis and collagenous colitis. *Semin Gastrointest Dis* 1999; **10**: 145–55.

76 Bowling T, Price AB, Al-Adnani M, Fairclough PD, Menzies-Gow N, Silk DBA. Interchange between collagenous and lymphocytic colitis in severe disease with autoimmune association requiring colectomy: a case report. *Gut* 1996; **38**: 788–91.

77 Jawhari A, Sheaf M, Forbes A, Kamm MA, Talbot IC. Microscopic colitis: widening the definition. *Gastroenterology* 1995; **108**: A843.

78 Zins BJ, Tremaine WJ, Carpenter HA. Collagenous colitis: mucosal biopsies and association with fecal leukocytes. *Mayo Clin Proc* 1995; **70**: 430–3.

79 Fernandez-Banares F, Salas A, Forne M, Esteve M, Espinos J, Viver JM. Incidence of collagenous and lymphocytic colitis: a 5-year population-based study. *Am J Gastroenterol* 1999; **94**: 418–23.

80 Zins BJ, Sandborn WJ, Tremaine WJ. Collagenous and lymphocytic colitis: subject review and therapeutic alternatives. *Am J Gastroenterol* 1995; **90**: 1394–400.

81 Bohr J, Tysk C, Yang P, Danielsson D, Järnerot G. Autoantibodies and immunoglobulins in collagenous colitis. *Gut* 1996; **39**: 73–6.

82 Fiedler L, George J, Sachar D, Kornbluth A, Janowitz H. Therapeutic outcomes in collagenous colitis. *Gastroenterology* 1996; **110**: A907.

83 Fine KD, Lee EL. Efficacy of open-label bismuth subsalicylate for the treatment of microscopic colitis. *Gastroenterology* 1998; **114**: 29–36.

84 Fasoli R, Talbot I, Reid M, Prince C, Jewell DP. Microscopic colitis: can it be qualitatively and quantitatively characterized? *Ital J Gastroenterol* 1992; **24**: 393–6.

85 Loft DE, Marsh MN, Sandle GI, *et al.* Studies of intestinal lymphoid tissue. XII. Epithelial lymphocyte and mucosal responses to rectal gluten challenge in celiac sprue. *Gastroenterology* 1989; **97**: 29–37.

86 Moayyedi P, O'Mahony S, Jackson P, Lynch DA, Dixon MF, Axon AT. Small intestine in lymphocytic and collagenous colitis: mucosal morphology, permeability, and secretory immunity to gliadin. *J Clin Pathol* 1997; **50**: 527–9.

87 Mullhaupt B, Guller U, Anabitarte M, Guller R, Fried M. Lymphocytic colitis: clinical presentation and long term course. *Gut* 1998; **43**: 629–33.

88 Naylor AR, Pollet JE. Eosinophilic colitis. *Dis Colon Rectum* 1985; **28**: 615–18.

89 Vitellas KM, Bennett WF, Bova JG, Johnson JC, Greenson JK, Caldwell JH. Radiographic manifestations of eosinophilic gastroenteritis. *Abdom Imaging* 1995; **20**: 406–13.

90 Tanigawa K, Sugiyama K, Matsuyama H, *et al.* Mesalazine-induced eosinophilic pneumonia. *Respiration* 1999; **66**: 69–72.

91 James SP. Remission of Crohn's disease after human immunodeficiency virus infection. *Gastroenterology* 1988; **95**: 1667–9.

92 Sharpstone DR, Duggal A, Gazzard BG. Inflammatory bowel disease in individuals seropositive for the human immunodeficiency virus. *Eur J Gastroenterol Hepatol* 1996; **8**: 575–8.

93 Kearney DJ, Steuerwald M, Koch J, Cello JP. A prospective study of endoscopy in HIV-associated diarrhea. *Am J Gastroenterol* 1999; **94**: 596–602.

94 Shepherd NA. Diverticular disease and chronic idiopathic inflammatory bowel disease: associations and masquerades. *Gut* 1996; **38**: 801–2.

95 Gratama S, Smedts F, Whitehead R. Obstructive colitis: an analysis of 50 cases and a review of the literature. *Pathology* 1995; **27**: 324–9.

96 Forbes A. Chronic radiation enteritis. In Nightingale J, ed. *Intestinal Failure.* London: Greenwich, 2001.

97 Azzena A, Litta P, Ferrara A, *et al.* Rectosigmoid endometriosis: diagnosis and surgical management. *Clin Exp Obstet Gynecol* 1998; **25**(3): 94–6.

98 Boulton R, Chawla MH, Poole S, Hodgson HJ, Barrison IG. Ileal endometriosis masquerading as Crohn's ileitis. *J Clin Gastroenterol* 1997; **25**: 338–42.

99 Satsangi J, Grootscholten C, Holt H, Jewell DP. Clinical patterns of familial inflammatory bowel disease. *Gut* 1996; **38**: 738–41.

100 Straus WL, Eisen GM, Sandler RS, Murray SC, Sessions JT. Crohn's disease: does race matter? The

Mid-Atlantic Crohn's Disease Study Group. *Am J Gastroenterol* 2000; **95**: 479–83.

101 Langholz E, Munkholm P, Davidsen M, Binder V. Course of ulcerative colitis: analysis of changes in disease activity over years. *Gastroenterology* 1994; **107**: 3–11.

102 Farrokhyar F, Swarbrick ET, Grace RH, Gent AE, Hellier MD, Irvine EJ. Long-term prognosis of ulcerative colitis. *Gut* 1999; **45**(Suppl V): A201.

103 Langholz E, Munkholm P, Davidsen M, Nielsen OH, Binder V. Changes in extent of ulcerative colitis. A study on the course and prognostic factors. *Scand J Gastroenterol* 1996; **31**: 260–6.

104 Gilberts ECAM, Greenstein AJ, Katsel P, Harpaz N, Greenstein RJ. Molecular evidence for two forms of Crohn's disease. *Proc Natl Acad Sci U S A* 1994; **91**: 12721–4.

105 di Mola FF, Friess H, Scheuren A. Transforming growth factor-betas and their signaling receptors are coexpressed in Crohn's disease. *Ann Surg* 1999; **229**: 67–75.

106 Sturm A, Schulte C, Schatton R, *et al.* TGF-β and HGF plasma levels in patients with inflammatory bowel disease. *Eur J Gastroenterol Hepatol* 2000; **12**: 445–50.

107 Biancone L, Viscido A, Cadau P, Caprilli R. Healing of the intestinal lesions in Crohn's disease. *Gut* 1999; **45**(Suppl V): A126.

108 Silverstein MD, Loftus EVV, Sandborn WJ, *et al.* Clinical course and costs of care for Crohn's disease: Markov model analysis of a population-based cohort. *Gastroenterology* 1999; **117**; 49–57.

109 Fockens P, Mulder CJJ, Tytgat GNJ, *et al.* Comparison of the efficacy and safety of 1.5 vs 3.0g oral slow-release mesalazine (Pentasa) in the maintenance treatment of ulcerative colitis. *Eur J Gastroenterol Hepatol* 1995; **7**: 1025–30.

110 Connell WR, Lennard-Jones JE, Williams CB, Talbot IC, Price AB, Wilkinson KH. Factors influencing the outcome of endoscopic surveillance for cancer in ulcerative colitis. *Gastroenterology* 1994; **107**: 934–44.

111 Ayres RC, Gillen CD, Walmsley RS, Allan RN. Progression of ulcerative proctosigmoiditis incidence and factors influencing progression. *Eur J Gastroenterol Hepatol* 1996; **8**: 555–8.

112 Makowiec F, Schmidtke C, Paczulla D, Lamberts R, Becker HD, Starlinger M. Progression and prognosis of Crohn's colitis. *Z Gastroenterol* 1997; **35**: 7–14.

113 D'Haens GR, Gasparaitis AE, Hanauer SB. Duration of recurrent ileitis after ileocolonic resection correlates with presurgical extent of Crohn's disease. *Gut* 1995; **36**: 715–17.

114 Best WR, Becktel JM, Singleton JW, Kern F Jr. Development of a Crohn's disease activity index. National Cooperative Crohn's Disease Study. *Gastroenterology* 1976; **70**: 439–44.

115 Harvey RF, Bradshaw JM. A simple index of Crohn's disease activity. *Lancet* 1980; **1**: 514.

116 Tromm A, Tromm CD, Huppe D, Schwegler U, Krieg M, May B. Evaluation of different laboratory tests and activity indices reflecting the inflammatory activity of Crohn's disease. *Scand J Gastroenterol* 1992; **27**: 771–8.

117 Schurmann G, Betzler M, Post S, Herfarth C, Meuer S. Soluble interleukin-2-receptor, interleukin-6 and interleukin-1B in patients with Crohn's disease and ulcerative colitis: preoperative levels and postoperative changes of serum concentrations. *Digestion* 1992; **51**: 51–9.

118 Vucelic B, Milicic D, Krznaric Z, *et al.* Akutphasenproteine im Serum zur Aktivitatsbeurteilung von Colitis ulcerosa und Morbus Crohn. *Acta Med Austriaca* 1991; **18**: 100–5.

119 Niederau C, Backmerhoff F, Schumacher B, Niederau C. Inflammatory mediators and acute phase proteins in patients with Crohn's disease and ulcerative colitis. *Hepatogastroenterology* 1997; **44**: 90–107.

120 Roseth AG, Schmidt PN, Fagerhol MK. Correlation between faecal excretion of indium-111-labelled granulocytes and calprotectin, a granulocyte marker protein, in patients with inflammatory bowel disease. *Scand J Gastroenterol* 1999; **34**: 50–4.

121 Sachar DB, Luppescu NE, Bodian C, Shlien TD, Fabry TL, Gumaste VV. Erythrocyte sedimentation as a measure of Crohn's disease activity: opposite trends in ileitis versus colitis. *J Clin Gastroenterol* 1990; **12**: 643–6.

122 Goebell H, Wienbeck M, Shomerus H, Malchow H. Evaluation of the Crohn's disease activity index and the Dutch index for severity and activity of Crohn's disease. An analysis of the data from the European Cooperative Crohn's Disease Study. *Med Klin* 1990; **85**: 573–6.

123 Acciuffi S, Ghosh S, Ferguson A. Strengths and limitations of the Crohn's disease activity index, revealed by an objective gut lavage test of gastrointestinal protein loss. *Aliment Pharmacol Ther* 1996; **10**: 321–6.

124 Miki K, Moore DJ, Butler RN, *et al.* The sugar permeability test reflects disease activity in children and adolescents with inflammatory bowel disease. *J Pediatr* 98; **133**: 750–4.

125 Powell-Tuck J, Day DW, Buckell NA, Wadsworth J, Lennard-Jones JE. Correlations between defined sigmoidoscopic appearances and other measures of disease activity in ulcerative colitis. *Dig Dis Sci* 1982; **27**: 533–7.

126 Baron JH, Connell AM, Lennard-Jones JE. Variation between observers in describing mucosal appearances in proctocolitis. *Br Med J* 1964; **1**: 89–92.

127 Walmsley RS, Ayres RCS, Pounder RE, Allan RN. A simple clinical colitis activity index. *Gut* 1998; **43**: 29–32.

128 Kennedy AP, Thompson DG, Robinison AJ, Wilkin D. Randomised controlled trial of a patient-centred guidebook: effect on quality of life in ulcerative colitis. *Gastroenterology* 2000; **118**: A213.

129 Mayberry MK, Probert C, Srivastava E, Rhodes J, Mayberry JF. Perceived discrimination in education and employment by people with Crohn's disease: a case control study of educational achievement and employment. *Gut* 1992; **33**: 312–14.

130 Duclos B, Planchon F, Jouin H, *et al.* Socioprofessional consequences of Crohn's disease. *Gastroenterol Clin Biol* 1990; **14**: 966–72.

131 Grimley CE, Walters S, Welch A, Hillenbrand P. The effect of inflammatory bowel disease on education employment and financial security in the United Kingdom. *Gut* 1999; **45**(Suppl V): A199.

132 Mayberry JF, Weterman IT. European survey of fertility and pregnancy in women with Crohn's disease: a case control study by European collaborative group. *Gut* 1986; **27**: 821–5.

133 Irvine EJ, Feagon B, Rochon J, *et al.* Quality of life: a valid and reliable measure of therapeutic efficacy in the treatment of inflammatory bowel disease. *Gastroenterology* 1994; **106**: 287–96.

134 Stewart AL, Hays RD, Ware JE Jr. The MOS short-form general health survey: reliability and validity in a patient population. *Med Care* 1988; **26**: 724–35.

135 EuroQol. The European quality of life tool. www.euroqol.org.

136 Hay JW, Hay AR. Inflammatory bowel disease: costs of illness. *J Clin Gastroenterol* 1992; **14**: 309–17.

137 Hanauer SB. The cost of inflammatory bowel disease. *Clin Ther* 1998; **20**: 1009–28.

138 Feagon BG, Larson LR, Vreeland MG, Bala MV. Annual cost of care for Crohn's disease patients. *Gastroenterology* 1999; **116**: A57.

139 Blomqvist P, Ekbom A. Inflammatory bowel disease: health care and costs in Sweden in 1994. *Scand J Gastroenterol* 1997; **32**: 1134–9.

140 Gregor JC, McDonald JWD, Klar N, *et al.* An evaluation of the utility measurement in Crohn's disease. *Inflamm Bowel Dis* 1997; **3**: 265–76.

141 Messori A, Brignola C, Trallori G, *et al.* Effectiveness of 5-aminosalicylic acid for maintaining remission in patients with Crohn's disease: a meta-analysis. *Am J Gastroenterol* 1994; **89**: 692–8.

142 Salter M. Sexuality and the stoma patient. In Myers C, ed. *Stoma Care Nursing.* London: Arnold, 1996.

143 Moody G, Probert CS, Srivastava EM, Rhodes J, Mayberry JF. Sexual dysfunction amongst women with Crohn's disease: a hidden problem. *Digestion* 1992; **52**: 179–83.

144 Moody GA, Mayberry JF. Perceived sexual dysfunction amongst patients with inflammatory bowel disease. *Digestion* 1993; **54**: 256–60.

145 Persson P-G, Bernell O, Leijonmarck C-E, Farahmand BY, Hellers G, Ahlbom A. Survival and cause-specific mortality in inflammatory bowel disease: a population-based study. *Gastroenterology* 1996; **110**: 1339–45.

146 Ekbom A, Helmick CG, Zack M, Holmberg L, Adami H-O. Survival and causes of death in patients with inflammatory bowel disease: a population-based study. *Gastroenterology* 1992; **103**: 954–60.

147 Probert CSJ, Jayanthi V, Wicks ACB, Mayberry JF. Mortality from Crohn's disease in Leicestershire, 1972–89: an epidemiological community based study. *Gut* 1992; **33**: 1226–8.

148 Mendelsohn RR, Korelitz BI, Gleim GW. Death from Crohn's disease. Lessons from a personal experience. *J Clin Gastroenterol* 1995; **20**: 22–6.

Medical therapy

The medical management of inflammatory bowel disease has recently entered a new era, the early promise of the novel immunomodulatory regimens translating into confirmed effective therapies. Nonetheless, corticosteroids, the 5-aminosalicylate (5-ASA) drugs (sulphasalazine and its successors) and azathioprine/6-mercaptopurine still constitute the mainstays of therapy. Primary nutritional therapy also has a place for some patients with Crohn's disease.

The remitting and relapsing course of inflammatory bowel disease, and the substantial rate of spontaneous improvement in the absence of therapy, would seem to argue for placebo-controlled trials, but the use of a placebo arm is acceptable only when there is no established treatment. The placebo response in ulcerative colitis has been re-explored in a thorough Medline review of 44 studies.[1] The clinical remission rate was 9.1 per cent (CI: 6.6–11.6) and the benefit rate was 26.7 per cent (CI: 24.1–29.2). Similar rates were observed for endoscopic and histological evidence. A number of study visits of three or more also improved response rates ($P = 0.05$). Spontaneous clinical improvement may be expected in around 30 per cent of episodes of active Crohn's disease.[2,3]

Corticosteroids

Corticosteroids remain a cornerstone in the medical management of patients with inflammatory bowel disease, providing rapid and effective relief of symptoms in acute exacerbations, though not usually accompanied by full remission on endoscopic or histological criteria. There is little difference between the response to hydrocortisone and to prednisolones when equivalent doses are compared (4 mg methylprednisolone: 5 mg prednisolone: 25 mg hydrocortisone), although there are some differences in their mineralocorticoid effects, which can occasionally be important. Intravenous therapy or adrenocorticotropic hormone (ACTH) may appear more efficacious than oral administration in resistant cases; this is probably an effect of the more direct route, and usually also a higher dose, rather than because of a switch between different steroids. A recent controlled trial in active Crohn's disease compared continuous intravenous infusion of 120 units/day of ACTH with hydrocortisone 300 mg/day.[4] There was no statistically significant difference, but there was numerical advantage to hydrocortisone (93 versus 82 per cent) and a tendency for the ACTH to act marginally faster in patients who had previously received steroids.

Mechanisms of action

The effects of steroids are mediated via their binding to cytosolic glucocorticoid receptors. This frees the receptors from the inactivating heat-shock protein 90, permitting their translocation into the nucleus to act on the glucocorticoid response element of the DNA to yield mRNA and a protein response.[5] The nuclear steroid–receptor complex inhibits activation of certain transcription factors, including binding lymphocyte AP-1 activator protein, which is then inhibited from producing (for example) mRNA for IL-2. Also, IκB is induced/stabilized, and hence NFκB (and its effects on TNF-α, etc.) is inhibited.[5] There is suppression of the 5-lipoxygenase-mediated metabolism of arachidonic acid,[6] and apoptosis of lamina propria lymphocytes may also be usefully stimulated.[7]

As some patients do not respond to steroid therapy, the reasons for resistance have been explored. Analysis of mRNA for the glucocorticoid receptor may be helpful in predicting responsiveness. Peripheral blood lymphocytes from all individuals appear to express the 477 base-pair mRNA for the alpha isoform of the receptor, but the 366 base-pair mRNA for the beta isoform was seen in only about 10 per cent of healthy volunteers and steroid-responsive patients with colitis, but in no less than 83 per cent of steroid-resistant patients. The sample size was too small for confident predictions but there is a strong suggestion that this could be clinically useful.[8] T-lymphocyte steroid resistance also appears to be an important factor in determining response to steroid treatment in patients with severe ulcerative colitis and may indeed be more predictive of outcome than disease severity.[9]

Efficacy

An early, partially controlled trial of 100 mg cortisone yielded a significantly better response than placebo in active ulcerative colitis (41 versus 16 per cent entering remission in 6 weeks), and with lower mortality in severe disease (16 versus 26 per cent),[10] but there has been no placebo-controlled trial in acute colitis since, or ever one in Crohn's disease. Response rates are now probably in the region of 70–80 per cent for both ulcerative colitis and Crohn's. The response to the first exposure to prednisolone in acute Crohn's disease was documented in a regional cohort: 80 per cent achieved a response, and 48 per cent complete remission.[11] Typical regimens of systemic steroids for moderate-to-severe exacerbations of inflammatory bowel disease comprise oral prednisolone 0.5–1.0 mg/kg body weight, with a suggested minimum of 30 mg daily, although as little as 0.25 mg/kg has been thought reasonable. It has, however, been shown that 40 mg is superior to 20 or 60 mg,[12] and that 40 mg taken as a single dose is superior to 10 mg four times daily.[13] Suggestions that alternate-day usage is as effective and leads to less growth retardation and adrenal suppression have not been confirmed.[14]

There are no good data to determine how long the initial dose should be maintained, and most gastroenterologists commence a reduction once response begins to be established in order to avoid unnecessary toxicity. I have favoured 7 days at the starting dose, reducing thereafter by 5 mg/week until weaning is complete, but both faster and much slower regimens have been advocated by others. It is, however, becoming clear that a steroid taper of some description is necessary. Thirty-five patients with active ulcerative colitis treated with 40 mg prednisolone for 2 weeks were then randomized to either a tapering course of prednisolone (reducing by a 5 mg daily dose every week) or similar placebo tablets in a double-blind manner.[15] At 8 weeks, 14 of 16 tapered patients, compared to 5 of 13 nontapered patients, were in remission. There are clearly difficulties in comparison as this is coloured by the initial response and the total steroid dose given, but if analysis is limited to the 25 patients who were in remission at 2 weeks, the results appear to hold good. Corroborative work would be useful.

Steroids contribute significantly to short- and long-term morbidity via their side effects. Issues specific to growth and osteoporosis are dealt with in Chapters 5, 6 and 7. Rates of other typical problems, chosen from a range of papers in the literature, indicate:

- central obesity, facial changes, and psychological manifestations in over 70 per cent;
- glucose intolerance, myopathy, easy bruising, acneiform rash, and sexual dysfunction in 50–70 per cent;
- oedema and opportunistic infection in 25–50 per cent; and
- the important but rarer complications of osteonecrosis, permanent neuropsychiatric disturbance, and subcapsular cataracts, each of which affect fewer than 2 per cent.

As steroids have been shown to be largely[16] or completely (most other studies) ineffective in maintaining remission, they should be withdrawn once the acute episode has settled. Some now take the view that steroids simply provide symptomatic control with no meaningful impact on the natural history of the inflammatory bowel disease. There are no data to refute this categorically, and indeed the failure of endoscopic criteria to correlate with clinical parameters of a steroid response in Crohn's suggests that it might be true.[17] There is, moreover, the very real problem of the patient who remains apparently steroid dependent.

Definitions of steroid responsiveness have been set for trial purposes, but are useful also for clinical guidance.[11] A steroid response comprises complete or partial clinical response without relapse within 30 days from completion of treatment. The steroid-dependent patient is one who achieves complete or partial clinical response and either relapses within 30 days after completion of treatment, or relapses with dose reduction, resulting in the use of prednisolone at doses of 15 mg or more for a year. The patient is termed steroid refractory if there is no response. In Crohn's disease, steroid dependence is more common in the younger patient who has coloanal disease without stenosis and who is a smoker.[18] No less than

32 per cent of one series of newly treated patients with Crohn's disease relapsed within 30 days or were unable to wean in 12 months. Of the initial responders, 45 per cent relapsed within a year, and only 42 per cent responded and remained in remission to 2 years.[11]

Topically active corticosteroids

When there is limited distal disease it is logical to employ topical therapy in the form of suppositories or enemas. It is to be expected that suppositories effectively treat the rectum and that enemas extend more proximally. Precise distribution is probably influenced by disease activity, but low-viscosity liquid steroid enemas can reasonably be expected to reach the splenic flexure within 15 minutes as judged by scintigraphic tracer scanning.[19]

Placebo-controlled trial data for the traditional steroids are not available, but there are many comparisons of the various agents and preparations, which typically yield response rates in the region of 40–50 per cent, and complete remission in 25–30 per cent.[20,21] It has seemed wise to favour steroids that are less well absorbed when comparable efficacy is documented. Nonetheless, all topical steroids have some potential for toxicity when used for prolonged periods, as up to 80 per cent of applied doses may be absorbed systemically. It is fortuitous that the degree of systemic absorption is directly related to the degree of inflammation and therefore diminishes as the patient comes into remission.[22]

Prednisolone metasulphobenzoate (Predfoam® or Predenema®) yields systemic levels significantly lower than those from a dose of prednisolone phosphate which achieves equivalent rectal tissue levels and therapeutic efficacy.[23] Budesonide, a prednisolone derivative, is poorly absorbed from the intestine, more rapidly metabolized in the liver and red blood cells, and is highly protein-bound in circulation, permitting little 'free hormone' action. It is now widely available as an enema (2 mg in 100 mL as Entocort®) and as foam (Budenofalk®: also 2 mg per application). Trials have demonstrated its superiority to placebo (19 per cent remission at 6 weeks, compared to 4 per cent; $P = 0.001$),[24] and at least equal efficacy to hydrocortisone acetate (125 mg as Colifoam®),[25] and prednisolone sodium phosphate (30 mg)[26] in the treatment of acute distal ulcerative colitis. Similar response rates are obtained from beclomethasone dipropionate enemas (3 mg/60 mL) compared with prednisolone sodium phosphate (30 mg/60 mL).[21] There is less suppression of endogenous cortisol secretion than from the older agents, but whether this is of major clinical advantage is somewhat questionable given the intention to confine steroid usage to the short-term management of the acute relapse.[20,22] Abstract data only are available for the effects of longer-term follow-up of topical budesonide.[27]

Orally administered budesonide in active Crohn's disease

The properties of budesonide could almost permit it to claim a role as a topical agent when given orally, but to aid maximal delivery to the terminal ileum and colon it has been coated (as Entocort® and Budenofalk®) with Eudragit®, the acrylic resin familiar to users of mesalazine. In a dose-ranging study in active Crohn's disease, doses between 3 and 15 mg daily were compared with placebo.[28] A 9 mg dose appeared optimal, there being no therapeutic gain, but appreciable increase in adrenal suppression with 15 mg. This dose was then compared with a tapering dose of prednisolone (starting at 40 mg daily).[29] The results indicate similar efficacy for the two agents. It should be noted that although there were no statistically significant differences in any of the measures of efficacy, in each case a modest numerical advantage lay with prednisolone. Adrenal toxicity from budesonide was certainly less, but not absent, in this study, which was too short term to provide information on other toxicological concerns. The Austrian/German results were very similar,[30] only one of the major studies suggesting

some advantage in efficacy to budesonide (60 versus 42 per cent remission at 8 weeks), but this was not significant.[31] Clinical impressions that budesonide is less effective in acute treatment are confirmed in a meta-analysis of 12 trials with a 'pooled rate difference' of –8.5 per cent for active disease compared with prednisolone.[32] Nonetheless, important adverse events occur acutely in 55 per cent of patients treated with prednisolone compared with only 33 per cent with budesonide.[29]

Orally administered budesonide in active ulcerative colitis

Oral budesonide has been compared with prednisolone in acute ulcerative colitis. In a 9-week double-blind trial of 72 patients, budesonide 10 mg was compared with prednisolone 40 mg, the dose being gradually tapered in both cases.[33] There were no significant differences in histological, endoscopic or clinical response rates, but again in each case a small numerical advantage lay with prednisolone. Plasma cortisol levels were not altered by budesonide, but were suppressed by prednisolone throughout the study period (albeit not significantly so at 9 weeks). It appears that a single daily dose of 9 mg is preferable to 3 mg thrice daily.[34] Somewhat less impressive results were recorded with fluticasone,[35] and work with this agent seems to have been discontinued.

Budesonide in maintenance of remission of Crohn's disease

Budesonide has also been assessed in the maintenance of remission in Crohn's disease. As a continuation of the therapeutic North American study into the remission phase, Greenberg *et al.*[36] studied patients on 3 or 6 mg budesonide in comparison to placebo. They found value in delaying the onset of relapse with both doses in the medium term, but this benefit was lost by follow-up to 1 year. A European maintenance study, also of 3 and 6 mg daily doses, showed benefit at 3 months only for the 6 mg dose, with an 81 per cent remission rate compared with 55 per cent and 56 per cent in the 3 mg and placebo groups, respectively ($P < 0.05$).[37] By 12 months only 41 per cent, 26 per cent and 37 per cent remained in remission, and all statistical advantage was again lost. As systemic side effects were few, the authors concluded that this represented a worthwhile therapeutic advance. I am not persuaded by this and would not select any steroid for true maintenance of remission inflammatory bowel disease. Whilst the patients in these medium-term studies were not steroid dependent, it would, however, be reasonable to draw from them further support for the use of budesonide in the steroid-dependent patient. Data on the effects (or lack of them) of budesonide on bone metabolism and the longer-term risks of osteopenia are so far few, but there is evidence that osteoblast activity is less influenced than by apparently equipotent doses of prednisolone,[38] which is clearly encouraging.

Aminosalicylates

Sulphasalazine has been used effectively in the treatment of ulcerative colitis since the early 1950s, with controlled trials demonstrating efficacy in treatment of acute colitis and in maintenance of remission.[39] Reductions in annual relapse rates of up to threefold were typical (for example from 71 per cent to 24 per cent[40]). There appeared to be no benefit in Crohn's disease, but studies using newer formulations of 5-ASA, which has been shown to be the principal active ingredient of sulphasalazine,[41] have shown more promise in prevention of relapse (see below).

Mechanisms of action
5-ASA (mesalazine or mesalamine in North America) is released from sulphasalazine by the azoreductase enzyme of colonic bacterial flora, and free drug is not normally thought to be available proximal to the caecum. How 5-ASA reduces intestinal inflammation in inflammatory bowel disease is not entirely clear, but its *in vitro* effects include inhibition of 5-lipoxygenase metabolism (diminishing the production of interleukins and inflammatory leukotrienes), suppression of platelet-activating factor, neutrophils and monocytes, chemotaxis, normalization of intestinal permeability, reduction of epithelial HLA-DR expression, stimulation of cytoprotective prostaglandins, and scavenging of free radicals. All these aspects are at least potentially relevant in life.[42] A direct influence on colonic mucosal flora is probably not important, however.[43]

Targeted delivery
Oral administration of plain 5-ASA is ineffective in inflammatory bowel disease because of proximal (mainly jejunal) absorption[44] and rapid metabolism. Sulphasalazine has a series of its own associated problems (see below), and alternative formulations of 5-ASA have therefore been developed. In each case it proves possible to use larger equivalent doses than has usually been the case with sulphasalazine, as fewer patients develop upper gastrointestinal intolerance. There is no oligospermia with the newer agents.

In normal controls, the intraluminal pH rises steadily from the stomach (pH 1–2) to approximately 7 in the terminal ileum, falling then to around 6 in the caecum,[45] lending logic to the use of pH-dependent release mechanisms for 5-ASA preparations. This has been adopted for several commercially available products. However, studies indicate that the lower small bowel and colon are more acidic in active inflammatory bowel disease (e.g. reference 46), and that colonic transit is faster.[47,48] While the pH-dependent approach may therefore be fallible, preliminary data indicate that it normally achieves what is intended.[49] We do not know the effect of other concurrent drug use such as proton pump inhibitors.

In 2000, sulphasalazine and at least eight other oral 5-ASA preparations were available around the world; their effects are very similar but probably usefully distinguishable, as shall be elucidated. Asacol® and Pentacol® are 5-ASA coated with an acrylic-based resin (Eudragit-S®) which dissolves rapidly above pH 7.0; this typically occurs in the region of the caecum and ascending colon. Eudragit-L® dissolves at pH 6.0 and is used to coat Claversal® and Salofalk®, with which release in the ileum is to be expected. Rowasa® is a hybrid with predominantly pH-dependent release. Pentasa® consists of microgranules of 5-ASA coated by a semipermeable ethyl cellulose membrane that releases 5-ASA steadily after tablet disintegration in the stomach, with enhanced release above pH 6.0: 5-ASA is made available throughout the small and large intestine. Pentasa® is the only 5-ASA preparation that is able to deliver useful quantities of drug to diseased areas proximal to the terminal ileum. Mesalazine will be taken, henceforth, to refer to these coated preparations.

Olsalazine (Dipentum®) is a 5-ASA dimer, the two molecules linked by an azo bond, which is broken by the same bacterial azoreductase that 'activates' sulphasalazine. Balsalazide (Colazide®) also has a 5-azo bond linking 5-ASA to an inert carrier (4-aminobenzoyl-beta-alanine), and is handled like sulphasalazine and olsalazine. The early publication record indicated comparable activity to other 5-ASAs and possibly a more favourable side effect profile.[50] It is evident, but surprisingly often neglected, that the 5-ASA preparations which depend on colonic bacteria for degradation of the azo bond cannot be effective in patients with colectomy and ileostomy. Too often sulphasalazine, olsalazine and balsalazide are still prescribed inappropriately and uselessly in this context.

Oral 5-ASA in active ulcerative colitis

Up to 60 per cent of patients with mildly to moderately active ulcerative colitis can be expected to respond to 5-ASA therapy alone. In a representative study, mesalazine 4.8 g/day produced 24 per cent complete and 50 per cent partial responses in mildly to moderately active ulcerative colitis compared with 5 per cent and 13 per cent in placebo controls ($P < 0.001$). There was numerical but not statistical advantage from 1.6 g/day.[51] Meta-analysis[52] yields an odds ratio (OR) of 2.0 (CI: 1.50–2.72) for superiority of mesalazine over placebo in active disease, and of 1.15 (CI: 0.83–1.61) for superiority over sulphasalazine.

Olsalazine appears similarly efficacious to coated 5-ASA preparations. Kruis *et al.* performed a blinded comparison of olsalazine and Claversal® in 172 patients with active colitis; 3 g daily doses of both drugs were used.[53] Their abstract indicates a somewhat higher frequency of adverse events from olsalazine, and little overall difference between the two agents, but a strong suggestion that olsalazine has an advantage in those with predominantly left-sided disease (58 versus 30 per cent attainment of remission).

Balsalazide 6.75 g daily (equivalent to 2.34 g mesalazine) has been compared with Asacol® 2.4 g daily, in a study of 101 patients with active colitis.[54] Topical steroids were allowed in the study protocol, which confuses things a little, but it is highly probable that the higher proportion of clinical and sigmoidoscopic remissions obtained (88 versus 57 per cent, and 62 versus 37 per cent, respectively at 12 weeks, and proportionately in the weeks before that), are of clinical as well as statistical significance ($P < 0.001$; $P < 0.05$). The responses obtained with balsalazide appeared also to be faster and associated with fewer side effects. A very similar 8-week study, so far only presented in abstract form, also showed a degree of advantage to balsalazide by virtue of a faster response.[55]

Oral 5-ASA in maintenance of remission of ulcerative colitis

5-ASA drugs help to maintain remission in ulcerative colitis,[39,40] and there is possibly a modest superiority of the newer agents over sulphasalazine

(OR: 0.85; CI: 0.64–1.15); longer-term follow-up is more persuasive with less evidence of toxicity.[56] Olsalazine and mesalazine have mostly been shown to be similarly effective in maintenance of remission, with one study significantly favouring olsalazine.[57] In this there was a lower relapse rate with olsalazine than with Asacol® in left-sided colitis (41.6 versus 70.4 per cent), presumed due to relatively enhanced delivery of 5-ASA to the left side of the colon. This study has, however, been criticized for its over-reliance on patient assessment and absence of sigmoidoscopic review. The relapse rate for mesalazine was also unexpectedly high, rates of no more than 50 per cent at 1 year being typical of other studies. It is also possible that olsalazine was favoured by the dosage schedule employed (1.0 g olsalazine versus 1.2 g Asacol®), given that the colonic concentration of 5-ASA after oral olsalazine is roughly double that when the same weight of mesalazine is given.[58]

A double-blind comparison of balsalazide 3 g daily (1.04 g 5-ASA) and Asacol® 1.2 g daily for 12 months in 99 colitics in remission favoured balsalazide. There were significantly better symptom scores and a lower number of relapses in the first 3 months (10 versus 28 per cent; $P = 0.035$) with balsalazide, but by 12 months 42 per cent of both groups had relapsed, and there was no difference in the side-effect profile.[59]

5-ASA: a dose response in ulcerative colitis?

Given continuing uncertainty as to the clinical relevance or otherwise of a dose response to 5-ASA and some concern about nephrotoxicity (see below), the Dutch Pentasa Study Group[60] examined both the efficacy and safety of daily doses of 1.5 g and 3 g of 5-ASA in the maintenance of remission in ulcerative colitis. More than 150 patients with ulcerative colitis in remission were randomized to one of the two doses and monitored to 12 months or to earlier relapse on clinical, endoscopic and histological criteria. The higher

dose of 5-ASA achieved a better 12-month remission rate on intention to treat – 67 versus 50 per cent. This difference just failed to reach statistical significance. A dose–response effect was also strongly suggested by a paper in which 4.8 g was more effective than 1.6 g in acute colitis, but it may be argued that the lower dose was subtherapeutic in this context.[61]

The appropriate duration of 5-ASA therapy in ulcerative colitis is debated, perhaps more by patients than by their doctors. There are strong suggestions that regular (and long-term) 5-ASA not only prolongs the relapse-free interval survival but also helps to reduce the risk of colonic neoplasia (see Chapter 8). Patients in prolonged remission nevertheless usually seek to stop maintenance therapy (or simply stop it on their own initiative). Aside from the issue of cancer risk, this becomes an increasingly reasonable proposition the longer the patient is from the last relapse. Two years of remission is suggested as a cut-off point for discontinuing maintenance therapy in ulcerative colitis, the nuisance (and hypothetical hazard) of therapy then perhaps outweighing clear benefit.[62]

5-ASA in Crohn's disease

Early studies failed to show worthwhile benefit from sulphasalazine in Crohn's disease, and studies of other 5-ASA preparations have mostly been too small to avoid type II error, but there are convincing positive data. Part of the difficulty results from the observation that a relatively large dose of 5-ASA seems to be required in Crohn's disease, there being a more obvious dose–response effect[63] than in ulcerative colitis (see above). A minimum maintenance dose of 2 g daily, and perhaps 4 g for acute therapy, may be necessary.

There have been multiple meta-analyses of the effects of 5-ASA therapy in Crohn's disease, which is testament first to the confusion and second to the recognition that any effect is numerically modest. There are three clinical scenarios for which data exist.

5-ASA for active Crohn's disease

Patients with active Crohn's disease have gained statistically significant advantage from a 4 g daily dose (relative to smaller doses or placebo) in only one single study.[64] Meta-analysis including other individually non-significant benefits appeared to support this usage, but this remains controversial as there are probably unpublished negative studies. There is, however, evidence to support an effect of similar potency to 40 mg methylprednisolone[65] with a numeric but non-significant advantage to a 4 g daily dose of a new microgranular Asacol® formulation. A recent literature survey concludes that at least 3 g/day is needed if there is to be therapeutic intent, and (more contentiously) that Pentasa® is only effective in small bowel disease, pH-dependent forms being more suitable for ileo-colonic disease.[66] There are no reliable data for topical application of 5-ASA in Crohn's disease.

5-ASA for Crohn's disease in medically induced remission

In a meta-analysis of 10 randomized controlled trials of sulphasalazine or mesalazine in the prevention of symptomatic disease relapse in quiescent disease (published up to 1993), Steinhart et al. concluded that treatment reduced the risk of clinical relapse at 12 months (relative risk: 0.77; CI: 0.64–0.92), but not significantly so at 3 or 6 months.[67] Subgroup analysis indicated that the benefit (all) lay with mesalazine (relative risk: 0.63; CI: 0.50–0.79).

A 48-week study that included patients with both medically and surgically induced remission supported this conclusion. No fewer than 293 patients were recruited (appropriately stratified) to a placebo-controlled study of 3 g mesalazine daily.[68] Relapse was defined from a Crohn's Disease Activity Index of > 150 and 60 points above baseline. Overall, mesalazine just failed to yield significant advantage (relapse rate 25 per cent versus 36 per cent; $P = 0.056$). Relapsing patients relapsed earlier if on placebo, and subgroup analysis revealed significant gains for patients with ileo-caecal–colonic disease and for females (relapse rates 21 versus 41 per cent, $P = 0.018$; and 19 versus 41 per cent, $P = 0.003$, respectively).

This benefit was not demonstrated in a comparable study of 5-ASA 3 g/day started immediately after a steroid-induced remission.[69] The trial was terminated when planned interim analysis showed a slightly higher relapse rate in the 5-ASA group, and the calculated probability of seeing a statistically significant difference by completing the study was minimal. Cumulative relapse rates at 6 and 12 months were 34 versus 31 per cent and 58 versus 52 per cent in 5-ASA patients and placebo patients, respectively, with no differences related to disease distribution.

Camma's meta-analysis (15 studies), performed before this last example, showed an absolute risk reduction of only 5 per cent for 5-ASA therapy after medically induced remission with a number-needed-to-treat of 20, and no statistical advantage.[70] This use is probably not clinically valuable.

5-ASA to prevent postoperative relapse of Crohn's disease

Evidence in support of the use of 5-ASA in prevention of postoperative relapse is somewhat more robust. Following the publication of a range of studies, including those which were positive,[71] or essentially neutral,[72,73] Camma's meta-analysis revealed overall benefit. In prevention of clinical relapse, there was an absolute risk reduction of 13 per cent (CI: –21.8 to –4.5 per cent), with value to one of every eight patients treated ($P < 0.05$).[70] A dose of at least 2 g daily is needed and it is suggested that benefit accrues only if the drug is started within 6 weeks of surgery. Nonetheless, this 13 per cent advantage means only the difference in clinical relapse rate at 1 year from approximately 45 per cent on placebo to 32 per cent on 5-ASA. Since this time, the European cooperative group have provided more neutral data using an 18-month 4 g Pentasa® regimen in over 300 patients.[74]

Cumulative relapse rates were 24.5 per cent with mesalazine compared with 31.4 per cent with placebo (not significant). However, those with isolated small bowel disease gained significant advantage (relapse rate 21.8 versus 39.7 per cent; P = 0.02). It is accordingly unreasonable to be too dogmatic about one's therapeutic strategy to the questioning patient who stands around a 55 per cent chance of remaining well to 1 year without medication and a 32 per cent chance of relapsing despite it! The GISSI group demonstrated that recurrence is more likely in those found to have a lower mucosal 5-ASA level at the time of relapse: 21.6 ng/mg tissue versus 70.9 in the ileum (P = 0.007) and 25.8 versus 60.3 in the colon (P = 0.010).[75] The authors are a little fey in their conclusions on results which suggest to me an issue of compliance. This might be taken into account when advising the postoperative patient.

Toxicity of 5-ASA drugs

The 5-ASA drugs have an excellent safety record and are among the very few drugs considered acceptable for use in pregnancy (see Chapter 5). However, more than occasionally, 5-ASA preparations can themselves be the cause of exacerbation of colitis, the associated worsening of the underlying disease leading potentially to confusion until the correct interpretation is reached.[76] Given the biochemical similarity with the non-steroidal anti-inflammatory drugs, and the potential for similar underlying mechanisms, this should perhaps be no surprise;[77] I estimate this risk to be around 1 per cent.

Problems peculiar to particular 5-ASA preparations

Up to 15 per cent of individuals are intolerant of the sulphapyridine moiety of sulphasalazine, and present with a typical drug rash or upper gastrointestinal symptoms, and very rarely with a Stevens–Johnson reaction;[78] the immunological problems seen with the drug in rheumatological

practice do not seem to be a problem. Predictable, reversible oligospermia is well recognized (see Chapter 5). Confusion may also arise because of the high eosinophil levels occasionally induced by sulphasalazine.[79,80]

Possible advantage for olsalazine shown over other 5-ASA preparations is limited by an osmotic diarrhoea provoked by the drug, which affects up to 10 per cent of patients, but may be minimized by taking the drug with food, and by commencing with a subtherapeutic dose and titrating up to the intended regimen over a week or two.[52]

Renal toxicity of 5-ASA

Increased usage of any drug, whether by increased numbers of recipients or by increased dose, raises anxieties about infrequent but important toxicity; 5-ASA is no exception. There has been concern that renal toxicity from 5-ASA may sometimes be responsible for end-stage renal failure with a need for renal dialysis or transplantation.[81,82] Debate continues as to the relative importance of idiosyncratic, dose-independent nephritis which is described (though very rare) with sulphasalazine, and of dose-dependent renal toxicity in which direct renal exposure to 5-ASA is more likely to be to blame.

Although there is a substantial literature and much clinical experience supporting the renal safety of the pH-dependent delivery systems, the systemic availability of 5-ASA is higher,[58] and renal failure is recorded more often with these agents.[82] This excess renal risk probably remains when corrected for the relative frequency of use of the different products, but is not of sufficient magnitude to warrant a major influence on choice of agent. Discussion with colleagues around the world suggests that the centres most concerned are those that have themselves seen and reported cases of renal failure.

Toxicity was actively sought throughout the Dutch Pentasa® study[60] and a probable or definite drug-related adverse event affected seven patients

(4 per cent), with no difference in the toxicity profile for the two doses used, or in the drop-out rate attributable to poor compliance. Pentasa® yields a high total circulatory 5-ASA concentration compared with other 5-ASA preparations, but relatively low free (non-acetylated) 5-ASA levels.[58] Two patients (1.3 per cent) developed modest and reversible renal impairment (one with mesalazine-related interstitial nephritis).

Prescribers of other 5-ASA preparations, worried that they are responsible for excessive or avoidable renal toxicity, will note that Pentasa® is also associated with renal problems quite frequently. If irreversible toxicity is, however, the result of sustained high, or peak, concentrations of free 5-ASA, then the results for Pentasa® (or, indeed, those for the agents dependent on colonic bacteria for 5-ASA release) are not necessarily wisely extrapolated to all pharmaceutical formulations. The particular concern with pH release systems is that there is the potential for release of a sufficiently large 'bolus' in the small intestine to overwhelm mucosal acetylation and thereby lead to a transient but high-concentration 5-ASA challenge to the kidney with each dose given. This prompted estimation of systemic 5-ASA and acetyl-5-ASA studied in a brief crossover study of olsalazine and mesalazine at recommended (not equivalent) doses in 15 patients. Plasma and urine levels of 5-ASA and its acetylated derivative were substantially higher with the mesalazine preparation (8.0 versus 1.2 μmol/L and 10.8 versus 2.8 μmol/L in plasma). There was considerable patient-to-patient variation and the clinical consequences are unknown.[83]

Whichever oral 5-ASA preparation is chosen, it must be remembered that it is likely to be employed for many years, and we should remain alert to the possibility of insidious nephrotoxicity developing after some years of treatment. There might be 'late' renal impairment with very prolonged use (10 years or more), for which data are not yet available. It is important that

prescribers audit their practice carefully, taking account of the renal dysfunction that may complicate inflammatory bowel disease itself, quite independently of any drugs used in its therapy.[84,85] Renal disease is discussed further in Chapter 6.

5-ASA and gastric emptying

The pharmacology of pH release mechanisms has come under scrutiny following suggestions that the Eudragit-coated preparations behave in the stomach as if solids, and leave very late in the gastric emptying process. Accordingly, the tendency for insightful gastroenterologists to increase compliance by advocating twice rather than three times daily dosage develops a scientific rationale. Hussain and colleagues have taken this a step further by comparing the effects of Asacol® when normal volunteers were given 1.2 g as a single daily dose as compared to a more conventional 400 mg thrice daily.[86] Disposition of native 5-ASA and its acetylated form was similar regardless of administration regimen, but clearly there are objections to the use of healthy volunteers and examination of only a 7-day study period. There should perhaps be relatively greater concern when considering the larger daily doses often used in North America.

Topical 5-ASA derivatives in ulcerative colitis

Given the distal nature of much ulcerative colitis and the low but real potential for systemic toxicity of oral 5-ASA, it is logical to consider topical therapy whenever possible. The extent to which mesalazine enemas reach the more proximal colon has been uncertain and based on extrapolation from studies of topical steroids.[18,87] Van Bodegraven et al. explored this scintigraphically in an examination of 31 patients.[88] The patients received one of three dose/volume regimens of liquid mesalazine (Salofalk® or Pentasa®) labelled with technetium, and had a repeat labelled enema at 12 weeks. Disease activity was not found to influence the distribution, but there was a non-significant tendency for the enema to reach a little more proximally in the active phase of illness. Extent of distribution was determined mainly by the volume of the enema, the 30 mL enema remaining mainly confined to the sigmoid, 60 mL reaching the descending colon in 15 per cent, and the 100 mL preparation reaching the descending colon in 25 per cent. Similarly, Campieri *et al.* demonstrated scintigraphically that a 20 mL foam preparation reached more proximally (mostly to around the splenic flexure) than a 10 mL foam and that 20 mL of foam might actually reach more proximally than a 100 mL liquid enema.[89] The foam also distributed more evenly around the colon.

It is notable and may be clinically important that the enema was not imaged in the rectum in the great majority of Van Bodegraven's patients (91–99 per cent), whatever the phase of illness or volume of enema; it may be logical to use concurrent suppository therapy in these patients.

Topical mesalazine in active colitis, and comparisons with topical steroids

Topical mesalazine is firmly established as an effective agent in the treatment of active proctitis and distal colitis, with a response rate typically in excess of 70 per cent over 3–6 weeks. A steadily widening range of products is available including Asacol® as foam and suppositories, and Pentasa®, ·Rowasa® and Salofalk® as both liquid enemas and suppositories. There do not appear to be important differences in efficacy between comparable products. A new gel formulation is also being evaluated, which may be better retained than foam.[90] It is not obvious why sulphasalazine should be marketed as an enema.

A 4-week study of more than 300 patients favoured Asacol® foam over Predfoam®, but fell short of conferring histological advantage.[91] The meta-analysis of this and six other trials (performed by Marshall and Irvine) lends further support for topical 5-ASA.[92] Rectal 5-ASA was significantly better than conventional topical corticosteroids for inducing remission symptomatically, endoscopically, and histologically, with highly significant pooled ORs of 2.42 (CI: 1.72–3.41), 1.89 (1.29–2.76), and 2.03 (1.28–3.20), respectively.

Where topical steroid foams are readily available, they may well remain many practitioners' first choice, given their undoubted efficacy, the wealth of clinical experience, and that some of the comparisons have been between relatively high doses of mesalazine (2 g daily) and more routine doses of prednisolone/hydrocortisone. In the UK, there is also a cost disincentive to the use of Asacol® foam instead of Predfoam® or Colifoam® (of the order of fivefold at year 2000 prices). A useful case is also presented by Mulder *et al.*[93] who argue that in difficult cases it is not only logical but also effective to combine the two drug types.

Topical versus oral 5-ASA in active colitis

Topical 5-ASA has been compared with oral preparations in a number of studies of patients with distal ulcerative colitis. There have been problems in interpreting these studies as it is difficult to be sure whether comparable doses are being administered to the area of interest, and whether any differences are because of a dose–response effect. A typical example of this problem was the favourable outcome from Rowasa® enemas (4 g) compared with oral therapy (2.4 g).[94] Campieri *et al.*[95] clarified things in a study of patients with ulcerative proctitis comparing 2.4 g orally with 1.2 g daily by suppository (400 mg t.i.d.). Results strongly favoured the rectal route at 2 and 4 weeks for clinical effect and histological improvement.

Although additional gain may be achieved from combining oral and topical 5-ASA,[94,96] there is also evidence that this is no better than using topical treatment alone.[97,98]

Topical versus oral 5-ASA in maintenance of remission in colitis

Topical 5-ASA has been shown to achieve remission in some patients who have previously been resistant to oral 5-ASA or to topical steroids.[22] It is also effective in maintenance of remission, administered daily as a liquid enema, foam or suppository. There is little gained from dose escalation,[99] and 1 g daily is not obviously inferior to 2 g or 4 g. A single daily dose of 1 g also appears superior to 500 mg twice daily.[100] It is probably sufficient to use intermittent administration and still outperform daily oral therapy,[101] aiming perhaps for alternate-night or thrice-weekly usage.[102] When enemas are employed, there is no major difference in efficacy between foam and liquid preparations. In most (but not all[103]) comparisons, patients have tended to prefer the foam formulation, and long-term compliance may therefore be improved. Little 5-ASA is absorbed when it is administered rectally and it may therefore be inferred that the above results generally reflect topical effects. I feel that the choice of route of administration may reasonably be left to the patient when the disease is entirely or predominantly distal.

Topical 4-ASA

Distal ulcerative colitis will also respond to topical 4-ASA (also known as para-aminosalicylic acid/PAS) with comparable results to topical prednisolone,[104] and to topical 5-ASA.[105] Clinical experience suggests, as for 5-ASA, that although the overall proportion of responsive patients is virtually identical, the particular patients who respond may differ, making a switch to an alternative topical regimen worthwhile in those who do not initially achieve remission.

Immunosuppressant therapy

Immunosuppressant drugs are valuable in refractory inflammatory bowel disease, in which they help to achieve and maintain clinical remission, reduce steroid use, and avoid surgery. Their usefulness has, however, been hampered by limited efficacy and, to some extent, toxicity. An increasing understanding of the mucosal immune response in inflammatory bowel disease is now permitting new agents to be targeted at particular, critical steps in immune activation.

AZATHIOPRINE AND 6-MERCAPTOPURINE

Azathioprine and 6-mercaptopurine (6MP) are purine analogues that competitively inhibit the biosynthesis of purine nucleotides. Their mode of action is incompletely understood but they are known to have selective suppressant effects on T cells. Once absorbed, azathioprine is almost entirely metabolized to 6MP, by sulphydryl compounds such as glutathione. The 6MP is then metabolized by thiopurine methyltransferase (TPMT) to 6-methylmercaptopurine (which may be immunoactive), by xanthine oxidase to the inactive 6-thiouric acid, or by a series of steps to active 6-thioguanine nucleotides. Deficiency of TPMT, or inhibition of xanthine oxidase (as with concurrent use of allopurinol), predisposes to accumulation of 6MP and the potential for severe bone marrow suppression.[106,107] Myelosuppression can occur in anyone when high doses of azathioprine or 6MP are employed, but is more likely in those with congenitally low TPMT activity.

Myelosuppression as a predictor of responsiveness?

It is proposed that efficacy might be dependent on the development of some degree of leucopenia.[108] Berg et al.[109] performed a retrospective study of 101 patients on 6MP. Of the 71 subjects who achieved complete remission on the drug, 65 per cent were leucopenic (although the definition of this is not given in the abstract) at some time, compared with 43 per cent of those in whom complete remission was not achieved. However, the two phenomena appeared unrelated as leuco-penia followed the attainment of remission in 50 per cent, and did not predict future remission. In another study, the course of 98 consecutive patients with refractory Crohn's disease treated with 6MP was examined according to whether leucopenia occurred (n = 51) or not. The induction of leucopenia was apparently not deliberate, but there were no real control data. The mean time to remission was 8.8 weeks for patients with leucopenia compared with 14.3 weeks for those without; the leucopenia was evidently not severe and was associated with no other toxicity. Other centres are less convinced that this phenomenon is of clinical relevance,[110] and it is difficult to know how it should influence practice, if at all. It is encouraging that a blinded prospective study is in progress.

TPMT genotype and enzyme activity

TPMT activity is subject to allelic polymorphism: approximately 90 per cent of Caucasians are homozygous for a high TPMT activity allele (*TPMT*1*), whilst around 10 per cent are heterozygous, and 0.3 per cent homozygous for variant alleles resulting in intermediate or low TPMT activity.[111] In a study of 106 predominantly Caucasian inflammatory bowel disease patients on azathioprine, a heterozygous genotype was detected in all patients with intermediate TPMT activity, and in none of those with high TPMT activity (all of whom were homozygous for *TPMT*1*).[107] Most of the heterozygotes had the *TPMT*1/TPMT*3A* genotype, and 2 had *TPMT*1/TPMT*3C*.

TPMT and 6-thioguanine – prediction of safety and efficacy?

The value of TPMT or 6-thioguanine levels to assist in the optimization of purine analogue dosage and, hence, response rates, has received a lot of attention recently. Final conclusions would be premature but there is an emerging consensus that the main role of 6-thioguanine levels is to give confidence that it is

safe to increase the dose of azathioprine or 6MP in non-responding patients.[112,113]

Even if plasma 6-thioguanine does correlate to a reasonably close extent with clinical response in some centres,[114] this is far from a universal observation.[115,116] Concomitantly, the activity of TPMT also proves a poor predictor of response. Red-cell TPMT activity in one study of 82 azathioprine-treated inflammatory bowel disease patients ranged from 5.3 to 20.2 nmol/h/mL on a mean dose of 1.5 mg/kg.[117] The response rate was 78 per cent (good in 54 per cent; partial in 24 per cent). Important side effects had occurred in 15 per cent (pancreatitis and neutropenia equally). TPMT levels did not predict a response to azathioprine or the risk of pancreatitis. Low activity of TPMT was, however, significantly associated with neutropenia in this and other studies, to an approximately fivefold excess.[107]

Azathioprine/6MP toxicity

Approximately 10 per cent of patients are intolerant of azathioprine and 6MP, side effects being mainly of a relatively trivial nature. Serious but idiosyncratic toxicities, including pancreatitis, hepatitis and hypersensitivity reactions, all of which recur on repeated administration, occur more rarely. Bone marrow suppression is dose related and reversible, and although it usually occurs in the first 6 months of treatment it can occur much later[118,119] and therefore necessitates regular 4–6-weekly monitoring of the white blood cell count while therapy continues. In the St Mark's review, only 5 per cent of patients developed myelosuppression.[118] In five cases (< 0.7 per cent) there were associated clinical manifestations, and it is probable that at least one death from sepsis was azathioprine related. If myelosuppression develops, it may be possible to retain therapeutic efficacy safely by reduction of dosage.

The overall frequency of major toxicity is low, with no attributable deaths in a 30-year audit from Oxford.[120] Azathioprine or 6MP had been used in

621 of 2205 inflammatory bowel disease patients for a mean of 634 days, yielding 1350 patient-years available for review. In 517 cases, the drug had been stopped by time of review, in 152 because of side effects (mostly nausea: 68), in 203 as planned withdrawal after defined duration, and in 113 for treatment failure. Only two patients developed pancreatitis and only 4.6 per cent had myelosuppression ($n = 29$) which was in the first 6 months in 41 per cent, but after 24 months in 6; most then stopped therapy.

There is also an interesting observation in respect of choice between azathioprine and 6MP. In the metabolism of azathioprine to 6MP, imidazole derivatives are released. It is suggested that, independent of TPMT status, these derivatives are the reason for much of the early upper gastrointestinal intolerance and flu-like symptoms, and render more explicable the experience that 6MP can be safely and effectively substituted in a majority (69 per cent) of these patients.[121]

The safety of azathioprine in pregnancy is considered in Chapter 5, and the possible risk of an increased incidence of malignancy is considered in Chapter 8.

Azathioprine and 6MP in chronically active Crohn's disease

Persuasive evidence for a role of azathioprine/6MP in the management of refractory Crohn's disease dates from Present's 1980 study in which induction of remission and steroid sparing were demonstrated.[122] In a 24-month placebo-controlled study of 83 patients (needing an initial mean daily prednisolone dose of 20 mg) 1.5 mg/kg of 6MP permitted full weaning from steroids in 55 per cent with improvement in 75 per cent, whereas only 36 per cent of the placebo group improved. The delay to response does, however, require comment, since in this study there was no significant difference from placebo until after 12 weeks. A more recent, South African, study of azathio-

prine (2.5 mg/kg) in steroid-treated patients with active disease[123] confirmed the delay (not significant at 12 weeks), and the response, with a highly significant difference in the proportion of patients in remission at 15 months (42 versus 7 per cent; $P = 0.001$). Perhaps more importantly still, there is good evidence that azathioprine (unlike steroids) not only improves the symptomatic response but is responsible for true mucosal healing.[124]

The 1995 meta-analysis of purine analogues in Crohn's disease was able to consider four studies of active disease, two of remission, and three in which both aspects were included.[125] Compared with placebo, azathioprine or 6MP therapy had an OR for response of 3.09 (CI: 2.45–3.91) in patients with active Crohn's disease. This was very much influenced by the New York data,[122] and there was greater benefit from 6MP than from the azathioprine that the other studies used (OR for azathioprine studies was only 1.45). Overall, a clear steroid-sparing effect was seen (OR: 3.69; CI: 2.12–6.42), and both higher cumulative drug dose ($P < 0.001$) and continuation of therapy for at least 17 weeks ($P = 0.03$) improved response rates.

In an attempt to speed the induction of a response to azathioprine in steroid-refractory Crohn's disease, a loading dose has been assessed in a placebo-controlled study.[126] Patients were randomized to a 36-hour infusion of azathioprine, 40 mg/kg, or placebo, and then all patients received oral azathioprine, 2 mg/kg, for 16 weeks. Although steady-state levels of 6-thioguanine occurred earlier with loading, there were no differences by 2 weeks in toxicity at any stage, or in the short- or long-term outcomes. At week 8, 25 per cent were in complete remission in the azathioprine-loaded group compared with 24 per cent in the placebo group. This strategy was no more effective in children.[127]

Purine analogues also appear to have a role in treatment of Crohn's-related fistulae (see Chapter 7). In an uncontrolled 6-month trial of 34 patients, a 39 per cent fistula closure rate was reported, with worthwhile improvement in a further 26 per cent, mostly in patients who had not already been treated surgically.[128] Other authors also document benefit to around 30 per cent of fistula patients[129] and on meta-analysis the OR for improvement of fistulae was 4.44 (CI: 1.50–13.20).[125] Nonetheless, the long mean times to response and the relatively low remission rates emphasize the continuing need for new therapeutic options here.

Azathioprine and 6MP in maintenance of remission in Crohn's disease

The long time to response in active treatment tends to blur the distinction between active therapy and maintenance with these agents, but several studies have confirmed benefit in maintenance of remission.[130,131] More recently, Lémann et al.[132] studied azathioprine in patients after 'curative' resection for Crohn's disease. As this was a retrospective analysis with only historical controls, the interpretation should be somewhat guarded. The authors' view that the clinical recurrence rate (26 per cent at 3 years) is better than with no maintenance therapy and of a similar order to that obtainable with 5-ASA seems reasonable, but whether controlled trial of a relatively hazardous agent is justified when a less toxic agent exists and may be of similar value must be considered carefully. A very large trial would be required to show differences between azathioprine and 5-ASA if Lémann's data are representative. It may no longer be legitimate to initiate placebo-controlled trials in this context. On meta-analysis, the overall OR for benefit proved to be 2.27 (CI: 1.76–2.93). Again, a higher dose ($P = 0.008$) and increased cumulative dose ($P = 0.01$) improved response.[125]

Azathioprine and 6MP in ulcerative colitis

Purine analogues have also been shown to be effective in induction and maintenance of remission in refractory ulcerative colitis, commencing with a study at St Mark's in 1982 in which 44 patients were randomized to azathioprine or placebo.[133] There was a clinical response and it was possible to achieve a significantly greater reduction in prednisolone dose by 3 months in the patients receiving azathioprine (mean prednisolone dose 6.7 mg versus 17.7 mg). Supportive data have come from other centres[134,135] and there is a significantly greater relapse rate in patients in whom the drug is subsequently withdrawn.[136] The New York group have reviewed their experience of 6MP in 105 chronic refractory ulcerative colitis patients.[137] Complete clinical remission was achieved in 65 per cent, partial remission in 24 per cent, and 11 per cent failed to respond. Following response, 35 per cent relapsed at some stage whilst on maintenance, compared with 87 per cent of those who discontinued 6MP.

Duration of therapy

Given continuing, and probably not entirely misplaced, concern about the long-term use of azathioprine, it behoves us to consider for how long therapy should be continued once remission is achieved. The data summarized above support its use for at least 12 months once the initial introductory phase is successfully negotiated. The data become less good thereafter, but the St Mark's data support use up to 24 months reasonably securely. Thereafter the data refer to relatively small numbers. Two North American surveys suggest that more or less indefinite therapy should be considered,[137,138] but only one was designed with this purpose. Bouhnik's study of 157 patients treated for more than 6 months is therefore helpful.[139] It is based on just over 40 per cent of all his group's patients exposed to azathioprine or 6MP. The cumulative relapse rates at 1 and 5 years were 11 per cent and 32 per cent (compared with 38 per cent and 75 per cent in those who, having achieved remission on the drug, stopped it more than 6 months after its commencement).

However, in those who stopped the drug more than 5 years after its initiation, there was no apparent disadvantage. Although this may simply be a small-number effect (12 continuing, 5 stopping) there were no relapses in those who stopped, compared to 2 in the 12 continuing, and for all other time brackets there was an obvious excess in those stopping, which failed to reach significance only in year 4, when 25 per cent of those stopping relapsed compared to 17 per cent of those continuing. The better American study (n = 120) examined the time to relapse in those who continued treatment compared with those who stopped treatment for reasons other than a relapse.[138] The cumulative probabilities of relapse at 1, 2, 3 and 5 years for those who continued and those who stopped therapy were 29 versus 36 per cent at 1 year; 45 versus 71 per cent at 2 years; 55 versus 85 per cent at 3 years; and 61 versus 85 per cent at 5 years. Extrapolating a little from the French and American data, I advocate a trial off azathioprine once more than 4 years of successful treatment have been completed.

A continuing audit of azathioprine use is run at St Mark's to judge the safety and appropriateness of its use outside a trial setting. Clinical guidelines were established some years ago (Table 3.1) against which the audit seeks to test compliance in regular clinical practice.

We find that indications for commencement and starting dose are implemented correctly and that hospital follow-up and haematological monitoring are excellent. Unfortunately, non-hospital haematological supervision leaves much to be desired.

CICLOSPORIN

Ciclosporin is a lipid-soluble fungal derivative with potent immunosuppressive effects, which acts primarily on T-cell function and proliferation, mainly by inhibition of IL-2 gene transcription, an effect mediated by blocking calcineurin activation of a nuclear factor in the T cells.[140] There is consequent loss of recruitment of cytotoxic cells and inhibition of cytotoxic lymphokines.[141] It has been widely used since the positive results reported for its use in fulminant ulcerative colitis,[142] but not without hazard.

Ciclosporin in Crohn's disease

Early uncontrolled, open studies of ciclosporin in Crohn's disease claimed impressive response rates within 5–10 days, followed then by a high late-failure rate. There are currently four published, randomized, double-blind, placebo-controlled trials of oral ciclosporin in refractory Crohn's disease. Brynskov *et al.*[2] reported improvement in

---

Table 3.1 Guidelines for azathioprine use in inflammatory bowel disease

1 Established inflammatory bowel disease
2 Failure to respond to steroid/5-ASA, or failure to wean from steroids, or need for systemic steroids > 4 months per year
3 Absence of need for early surgery
4 Prescription of 2 mg/kg
5 Regular clinical review
6 Full blood count every clinic visit and every 4–6 weeks
7 Dose reduction/stop if toxicity (total leucocytes < 3.5, or neutrophils < 1.5)

50 per cent of treated patients compared with only 32 per cent in controls. Although this was significant, only 19 per cent of the responding patients retained their improvement to 6 months after tapering and discontinuing the drug. The study by Jewell *et al.*[143] was more disappointing, even with continuing maintenance therapy. The Canadian Crohn's Relapse Prevention Trial Investigators[144] reported on their multicentre, double-blind, placebo-controlled trial of low-dose ciclosporin in which a total of 305 patients were entered. Actively treated patients had a worse symptomatic outcome than the placebo group, and there was no reduction in requirement for other medication. Very similar conclusions come from the fourth study,[145] and a meta-analysis concludes that it is of no value in Crohn's disease.[146] While it is possible that a better response might be obtained with higher doses, toxicity precludes this as a long-term measure (see below). A role may exist for the patient with fistulous disease, to judge from an uncontrolled study of 16 such patients.[147] All had failed on standard therapies, and were started on 4 mg/kg by continuous intravenous infusion. Fourteen patients showed some response, and seven fistulae closed. There was substantial toxicity, and a high relapse rate when parenteral therapy was discontinued. The authors concluded that intravenous ciclosporin was effective in fistulating Crohn's disease, but that its future role should be determined by controlled trial. This is probably an appropriate conclusion for the use of the drug in Crohn's in general, despite the occasional apparently dramatic anecdotal response. Its use is not currently justified outside formal clinical trials.

Ciclosporin in ulcerative colitis

The initial promising results from an open pilot study of intravenous ciclosporin in fulminant ulcerative colitis have subsequently been strongly supported by the same group. A dual-centre controlled trial was designed to include 40 patients failing to respond to 5 days of high-dose intravenous steroids.[142] Fulminant colitis was defined from the revised Oxford criteria[148] (see also Chapter 4). The patients were randomized to receive either intravenous ciclosporin 4 mg/kg as a continuous infusion together with continued high-dose steroids, or to continue conventional therapy alone. The study was stopped prematurely on statistical and ethical grounds after only 20 patients had been entered. Nine of 11 patients given ciclosporin responded as compared to none of the nine continuing conventional therapy alone. This improvement was maintained in over 60 per cent of patients at 6 months after discharge from hospital.

The Chicago group have since published on their experience of 5 years' use of ciclosporin in severe ulcerative colitis.[149] All patients were treated with 4 mg/kg/day intravenously. Of 42 patients, 36 (86 per cent) responded and 31 transferred to oral ciclosporin (8 mg/kg/day) for an overall mean of 20 weeks. The six complications encountered resolved with drug withdrawal. Ten initial responders had interval colectomies after a mean of 6 months. Many of their patients were also given azathioprine/6MP and these patients did better than those managed without. The quality of life in those successfully treated with ciclosporin was better than in those receiving surgery,[150] but this is arguably a flawed comparison, as like is not compared with like.

A comparable 6-year study from Oxford was less bullish.[151] From 216 patients with fulminant colitis, 84 failed to respond to conventional medical measures. Colectomy was performed forthwith in 34 (40 per cent), and 50 received ciclosporin (4 mg/kg by continuous slow infusion). Remission was achieved in 28 patients who went on to oral ciclosporin (5 mg/kg). However, 8 of the 28 later relapsed and needed colectomy. The short-term efficacy of 56 per cent therefore falls to 40 per cent in the longer term (mean follow-up 19 months). (The results of interval surgery did not, however, appear to be compromised by the prior use of ciclosporin.) In an admittedly much smaller American survey, all of the patients required colectomy within a year![152]

The St Mark's data correspond closely to those from Oxford, and I suspect that this may reflect selection criteria as our patients and those in Oxford have to 'earn' their ciclosporin by failing intensive conventional therapy over (normally) 3 days (see Chapter 4). If patients are less optimally managed initially, or are started on ciclosporin sooner, then one would expect better responses overall. The current practice at St Mark's mandates an agreement between all parties that ciclosporin is a short-term measure aiming to avoid surgery, but that this pharmacological intervention will not be permitted to delay surgery in the patient who continues to deteriorate or in whom there is no obvious response to medical therapy by a further 5–7 days (10–12 days in total). There is no place for ciclosporin in the management of patients with complications such as megacolon, perforation or major haemorrhage.

Ciclosporin enemas have also been assessed in refractory ulcerative proctitis, and here prove no better than placebo.[153]

Monitoring ciclosporin, toxicity and potential long-term use

To date there are no controlled data to determine whether ciclosporin has a role in maintenance or in the chronically active steroid-dependent patient. Most specialist centres are aiming to avoid such use, preferring to transfer patients who have responded to the drug in fulminant disease onto more established maintenance regimens – particularly azathioprine/6MP.[149]

One Australian centre has, however, explored the use of oral ciclosporin in the management of chronically active ulcerative colitis with moderately good results.[154] Nine of 13 patients (and 6 of 15 with Crohn's colitis) showed a clinical response within 4 weeks. This was maintained after

ciclosporin withdrawal (after mean of 9 months) in only 18 per cent.

Toxicity is relatively frequent even in short-term use and is mainly dose related, there being a narrow therapeutic index. Reversible nephrotoxicity, hyperkalaemia, hyperuricaemia, hepatotoxicity, hypertension and seizures are not unusual despite careful use,[142,154,155] and hypertrichosis, gingival hyperplasia, tremor and paraesthesiae are all common and of great concern to patients. The short-term control documented in six of seven patients in one small open study in Crohn's disease (abstract only) is heavily counterbalanced by the death of one of the six from opportunistic infection.[156] Caution in respect of possible coincidental cytomegalovirus infection is also appropriate.[157] The New York and Chicago groups have the most cumulative data for ciclosporin in inflammatory bowel disease, and the former have reported major toxicity in around half of all patients treated – some recorded only in abstract form.[155,158] There were two deaths – one from septic shock and one from massive duodenal haemorrhage – and seven life-threatening infections. Fits occurred in three patients, attributed in part to low cholesterol levels. No less than 51 per cent had paraesthesiae, 43 per cent had hypertension, and 42 per cent had hypomagnesaemia. Renal impairment occurs in up to 10 per cent of inflammatory bowel disease patients receiving the drug[159] and in fully half of some series.[154] Deaths from opportunistic infection with *Pneumocystis* pneumonia have also been reported in London and Brussels[160,161] and overwhelming sepsis has also been the main indication for surgery.[152] The possible relevance of ciclosporin therapy to a subsequently increased risk of neoplasia is considered in Chapter 8.

It is recommended that ciclosporin is not given if the plasma cholesterol is less than 3 mmol/L as the Cremophor lipid solubilizer present in the infusion is then prone to cause fitting (especially if the plasma magnesium is low or borderline). Many units prescribe prophylaxis for *Pneumocystis* pneumonia whilst the patient is on high-dose steroids and ciclosporin – this is a wise but untested precaution.

Whole blood levels (not plasma) should be adjusted to 100–150 ng/mL in chronic low-dose oral therapy and definitely to no more than 200–300 ng/mL in high-dose intravenous therapy, as measured by high-performance liquid chromatography, or monoclonal antibody radioimmunoassay. The intestinal absorption of the drug is affected by active intestinal disease and short bowel (and by cholestasis), and dietary factors such as grapefruit juice (but not other fruit juices) can significantly affect blood levels.[162] This may account in part for the poor results in most studies of Crohn's disease if insufficient active agent has been available.

Given at least four fatalities from ciclosporin immunosuppression-related opportunistic infection, options for improving the safety profile of ciclosporin have been examined. There are uncontrolled Italian data suggesting that a 2 mg/kg regimen might be effective and Belgian data in favour of ciclosporin monotherapy, thereby avoiding the additive risks of ciclosporin and high-dose steroids. A controlled trial is now in place comparing 2 mg/kg with 4 mg/kg and the first interim analysis is encouraging.[163] We should certainly not be killing patients in a well-intentioned attempt to save colons.

METHOTREXATE

Methotrexate is a dihydrofolate reductase inhibitor that interferes with normal DNA synthesis. It has immunosuppressive and anti-inflammatory properties, and has accordingly been widely used in conditions such as psoriasis and rheumatoid arthritis, as well as in oncological practice. Because it is abortifacient and toxic to the skin, it requires careful handling, with many UK pharmacies preferring to issue parenteral supplies in prepared syringes to special order.

Methotrexate in active Crohn's disease

In 1989 Kozarek *et al.*[164] reported the results of an open trial of 12 weeks of methotrexate in patients with refractory Crohn's disease (*n* = 14) and ulcerative colitis (*n* = 7). There was an apparent short-term response in the majority of both groups of patients, allowing significant reduction in steroid dosage, which was then sustained by maintenance therapy in two-thirds of the responders to 72 weeks. Modigliani's group have been using methotrexate for longer than most, and continue to provide clinical data on its (uncontrolled) use in patients resistant to other forms of therapy.[165] A 72 per cent success rate is claimed at 3 months but this falls to 42 per cent at 12 months. Previous failure to respond to azathioprine/6MP does not seem to preclude response to methotrexate. Their protocol gives 25 mg intramuscularly each week for 3 months (a relatively high dose for use other than in neoplasia therapy), and then switches to oral administration, reducing gradually to a minimum dose of 7.5 mg weekly. They report a continuing low incidence of important toxicity in these and in 31 patients with Crohn's disease continuing the drug on an uncontrolled basis for longer periods (at least 7 months, median 19 months), only 16 per cent of whom had to discontinue the drug.[166]

A controlled trial from North America subsequently reported on 141 patients with active Crohn's disease, all of whom were brought to a common daily dosage of 20 mg prednisolone, either by weaning down to this dose or by increasing a lower maintenance dose.[167] A steroid-weaning protocol was then followed for the study period. Half were randomized to receive intramuscular methotrexate 25 mg each week for 16 weeks. The end points comprised Crohn's activity and degree of weaning from steroids. Remission was achieved in 39.4 per cent of those given methotrexate compared with only 19.1 per cent in those given placebo (RR: 2.1; CI: 1.1–3.5), and with significantly greater reduction in final prednisolone dose. The relatively poor results are probably accounted for by the prior severity of disease (all patients requiring prednisolone at a dose of at least 10 mg/day). Methotrexate was not associated with substantial toxicity in this relatively short-term study, although there was a deterioration in liver function parameters in 7 per cent, and nausea led to withdrawal from the drug in 6 per cent (total withdrawals 17 versus 2 per cent in the placebo arm).

As the optimal dose and route of methotrexate are not known, a 16-week randomized, single-blind comparison of subcutaneous methotrexate, 15 or 25 mg/week, was performed in 32 steroid-dependent patients (with Crohn's disease or ulcerative colitis).[168] Patients who did not respond to 15 mg/week were studied for an additional 16 weeks on 25 mg. Marginally (and not statistically) more patients responded to the lower dose in each group by 16 weeks (39 versus 33 per cent). Methotrexate blood levels predicted neither efficacy nor toxicity.

Methotrexate in maintenance of remission in Crohn's disease

A remission phase continuation of the North American treatment study engaged 23 of the same group of patients and an additional 53 from open-label usage. Once in remission, they entered a double-blind, placebo-controlled trial, using 15 mg/week also given intramuscularly.[169] By 40 weeks, twice as many in the placebo group had relapsed (CDAI increase of > 100 and/or need for new therapy) (71 versus 35 per cent relapse rate; P = 0.015). All of the secondary end points (steroid use, mean CDAI, IBDQ, adverse events) were also in favour of the treatment arm. Most of the relapses occurred within 8 weeks of commencing placebo and about half of those re-treated again responded. There were no important

adverse events in the actively treated patients. Methotrexate is known to be absorbed proximally and comprehensively in other conditions and there is debate but remarkably few data in respect of its possible oral use in Crohn's disease.[170] The impression at St Mark's is that oral therapy is effective in a majority of those who respond to intramuscular treatments and (given what may be a considerable logistic exercise to do with parenteral supplies) that this is a reasonable starting point, but with a switch to parenteral therapy if there is no response within 4 weeks.

Methotrexate in ulcerative colitis

Methotrexate has been less encouraging in ulcerative colitis than predicted from the early data from the Canadian and French groups. A careful double-blind trial from Israel (n = 67) demonstrated that a weekly oral dose of 12.5 mg in steroid-resistant/dependent patients had no therapeutic effect over a 9-month study period.[171] It might be argued that the dose was inadequate, but it is most unlikely that malabsorption was the reason in colitic patients. Poor results were also seen in a study in which 15 mg orally was given in addition to prednisolone.[170] There is therefore no current justification for the use of this drug in ulcerative colitis.

Safety of methotrexate in inflammatory bowel disease

The traditional advice that a liver biopsy should be performed before methotrexate therapy is not warranted in inflammatory bowel disease patients with normal liver function, but regular estimation of hepatic biochemistry and coagulation status while on the drug is probably wise, with consideration given to liver biopsy once a total dose of 2 g has been given.[172] With the regimens currently being promoted this is not likely to occur much before 4 years of therapy (the Lémann regimen rarely leads to more than 750 mg being given even in the first year). There is no confirmation that supplementation with folic acid is necessary, nor conviction that it might not reduce the potential therapeutic effect. The positions with regard to pregnancy and possible risk of malignancy are considered in Chapters 5 and 8.

OTHER IMMUNOSUPPRESSANTS

Tacrolimus

Tacrolimus (previously FK-506) is a macrolide with potent immunosuppressive activity. It has similar mechanisms of action to cyclosporin and has gained a major role in organ transplantation. Extrapolation from its use in patients undergoing small bowel transplant suggests that it may have a role in inflammatory bowel disease, and preliminary results suggested some benefit in chronic Crohn's fistulae and pyoderma gangrenosum.[173]

The Mayo Clinic have published their experience of combination treatment with tacrolimus and either azathioprine or 6MP in 11 patients with Crohn's-related perianal fistulae treated for a mean duration of 22 weeks.[174] The initial oral dose of tacrolimus ranged from 0.15 to 0.31 mg/kg/day. All 11 patients improved, and seven had a complete response. The mean time to improvement was 2.4 weeks, and to complete response 12.2 weeks. Adverse events included nausea, paraesthesiae, nephrotoxicity and tremor. Higher initial doses appeared to increase the risk of nephrotoxicity without improving clinical response.

There are further preliminary, uncontrolled abstract data in favour of tacrolimus 0.1–0.2 mg/kg/day in steroid-dependent Crohn's disease,[175] and for intravenous use (0.01–0.02 mg/kg/day switching to oral at 7 days) in a group of 31 inflammatory bowel disease patients, most of whom had ulcerative colitis.[176]

Mycophenolate

Mycophenolate mofetil is a lymphocyte proliferation inhibitor that reduces IFN-γ but not TNF-α.

It is effective as a transplant immunosuppressive and has been thought of value in rheumatoid arthritis, pemphigus and psoriasis. There was a positive report from a very small, open study in recalcitrant Crohn's disease,[177] and in a controlled but unblinded trial of 70 steroid-dependent Crohn's patients it yielded a comparable and perhaps favourable outcome in comparison to azathioprine.[178] There was little toxicity.

There are other supportive abstracts, but the positive effects may be short-lived[179] or absent,[180] and toxicity may include an epithelial-stripping colitis and lower gastrointestinal bleeding.[180] Whatever its scientific merits, it appears that the pharmaceutical company responsible for the drug has decided that it is not commercially viable, as it has unilaterally curtailed a multicentre trial that had the capacity to determine the truth of these issues.

Transplantation

Intestinal transplantation for short bowel syndrome is mentioned in Chapter 7, but forms of marrow and stem cell transplantation to tackle the immune defect underlying Crohn's disease may also be pertinent. Six patients with Crohn's disease (three of whom also had sclerosing cholangitis) who underwent bone marrow transplantation for coincidental leukaemia were reviewed in Seattle. There was one early septic death but the other five were followed for 4.5–15.3 years (median 8.4) and four of the five remained in complete remission as regards their Crohn's.[181] There are other supportive single case reports,[182,183] including one who had confirmed normal endoscopic appearances on no therapy 58 months after transplant.[183] It is considered too controversial to embark on allogeneic transplantation for Crohn's disease itself at present, but there is interest in stem cell transplantation for a variety of other benign immunological disorders, and good results may well move the gastroenterology community in this direction.

Antibiotics in Crohn's disease and ulcerative colitis

Antibiotics have a clear role in the management of certain of the complications of inflammatory bowel disease but their role in primary therapy is less certain. A number of broad-spectrum antibiotics have been evaluated in both ulcerative colitis and Crohn's disease. There is some evidence (mostly from small, uncontrolled studies) demonstrating efficacy for various agents, and rather better evidence for the use of metronidazole and ciprofloxacin.

METRONIDAZOLE

Metronidazole is licensed as an antimicrobial with action against anaerobes and protozoa but it is probable that it also has independent anti-inflammatory actions. It is frequently used for management of perianal Crohn's disease given an expected benefit in two-thirds of recipients.[184] An earlier study in the UK was less enthusiastic; despite doubling the response rate at 2 weeks compared with placebo (from 35 to 67 per cent or 71 per cent depending on whether co-trimoxazole was also used), this effect was not sustained to 4 weeks.[185] Lasting benefit is probably achieved in fewer than one-third of patients.[186]

Aside from its probable role in perianal Crohn's, limited but significant benefit accrued from metronidazole given for a month or more at a dose of 10 or 20 mg/kg for active ileocolonic Crohn's disease (but not in disease affecting the small bowel alone).[3] Nearly half the patients left the study prematurely, 16 per cent because of side effects. There was a numerical advantage in reduction of CDAI to the higher dose.

Finally, in a controlled trial of 60 patients undergoing terminal ileal resection given a 3-month course of metronidazole (20 mg/kg) or placebo starting within 1 week of surgery, there was a statistically significant reduction in clinically apparent postoperative recurrence at 1 year (4 versus 25 per cent), but this was not maintained to 2 or 3 years.[187] Toxicity, particularly peripheral neuropathy, also remains a concern. In one study employing nerve conduction studies, 85 per cent of treated patients had abnormalities, 46 per cent were symptomatic, and in 11 per cent the neuropathy was not reversible on discontinuing the drug.[188]

CIPROFLOXACIN

Ciprofloxacin (500 mg b.i.d. or 2 g b.i.d., for 6 weeks) has been compared to Pentasa® in active Crohn's disease.[189] The study was small and incompletely blinded. There was a relatively high drop-out rate, mostly for disease progression rather than for side effects; remission was achieved in 56 per cent with ciprofloxacin and 55 per cent with the mesalazine. A 6-month double-blind, placebo-controlled trial of ciprofloxacin in 83 patients with moderate-to-severe ulcerative colitis, given in addition to conventional therapy, demonstrated a reduction in treatment failures from 44 per cent in the placebo group to 21 per cent in the ciprofloxacin group ($P = 0.02$).[190] There was also an associated reduction in the need for colectomy. Data from a blinded placebo-controlled trial performed in fulminant colitis, however, showed no difference in response rate or need for surgery with ciprofloxacin 250 mg orally twice daily.[191] An effect may have been masked by concurrent high-dose steroids or overlooked because the antibiotic regimen itself was inadequate (dose and/or route). There is as yet no mandate for routine use of antibiotics in ulcerative colitis, whether fulminant or not.

OTHER ANTIMICROBIAL AGENTS IN ULCERATIVE COLITIS

Burke *et al.*[192] reported long-term symptomatic and histological improvement in patients with refractory extensive colitis treated with a 1-week course of oral tobramycin. Some 90 per cent of their patients were able to discontinue steroids, but relatively few subsequent trials have proved supportive. Amongst those that have, Malagelada's group have explored the use of co-amoxiclav in a Eudragit-coated delayed-release form.[193] When 3 g/750 mg was given daily to acute colitics, potentially beneficial changes were demonstrable in the cytokine content of rectal dialysates, together with suggestive clinical differences of a magnitude to warrant formal clinical trial.

Concurrent cytomegalovirus infection may be a cause for the apparent intractability of ulcerative colitis; useful responses to antiviral therapy can be expected.[194] A similar circumstance may arise with pouchitis.[195]

ANTITUBERCULOUS THERAPY AND OTHER ANTIBIOTICS IN CROHN'S DISEASE

One early study[196] using a variety of broad-spectrum antibiotics given continuously for 6 months indicated symptomatic improvement in 93 per cent of patients with Crohn's disease. Radiological improvement was seen in 57 per cent, and 40 per cent were able to discontinue steroids; it is unlikely that these impressive results were the direct consequence of antibiotics alone, given the inability of others to replicate this success.

Various antimycobacterial regimens have been evaluated in the treatment of Crohn's disease (in part to test the hypothesis that *Mycobacterium paratuberculosis* is of aetiological relevance)[197] (see Chapter 1). Although debate continues as to whether the result of inappropriate regimens or inappropriate logic, the early published results were disappointing. *M. paratuberculosis* has much in common with the relatively non-aggressive opportunistic mycobacteria, and the therapeutic regimens developed for AIDS patients have now accordingly been applied in Crohn's disease. *In*

vitro data support a combination of rifabutin with streptomycin, and an oddly constructed double-blind trial of 51 patients studied over 2 years (with 16 weeks of almost daily streptomycin injections) demonstrated improvements in those receiving streptomycin and rifabutin compared with those receiving streptomycin alone.[198] Remarkably, only 27 per cent of the patients failed to complete the study. The magnitude of the apparent benefit from the two antibiotic regimens is difficult to judge as conventional therapies were continued and the overall response rates are within the range typical for Crohn's disease treated more conventionally. Despite an abstract in 1996 and the considerable interest in the topic, this has still not been fully published.

The combination of rifabutin and ethambutol was ineffective in an open study in Belgium in which most patients had 12 months of therapy and all had 6 months.[199] No pharmacologically 'clean' study yet demonstrates significant benefit. Trials using newer drugs and regimens continue, including an open study of rifabutin (300 mg or 450 mg daily), clofazimine (2 mg/kg) and clarithromycin (250 mg t.i.d.) in 20 patients with resistant disease. Twelve patients responded clinically to 6 months of therapy.[200] Workers at St George's Hospital in London have been enthusiasts for the mycobacterial hypothesis and have reported on 52 of their patients, 19 of whom were initially on steroids.[201] Unfortunately, the study is entirely uncontrolled and patients received several different regimens (rifabutin in combination with clarithromycin or azithromycin, treated for a wide range of different intervals: 6–35 months). Six were intolerant of the medication and had to be excluded. Clinical and inflammatory parameters improved over 2 years of follow-up, but it is very difficult to know whether this represents a difference from what might be expected with placebo. It is also worth remembering that tacrolimus (see above) is a macrolide, and that any gain from use of clarithromycin and similar drugs may be an immunomodulatory effect rather than an antimicrobial one.

Probiotics and prebiotics

There is a great deal of interest, not least from patients, in the possibility that knowledge of the importance of the gut flora in inflammatory bowel disease as demonstrated in cell culture and animal models (see Chapter 1) might lead to therapeutic advances. There are two main strategies: the use of probiotics – live organisms chosen to repopulate the intestinal lumen with a more favourable flora; and the use of prebiotics – the supply of nutrients for the microflora to encourage a more favourable milieu by nutrient selection.[202] There has been much written, not least in favour of oral administration of helminth eggs, but little in the way of scientifically verifiable data.

Five main groups of organisms have been considered for use as probiotics:

- *Lactobacillus*, including GG (*rhamnosis* and *casei*), *salivarius* and *acidophilus*;
- *Bifidobacterium*, especially *bifidum*;
- *Streptococcus thermophilus*;
- *E. coli* species, especially Nissle 1917;
- *Saccharomyces boulardii*.

There are some human data for all. Their characteristics vary somewhat as (for example) lactobacilli survive well in the gut and have an immune-modulating effect but little effect as antimicrobials, whereas bifidobacteria are better at bacterial killing but less influential on the immune response. The postulated mechanisms include competitive exclusion of luminal-aggravating factors including enhancement of mucosal barrier integrity, and improvement in mucins, stimulation of the immune system enhancing the Th2 response, and an antimicrobial effect, which includes effects on luminal pH and peroxide levels, as well as a direct bactericidal effect. The rationale for human use is supported by data showing (*inter alia*) reduced levels of bifidobacteria[203] and bifidobacteria and lactobacilli[204] in Crohn's disease, and a number of other abnormalities in ulcerative colitis.

PROBIOTICS IN INFLAMMATORY BOWEL DISEASE THERAPY

Single agents

A total of 120 patients with inactive ulcerative colitis were included in a double-blind, double-dummy study comparing mesalazine 1500 mg daily with an oral preparation of viable, non-pathogenic *E. coli* strain Nissle 1917 (Serotype O6: K5: H1) for 12 weeks.[205] Relapse rates were 11.3 per cent with mesalazine and 16.0 per cent with *E. coli* Nissle 1917, and there were no other apparent outcome differences. The probiotic regimen was well tolerated and no serious adverse events were reported.

The same agent was used in a controlled trial comparison with mesalazine in 120 patients with active ulcerative colitis who were followed into remission.[206] The study is arguably confounded by the preliminary use of oral gentamicin in all subjects for 1 week. Seventy-five per cent of patients in the mesalazine group attained remission compared with 68 per cent in the *E. coli* group (NS). A disappointing 67 per cent of *E. coli*-treated patients relapsed within a year, but there was also a startlingly high relapse rate in the mesalazine-treated arm (73 per cent at 12 months), which renders the study unrepresentative and difficult to place within the generality of ulcerative colitis studies.

Saccharomyces boulardii 1 g together with mesalazine 2 g was compared to mesalazine 3 g daily for 6 months in patients with Crohn's disease in remission.[207] Relapse occurred significantly less often (1/16 versus 6/16; $P = 0.04$) in the probiotic group, but this was a small open study and confused by the similar but not identical mesalazine doses.

Multiple agents

Daily administration of 100 mL of a yoghurt-type ferment was assessed in an open controlled trial of 21 subjects with active ulcerative colitis treated otherwise in conventional fashion.[208] Relevant bifidobacteria were recoverable from stools of treated patients. At 1 year there were cumulatively fewer relapse episodes in treated patients, but this does not reach statistical significance and can be considered only interesting preliminary data.

Campieri and his group have pioneered work with a mixture of potentially pertinent bacteria (three strains of bifidobacteria, four strains of lactobacilli and one strain of *Streptococcus salivarius thermophilus*) termed VSL#3. In preliminary work 20 patients with ulcerative colitis in remission but intolerant of 5-ASA drugs received 3 g of this cocktail twice daily for 12 months.[209] Stool cultures changed in line with expectations for effective colonization and 75 per cent remained in remission.

Their further work has included postoperative Crohn's disease patients[210] in a non-blinded study in which 40 patients received either the non-absorbed antibiotic rifaximin 1.8 g/day for 3 months and then VSL#3 for 9 months, or mesalazine 4 g/day for the full 12 months. There were better numerical results in the antibiotic/probiotic group.

PREBIOTICS

Probiotic therapy is probably safe most of the time but is not without risk. At least one liver abscess has been described with *E. coli* Nissle, and there are several examples of fungaemia with *Saccharomyces* species.[211] This has been a further stimulus to see if similar amendments in gut flora can be achieved with a range of oligosaccharides used as prebiotics as fermentable dietary fibre, i.e. source of short-chain fatty acids (especially butyrate and acetate).

In a randomized, but open, clinical trial of *Plantago ovata* seeds 20 g (dietary fibre) as compared with mesalazine 1.5 g in maintaining remission in 102 patients with ulcerative colitis, the relapse rate at 12 months (40 per cent) was comparable to that with mesalazine 1.5 g daily (35 per cent) and numerically superior if both were given (30 per cent).[212] More work appears to be warranted.

A small volunteer study indicates that lactulose 10 g daily for 6 weeks leads predictably to an increase in faecal bifidobacterial counts, and a substantial increase in the ratio of bifidobacteria to anaerobes (from 4 to 50).[213] There were (somewhat surprisingly) no changes in faecal pH and, at this dose, little change in bowel function. Whether this can explain the benefit seen in some patients with constipation proximal to distal colitis remains to be seen.

Nutritional therapy in inflammatory bowel disease

A detailed account of nutrition in inflammatory bowel disease is beyond the scope of this volume, but some discussion of its therapeutic role is important. Nutritional intervention is crucial in malnourished patients, and most of all in children, in whom permanent growth retardation will result if it is neglected (see also Chapter 5). The patient with Crohn's of the small bowel is particularly at risk. This use of nutritional measures should be distinguished from primary nutritional therapy, in which a nutritional regimen is used as the therapy (as opposed to providing nutritional support or treating malnutrition) (see also the section on short bowel syndrome and intestinal failure in Chapter 7).

ULCERATIVE COLITIS

Colitic patients tend to eat more protein and carbohydrate than controls[214] and some 64 per cent may have food intolerances (compared with 14 per cent of controls using the same criteria).[215] 'Normalization' of the diet might appear worth testing, and modification of the colonic bacterial flora can certainly be achieved by dietary manipulation (see above). It is difficult to give advice that will be of general value, but it is worth recognizing this influence, and encouraging patients to make their own manipulations. Reduction in consumption of milk products is more likely to be helpful than most other well-defined changes,[216] and supplementation of the diet with omega-3 fatty acids[217] or a malted dietary source of antisecretory factor[218] have provisional data in their favour. Many patients find that dietary modification has a major impact on their symptoms, but primary nutritional therapy has not yet been shown to have a major place in ulcerative colitis.

CROHN'S DISEASE

There is, on the contrary, an expanding literature indicating a role for dietary therapy in selected patients with Crohn's disease. Patients with Crohn's are generally found to eat more carbohydrate, especially in the form of sugar,[214,219] but there is no evidence that sugar restriction is therapeutically valuable.[219] Food intolerance is present in around two-thirds of patients[215] with a wide range of suspect foods, including wheat and dairy products, but this does not constitute true food sensitivity as it can rarely be confirmed on blinded testing.[220]

NUTRITIONAL THERAPY FOR ACTIVE CROHN'S DISEASE

Exclusive parenteral nutrition encompassing 'bowel rest' yielded a 65–95 per cent response rate in patients with refractory Crohn's disease. However, it has subsequently been realized that elemental, 'pre-digested', and polymeric liquid formula diets can have similar efficacy to exclusive parenteral feeding in inducing remission.[219,221] It remains unclear whether nutritional repletion, relative bowel rest, or other factors explain these improvements.

Much of the supportive literature for nutritional therapy comes from a small number of enthusiastic centres (reviewers including Silk,[222] O'Morain[223] and Giaffer[224]), and analysis of results by strict 'intention to treat' has not always been volunteered. One is compelled to estimate a likely placebo response, as there are no placebo-controlled trials, so the 30 per cent or so of Crohn's patients who will go into remission without specific intervention in most therapeutic settings should be kept in mind. In the 10-year retrospective Northwick Park study published in 1990, nutritional therapy appeared to offer clear advantage, with remission being achieved in 96 of 113 acute Crohn's episodes (in patients with no previous surgery).[225] Only 22 per cent relapsed within 6 months, as did a further 9 per cent per year thereafter.

Controlled (though inevitably unblinded) comparisons of nutritional therapy with steroid therapy permit a more objective view. O'Morain's landmark paper of 1984 found no difference between the two therapies in 21 Crohn's patients.[226] The same conclusion is reached by most of the other studies.[227–233] Only the 4th European Crohn's Study,[234] which included 55 patients, found a significant difference, and this was in favour of prednisolone.

If nutrition and steroids are truly therapeutically equivalent, it would be appropriate always to choose the former on safety grounds. It is therefore especially pertinent to examine the relative ease of use and the degree of compliance in routine use of these two options. The high drop-out rate for continuing enteral nutritional therapy, whether given orally or by overnight nasogastric intubation, is therefore an important factor. As examples from two nutritionally orientated centres, we find failure to complete maintenance studies in 33 per cent and 55 per cent of patients even though the 42 and 78 patients respectively recruited had personal experience of the benefits of exclusive elemental feeding, having obtained their initial remissions in this way.[220,235] It is also striking that, despite the authors' enthusiasm for primary nutritional therapy, in the East Anglian study of 228 eligible subjects only 136 were recruited (with a 57 per cent response rate).[235] The key to this issue thus lies in comparisons by intention to treat.

Griffiths et al.[221] have performed a meta-analysis which included eight randomized controlled trials of steroids versus nutritional therapy ($n = 413$) and identified clinical remissions in 80.5 per cent of those receiving steroids compared with 56.8 per cent of those on nutritional therapy (OR: 0.35; CI: 0.23–0.53). If remission was achieved, the relapse rate at 12 months was the same for both therapies (65 per cent and 67 per cent). This does, nevertheless, clearly support the view that nutritional therapy is more effective than placebo. The literature suggests that those with colonic Crohn's are less likely to respond than those with predominantly ileal involvement, but there is little clarity in respect of the patient with extensive and proximal small bowel disease – who is equally in most need of non-surgical options if resection leading to short bowel syndrome is to be avoided. Sadly, those with the most proximal disease are also those least likely to tolerate enteral regimens for the necessary time.[236]

It is possible that different nutritional regimens have different chances of inducing remission, and the data have accordingly been assessed according to the nature of the nutritional regimen. Elemental nutrition does not appear to offer an advantage over semi-elemental or polymeric feeds; there is, in fact, a non-significant trend in the opposite direction, an OR of 0.87 favouring non-elemental feeds (which may reflect better tolerability and better compliance). More recent studies have addressed this directly.

It has been thought that the lipid content of feeds might explain the differences (why, for example, there should be a discrepancy between the two elemental formulations most tested). Some surprising results have emerged and the full papers are awaited with interest. In the UK, a double-blind comparison of high and low concentrations of long-chain triglycerides has been performed in active Crohn's disease.[237] The polymeric feeds were whole protein and with equal total fat content, and were given exclusively for 3 weeks. The remission rates for both feeds were low but proved numerically better in the patients given more long-chain triglycerides (33 versus 25 per cent; $P = 0.8$; 68 versus 65 per cent by treatment given). A double-blind multicentre European trial compared two forms of exclusive polymeric enteral nutrition with prednisolone 1 mg/kg/day in active Crohn's disease.[238] Both feeds provided 35 g fat per 1000 kcal, which in one was 80 per cent as oleate, whereas the other was based on linoleate (50 per cent). The remission rate for prednisolone was 79 per cent, and 63 per cent for the linoleate feed, but a strikingly poor 27 per cent for the oleate-based feed; the lipid formula is evidently important. Also (unusually) there were better results in those with colonic disease. Short-chain fatty acids are considered below.

The hypotheses in respect of sensitivity to titanium and other metals (see Chapter 1) are now being tested by specific diets designed to be low in microparticles. Only provisional data so far exist but these are positive.[239]

NUTRITIONAL THERAPY FOR MAINTENANCE OF REMISSION IN CROHN'S DISEASE

The greater commitment required of the patient for nutritional therapy coupled with a tendency for a slower induction of remission, lead most gastroenterologists to continue to favour systemic steroids as first-line treatment for acute relapses of Crohn's in the adult. There should be no doubt, however, that they can be effective in some patients who have failed on steroids, in those in whom steroids are strongly contraindicated, and when steroids are refused by the patient. Whether there is a place for exclusion diets, with systematic slow reintroduction of foods once remission has been achieved – advocated as effective in maintenance of remission in inflammatory bowel disease[240] – remains ill-defined; these diets are difficult to implement even in patients brought to remission by nutritional therapy. Although food sensitivities remain evident after nutritional treatment of Crohn's disease, they are very variable, are often transient, and are ultimately of insufficient importance to warrant putting patients through the rigours of an elimination diet.[220]

There is evidence that continued use of supplementary defined liquid enteral nutrition may help to maintain remission in Crohn's disease.[241] This was an uncontrolled paediatric study, and has been followed by a year-long comparative study in 35 adults.[242] One group continued a normal unrestricted diet whilst the treatment group were expected to take additional elemental feed (Elemental 028 Extra®) to provide at least 35 per cent of usual energy intake. There was a significantly greater proportion still in remission at 12 months in the treatment group (48 versus 22 per cent by intention to treat; 60 per cent by treatment taken; $P < 0.05$). These are observations of real practical value, since it has been difficult to give meaningful advice on whether nutritional therapy should be continued once remission is achieved, given that the patient will then wish to recommence eating, coupled with our knowledge from the East Anglian study that continued food avoidance is not a long-term answer. Dietary supplements may be considered legitimate if not mandatory, and should certainly be encouraged in the patient who is still malnourished.

Fish oils, fatty acids and eicosanoids

Prior to the European nutritional study described above,[238] it had been thought that avoidance of linoleate was crucial to the therapeutic response.[243] This seemed logical as linoleic acid is a key precursor of arachidonic acid and thus of inflammatory eicosanoids such as leukotriene B4 (LTB4), thromboxane A2 and prostaglandin E2. Other dietary methods of reducing eicosanoid synthesis have also been considered in both Crohn's disease and ulcerative colitis. Fish oils, which contain large amounts of eicosapentanoic acid, divert eicosanoid metabolism towards B5 and prostaglandin E3, which are much less inflammatory than B4 and prostaglandin E2.[244] It is possible that useful inhibition of cytokines can also be achieved, and inhibition of platelet aggregation promoted. It may be noted that several of the more standard therapeutic manoeuvres (5-ASA, azathioprine, cyclosporin) have significant, normalizing influences on the eicosanoid content of colonic mucosa.[245]

FISH OIL THERAPY

In a multicentre, double-blind, crossover trial of eicosapentanoic acid in active ulcerative colitis, there was a significant reduction in rectal dialysate leukotriene B4 levels, associated with clinical and histological improvement during the treatment period.[246] The Nottingham group also showed modest benefit from fish oil supplementation in active colitis but no advantage in maintenance.[247]

The Italian study of fish oil therapy was a more substantial two-centre Italian evaluation of a lipid concentrate in Crohn's disease maintenance.[248]

The active preparation included 1.8 g 40 per cent eicosapentanoic acid, and 0.9 g 20 per cent docosahexanoic acid, each day for 12 months, in comparison with a mixed-acid triglyceride of fractionated fatty acids (60 per cent caprylic, 40 per cent capric acid). Compliance was surprisingly good with only 4 of 39 patients ceasing active therapy because of side effects (diarrhoea). At 1 year, and by intention to treat, 59 per cent of the treated group remained in remission compared with only 26 per cent of the control group ($P = 0.003$). Multivariate analysis indicated that the results could reasonably be attributed only to the specific therapeutic intervention. This response is equivalent to that predicted for 5-ASA regimens and now deserves comparative study.

SHORT-CHAIN FATTY ACID THERAPY

Short-chain fatty acids are released from dietary fats by anaerobic bacteria and (particularly in the case of butyrate) are physiologically important colonocyte nutrients.[249] Good evidence now exists that their absence in the defunctioned colon is an important factor in the development of diversion colitis (see Chapters 1 and 4), supported by a rapid response of some affected patients to short-chain fatty acid enemas.[250,251]

Short-chain fatty acids are also depleted in ulcerative colitis, attributed (at least in part) to the effects of functionally abnormal anaerobic bacteria producing excess sulphur mercaptides[252] (see Chapter 1), and have accordingly been used therapeutically in enema form. In a randomized trial in patients with acute distal colitis Senagore et al.[253] demonstrated a remission rate equivalent to that for topical steroids or mesalazine, with an overall 80 per cent response rate. Topical butyrate (80 mL of 80 mmol/L twice daily) in combination with topical 5-ASA (4 g) was also more effective in refractory distal colitis than 5-ASA alone (25 versus 4 per cent response).[254]

The attraction of using a natural agent with assumed low toxicity is offset by the current lack of availability of fatty acid preparations, the pharmaceutical difficulties resulting from their volatility, and their unpleasant smell. In the face of these difficulties and two similar trials with less promising results,[255,256] this is not a strategy that is currently recommended at St Mark's. Whether the apparent effect of short-chain fatty acids in reducing the degree of proliferation in colitic rectal mucosa[257] has any bearing on risk of neoplasia such as to suggest a prophylactic therapeutic role remains to be seen.

Similar mechanisms to those of the free fatty acids may also underlie the effect of topical arsenicals in the form of acetarsol – an agent of proven equivalence to topical steroids.[258] There is an appropriately high degree of caution in utilizing an arsenic-containing agent, but the short- and medium-term risks are low.[259] Uncertainty remains in respect of the long-term cancer risk, and the drug, which is not generally available, cannot be recommended.

LEUKOTRIENES

Leukotriene B4 (generated by the action of 5-lipoxygenase on arachidonic acid) has been shown to play a central role in the inflammatory cascade in inflammatory bowel disease, with elevated levels detected in the colonic mucosa of patients with active ulcerative colitis, but not in steroid-treated, quiescent disease.[260,261] Several 5-lipoxygenase inhibitors now exist including zileuton (A-64077), which inhibits 5-lipoxygenase without an effect on cyclo-oxygenase or phospholipase A, but with inhibition of LTB4 production from neutrophils. Early results from zileuton suggested promise[262] comparable to the good results being recorded in respiratory disorders. Unfortunately, an 8-week randomized, double-blind, controlled trial showed poorer results than placebo in ulcerative colitis and remains unpublished.[263] In maintenance of remission, zileuton is no better than placebo.[264]

It is unlikely that this will be further developed for therapeutic use.

A LT receptor antagonist appears effective in a rabbit immune colitis model, but human studies are still in their earliest stages.[197] Verapamil, a calcium channel blocker, has been shown to reduce LTB4 release and accelerate healing in experimental colitis in the rat. This is probably because 5-lipoxygenase is calcium dependent; the use of calcium channel blockers warrants study in man.[265]

PROSTAGLANDINS

Prostaglandins have a protective role in the normal gastrointestinal tract, contributing to microvascular integrity and mucus production. Their inhibition is linked to the general tendency of non-steroidal anti-inflammatory agents to worsen inflammatory bowel disease, and there are good laboratory data to indicate that prostaglandin analogues can actively suppress cytokine-mediated inflammation.[266] It would seem logical to explore their therapeutic use. Unfortunately, misoprostol (one such agent) causes secretory diarrhoea in some patients, and has the potential to exacerbate proctitis.[267] The undoubted efficacy of the 5-ASA drugs (which are, after all, a form of non-steroidal) contributes further paradox in this regard.

Thromboxane synthesis inhibitors and antagonists

Thromboxanes are produced in excess in both ulcerative colitis and Crohn's disease.[268–270] They are produced by activated neutrophils, mononuclear cells and platelets. Increased mucosal permeability may be the trigger to their release, through allowing entry of bacterial antigens (such as lipopolysaccharides) which induce neutrophil activation. Ridogrel and picotamide both inhibit thromboxane A2 synthesis and competitively block its receptors; ridogrel also blocks receptors for prostaglandin endoperoxide at higher dose. They were thought to have a potential role in inflammatory bowel disease, given the demonstration of reduction of thromboxane A2 and concomitant increase in thromboxane B2 in incubated biopsy material from patients with both ulcerative colitis and Crohn's disease.[270] Picotamide also has important effects on platelet function and a fibrinolytic effect, and both agents stimulate production of prostacyclin. They were effective in experimental models of colitis, but despite encouraging preliminary human studies,[271] the outcomes were not sufficiently convincing to sustain commercial interest and support.

Cytokine manipulation

Inhibition of TNF-α has dominated the cytokine arena for the past few years, and rightly so, but there are other manipulations of cytokines that might also usefully be considered.

INTERLEUKIN-10

The putatively inadequate IL-10 response in inflammatory bowel disease (see Chapter 1) has led to hope that supplementary, therapeutic IL-10 might be beneficial. Initial promise from an open study of topical IL-10 therapy in resistant distal colitis[272] has prompted further trials both in ulcerative colitis and Crohn's.

An extended, placebo-controlled phase II study has now been completed in 45 patients with steroid-resistant Crohn's disease.[273] IL-10 was given daily for 7 days and the patients were followed for 4 weeks. Tolerance was good and, combining the different doses used, there was an overall clinical response at 3 weeks in 50 per cent, compared to 23 per cent in the placebo group. Larger and more definitive trials in milder chronic

Crohn's disease have been completed and indicate advantage over placebo.[274] There is a bell-shaped dose–response curve, doses above 5–8 µg/kg being less effective (probably because of induction of TNF-α by these higher doses).

INTERLEUKINS 2, 11 AND 12

Blockade of the IL-2 receptor with daclizumab, which is an IgG1 antibody, appears useful in prevention of renal transplant rejection,[275] and it is possible that it might be useful in Crohn's disease.

Although closely related to IL-6, IL-11 is probably cytoprotective, and has been shown to down-regulate TNF-α and IL-1β production by macrophages. A small dose-ranging, placebo-controlled trial in Crohn's disease suggests benefit at a dose of 16 µg/kg five times weekly by subcutaneous injection.[276] More definitive trials in comparison to placebo and to systemic steroids are in progress.

IL-12 is overtly inflammatory and is over-expressed in inflammatory bowel disease. An antibody directed against IL-12 is poised for trial evaluation.[277]

INTERFERONS

Interferon-alpha (INF-α) has some anti-inflammatory properties as well as the better known antiviral effects. It has been assessed in a small controlled trial (n = 32) in comparison with prednisolone enemas in ulcerative colitis.[278] Patients received either INF-α-2a subcutaneously (week 1: 9 MIU three times a week; week 2: 6 MIU; week 3–12: 3 MIU) or daily prednisolone enemas 25 mg for 30 days. INF-treated patients showed a clinical response and histological improvement, similar in magnitude to that of the steroid. The study was, however, unblinded and the impact of frequent injections on symptoms is unknown.

A very small pilot study of interferon-gamma (INF-α) has been conducted in active Crohn's disease, and an apparent useful effect on C-reactive protein (CRP) levels was seen, but without sufficient clinical response to warrant further study in the absence of stronger supportive laboratory data for its logical use.[279] Studies with interferon-beta (INF-β) are said to be in progress.

TRANSCRIPTION FACTORS

Antisense oligonucleotides are short sequences of nucleotides designed to be complementary to the messenger RNA of interest (so are effectively little chunks of DNA). They are intended to bind to mRNA within the cell and thereby prevent translation of RNA to protein synthesis. Antisense technology has been explored to inhibit the expression of transcription factors. Nuclear factor kappa B (NFκB) has a key role in the control of expression of a number of pro-inflammatory cytokines. In the case of TNF-α, NFκB appears to have a role in a positive feedback loop. When TNF-α binds to its cell surface receptor, inactive NFκB (IκB) is activated and moves to the nucleus where it then binds to a series of gene promoters, resulting in (*inter alia*) the production of more TNF-α. There are very high levels of NFκB in inflamed tissues from patients with Crohn's disease. Intracolonic administration of an antisense nucleotide to NFκB appears effective in a mouse colitis model,[280] and clinical trials are awaited.

INHIBITION OF TNF-α IN CROHN'S DISEASE

It has seemed logical to tackle TNF-α specifically because of its apparent primacy amongst cytokines, its possible role in the pathogenesis of inflammatory bowel disease and particularly the vigorous Th1 reaction of Crohn's disease.[281–283] Animal models in which the introduction of antibody to TNF-α downregulated Th1 cells and not only prevented colitis, but also ameliorated established disease, set the scene for the development of a series of antibodies suitable for therapeutic use and the dramatic first pilot study in Crohn's disease.[284]

INFLIXIMAB: THE CROHN'S DISEASE TRIALS

The first double-blind, placebo-controlled, dose-ranging trial of infliximab included 108 patients with moderate-to-severe active Crohn's disease (CDAI 220–400).[285] Trial allocation was well balanced in terms of all the usual parameters (except that there were more patients in the placebo group with isolated ileal disease). Patients received a single infusion (0–20 mg/kg) and were followed for 12 weeks. At 4 weeks, clinical responses were recorded in 65 per cent and remission (CDAI < 150) was achieved in 33 per cent of infliximab recipients compared with only 17 per cent and 4 per cent of those on placebo ($P < 0.001$ and $P = 0.005$, respectively). By 12 weeks, the differences were less marked but persistent, with 41 per cent of the infliximab-treated patients showing a (continued) clinical response compared with 12 per cent of the controls ($P = 0.008$). The 5 mg/kg dose appeared most efficacious and there was not a conventional dose–response curve (results for 20 mg/kg approximated to the mean for all three doses with least benefit seen in patients receiving 10 mg/kg). Toxicity was minor and largely of the flu-like nature expected (75 per cent of patients versus 60 per cent of controls). Antibodies to DNA appeared in 3 per cent, and 6 per cent developed antibodies to infliximab, now known as HACA (human anti-chimeric antibodies); neither seems to be of great clinical consequence. This trial had immense influence in accelerating the licensing of the drug in the USA and subsequently in Europe, but it is clear that questions remain, not least in respect of the dose–response characteristics and its duration of action.

Following on from the single infusion study and before its results were known in any generalizable way, another multicentre trial recruited 73 patients who had already selected themselves as responders to infliximab by showing a clinical response (reduction in CDAI of at least 70) to a single infusion.[286] They therefore represent around two-thirds of the 'difficult' Crohn's disease population for whom infliximab will have been considered and this should be borne in mind when response rates in the retreatment study are examined. Recruited patients received a further four infusions of 10 mg/kg or placebo at 8-week intervals (the first of these 12 weeks from the initial response-defining infusion). Serum infliximab levels remained detectable throughout, but there was little immunogenicity. The placebo group had an initially lower CRP and more males but balancing was otherwise good. During the trial period, 33 per cent of the placebo group dropped out because of disease progression/loss of efficacy, compared with only 11 per cent of those receiving infliximab. Two patients developed DNA antibodies, and another developed steroid-responsive lupus. There was one lymphoma at 9.5 months. At 32 weeks, 62 per cent of the treated group were still in remission compared with 37 per cent of those on maintenance placebo ($P = 0.16$). It may be unfortunate that 10 mg/kg was chosen given the subsequent observations from the 'prior' Targan study. In respect of maintenance of full remission, infliximab scored better. Only 38 per cent were in remission (as opposed to being responders) at entry; this figure improved to around 60 per cent for most of the trial period, finishing at 53 per cent at week 32. The controls deteriorated from 44 per cent to 20 per cent at week 32 ($P < 0.013$). Individual analyses of the CDAI, the IBD Questionnaire, or laboratory markers yield concordant results. Patients who were on azathioprine or 6MP before and during the infliximab period had a better clinical outcome (75 per cent response rate) than those who were not (50 per cent). This has been extrapolated to a cause and effect relationship by various experts, but without statistical support for benefit ($P = 0.17$) and arguably unwisely, given that this was a *post hoc* subgroup analysis that was not part of the study design.

A smaller European double-blind, placebo-controlled, dose-ranging study trial of 30 patients with active Crohn's disease provided useful information, the special aspect being the inclusion of ileocolonoscopy at entry and 4 weeks after a single infliximab infusion (5, 10 or 20 mg/kg), with scoring by the Crohn's Disease Endoscopic Index of Severity (CDEIS) and histologically.[287] Small numbers make conclusions insecure but mean CDEIS fell from 13.0 to 5.3 ($P < 0.01$) for all doses of infliximab compared with no change in the placebo group (but in whom initial score was only 8.4). There was close correlation between CDAI and CDEIS. Histologically, there was loss of inflammatory infiltrate in colonic biopsies from treated patients and improvements in the Leuven numerical score (from 8.8 to 2.7 compared with 11.0 to 9.0 in the placebo group), but architectural abnormalities remained. There were only four treated patients and three controls with paired ileal biopsies but a similar trend was seen (7.7 to 3.3 versus 9.2 to 8.7). Three patients with prior stenosis appeared no worse from this viewpoint, but one with ulcerated stenosis had progressed to a frank (non-ulcerated) stricture, and a fifth who had no stenosis prior to infliximab developed a tight rectal stricture which necessitated multiple dilatations.

As infliximab is relatively invasive and expensive, it is important for us to seek means of predicting those who will respond and of anticipating relapse. Schreiber's group have studied 22 patients with acute Crohn's disease treated by a single infusion. All were refractory to steroids and immunosuppressants, and had severe and accessible inflammation.[288] Mucosal levels of activated nuclear NFκB-p65 decreased within 2 weeks of infusion in all patients, 20 of whom had a clinical response. Relapses (increase of CDAI of > 50 to > 150) occurred in 25 per cent by week 4, and 90 per cent by week 16. As patients relapsed, their levels of TNF-α rose, but increased levels of activated mucosal NFκB-p65 were demonstrable at least 2–4 weeks prior to clinical or endoscopic features. This phenomenon has the potential to be clinically useful. Numerous genetically based tests are under evaluation to the same purpose; considerable controversy surrounds this at present.[289,290]

In a rather complex financial model (Markov method) based on an average US costing of $2245 per treatment (drug and administration), and incorporating published response rates, there is evidence for net cost benefit from infliximab if the quality of remission (when achieved) is as good as surgical remission in one-third of treated patients.[291] If only a quarter get a response of this quality, then surgery remains 'cheaper' in terms of quality-adjusted life years (see Chapter 2).

INFLIXIMAB COMMENTARY

Tens of thousands of infliximab infusions have now been administered, amounting to more than 10 per cent of all Crohn's disease patients treated in some centres. The short-term safety record is becoming more secure. The risk of lymphoma is not a major concern (see Chapter 8). The serious infection risk is now said by its manufacturers to be lower than in placebo-treated patients. It should not, however, be used in the presence of active sepsis (see also Chapter 7). Discussion of the risk of promoting intestinal obstruction is hampered by exclusion of patients at higher than average risk from trial recruitment to avoid 'losses' from early surgery, but there is more than anecdotal evidence to suggest that it is a real issue.[292] Of ten cases reported from a single busy centre (unfortunately, no denominator is given in the abstract), four were known to have strictures and their obstruction was at this site, but a variety of sites were implicated in the other six. All required surgery.

Most of the other data in respect of infliximab use are based on clinical experience whilst we await the outcome of studies looking at repeated (semi-prophylactic) infusions and the influence of combining therapy with longer-term disease-modifying agents such as azathioprine. Until then there is a clinical consensus that the limitations of the licensed indications are appropriate. There appears little point in giving more than two doses if there has been no response, but commencement on azathioprine before or at the time of infliximab infusion is wise so long as the patient is not intolerant (even if there has previously been therapeutic failure).[286,293] Delayed or severe hypersensitivity is widely considered a contraindication to further exposure to infliximab.

CDP571

There are, to date, three reported studies of the more humanized CDP571 IgG4 antibody to TNF-α. The British multicentre study in patients with active Crohn's disease (CDAI > 150), was relatively small, and fell short of a true placebo-controlled trial, but there was a significant response by standard criteria at 2 weeks in patients receiving a single 5 mg/kg infusion in comparison with the baseline values.[294] Only a minority of patients achieved a full remission, and the effect did not appear to last as long as that quoted for infliximab; by 4 weeks the response had largely evaporated. Despite the more humanized antibody, several patients developed antibodies directed against CDP571.

A subsequent large and complex study in active Crohn's disease compared 10 mg/kg with 20 mg/kg in a double-blind, placebo-controlled trial. All patients had an initial infusion and follow-up infusions at 8 and 16 or at 12 weeks.[295] All follow-up infusions were of 10 mg/kg. Response was defined from a fall in CDAI of > 70 and a good response from a fall of > 100. The placebo response and good response were 27 per cent and 14 per cent, respectively, compared with 45 per cent and 30 per cent for all CDP571 regimens (P = 0.023). There are odd discrepancies between the 10 and 20 mg/kg dosages with some parameters being better with one and some with the other. There was an impression that fistulae were helped. Adverse events were many but minor (87 versus 69 per cent in the placebo group). Nine per cent developed an anti-idiotype antibody and 12 per cent (versus 7 per cent controls) had an infusion reaction.

CDP571 also appears to be effective in steroid-dependent (15–40 mg prednisolone or 9 mg budesonide) Crohn's patients in remission. Weaning from steroid was significantly more successful in a 16-week, double-blind, placebo-controlled trial of 20 mg/kg initially and then 10 mg/kg at week 8.[296] At 16 weeks, 43.6 per cent were in remission and off all steroids compared with 21.9 per cent of the controls (P = 0.049). Safety was good with only 2.6 per cent developing anti-idiotype antibodies, and 15 per cent (versus 9 per cent) infusion reactions.

A third TNF antibody (DE27) does not yet appear to have been evaluated in Crohn's disease.

ETANERCEPT

Etanercept is a genetically engineered fusion protein comprising two identical recombinant chains of the human extracellular TNF-receptor p75 component fused to the Fc domain of human IgG1. It is known to bind TNF-α and also lymphotoxin (which infliximab does not) but has less effect on E-selectin and cell trafficking than does infliximab. Clinical trials have shown safety and, with 25 mg given subcutaneously twice weekly, considerable benefit over placebo in otherwise non-responsive rheumatoid arthritis,[297] an indication for which it is now licensed in the USA. There are very few data in Crohn's disease as yet, but a 12-week open pilot study of 25 mg twice weekly in 10 patients with resistant Crohn's disease failing on prednisolone, azathioprine or methotrexate has been reported.[298] The agent appears safe and about 50 per cent of patients appear to show a response, clinically and biochemically; endoscopic responses were not recorded.

THALIDOMIDE

TNF-α may be manipulated by means other than neutralizing antibodies. Thalidomide is a potent antagonist of TNF-α, mainly through enhanced degradation of TNF-α mRNA (and inhibition of angiogenesis),[299] and given its efficacy in mucosal ulceration in HIV disease, and in Behçet's disease, it has been logical that its effects have been examined in Crohn's disease. Clearly the risk of phocomelia will always preclude its use in all but the most carefully selected female patients.

In an open dose-ranging study, safety, tolerance and efficacy of low-dose thalidomide were evaluated for treatment of moderate-to-severe, steroid-dependent disease in 12 males. All were dependent on at least 20 mg prednisolone, to which was added either 50 or 100 mg thalidomide each night.[300] Steroid doses were tapered only after 4 weeks. There appeared to be clinical value from the addition of the drug; all patients were able to reduce steroids by at least 50 per cent, and 44 per cent discontinued steroids entirely. Side effects were mostly mild and transient, with drowsiness the most common, but peripheral neuropathy, oedema and dermatitis were also seen.

A second open study included 22 patients (6 female) with refractory Crohn's disease, who received thalidomide, 200 mg (or 300 mg in four cases) at night.[301] Only 14 patients completed 12 weeks of treatment, but all of these met reasonably conventional criteria for clinical response, and 9 achieved clinical remission.

The third small study yielded similar results from 200–300 mg daily for a median of 14 weeks,

which were accompanied by endoscopic improvement in responders.[302] Two (29 per cent) discontinued therapy because of chronic fatigue and dizziness, and two developed sensory neuropathy which reversed symptomatically with drug withdrawal.

There are also some positive results from a pilot study of thalidomide in ulcerative colitis.[303]

PENTOXIFYLLINE/OXPENTIFYLLINE

It is also possible to inhibit TNF-α with oral pentoxifylline, but although an open study of 1.6 g daily in 16 steroid-dependent Crohn's patients confirmed its suppressant effect on TNF-α secretion from *ex vivo* stimulated monocytes, no effect on any of the standard measures of disease activity (CDAI, CRP, endoscopic score) could be demonstrated.[304]

INHIBITION OF TNF-α IN ULCERATIVE COLITIS

Antibody to TNF-α is effective in several animal models of ulcerative colitis, including the colitis of the tamarin monkey. Six cotton-top tamarins with confirmed ulcerative colitis received repeated doses of CDP571. Disease was assessed by measuring body weight, faecal volume, and scoring rectal biopsies.[305] All six animals improved.

TNF-α antibodies have also been used to apparently good effect in small open studies of human ulcerative colitis, CDP571 in mild-to-moderate disease,[306] and infliximab in severely ill, steroid-refractory patients.[307] In the former, 15 patients received a single infusion of 5 mg/kg. This was well tolerated and there was a reduction in the disease activity score at 1 and 2 weeks. In the 15 more seriously ill patients treated with infliximab 5 mg/kg, there were responses but the study was terminated prematurely because of poor recruitment. Anecdotal support for infliximab in severe but perhaps not in fulminant colitis exists and my group is part of a three-centre controlled trial which is now in progress to clarify things.

Intravenous immunoglobulin, T-cell apheresis and mono-clonal antibodies to CD4 cells

Intravenous immunoglobulin has been used in preliminary open-label studies in refractory inflammatory bowel disease,[308] but there are no confirmed data, and its relative invasiveness and uncertain risks have prevented therapeutic enthusiasm.

T-cell apheresis, using differential centrifugation, has been assessed in patients with chronic resistant Crohn's disease in an open trial,[309] interpretation of which is complicated by the simultaneous administration of parenteral nutrition.[309] However, long-term remission with steroid withdrawal in 64 of 72 patients is recorded. The French GETAID group have reported similarly good results from a controlled study of T-cell apheresis in 28 Crohn's patients recently brought to remission by steroids.[310] Steroid tapering and relapse rates were determined. The study group received lymphapheresis (9 procedures within 4–5 weeks) and all 12 achieved full weaning from steroids compared with only 5 of 12 controls (not significant). No adverse effects were seen but there was a high rate of relapse in 18 months of follow-up after treatment (83 per cent in the lymphapheresis group and 62 per cent in the control group).

A Japanese group have examined a similar technique in an open study of 45 patients with active ulcerative colitis.[311] The apheresis unit was equipped with a leucocyte-removal filter and was administered at 1-week intervals in 5 weeks of intensive therapy and at approximately 1-month intervals during 5 months of maintenance therapy; around 95 per cent of all passaged white cells

were removed. Heparin was thought unlikely to have contributed to the effect. Only prolonged remission would justify the invasiveness and costs of such regimens, and it is unlikely that apheresis will ever have more than a peripheral place in inflammatory bowel disease management. Confirmatory data from other centres are also notably absent.

Initial studies using a chimaeric anti-CD4 antibody in patients with active Crohn's disease yielded clinical remission in 10 of 12 patients (83 per cent), with complete steroid withdrawal in two-thirds.[312] Remissions, however, were not long lasting. In two further preliminary studies in severe Crohn's disease using anti-CD4 monoclonal antibodies, the therapeutic gains were not impressive[313,314] and, although the sustained suppression of CD4 cells was sufficient to cause concern, there was again little evidence for sustained benefit even in those with an initial good response.

Heparin, adhesion molecules and growth factors in inflammatory bowel disease therapy

HEPARIN

Actions and potential mechanisms

Heparin is best known as an anticoagulant but, like its endogenous equivalent heparan, has important other properties. The anticoagulant effects on thrombin themselves produce secondary inhibition of neutrophil activation and limit pathological increases in endothelial permeability. There is also inhibition of neutrophil elastase which reduces the ability of these cells to penetrate endothelium, associated with inactivation of a range of cytokines and binding of lactoferrin.

An apparent congenital absence of enterocyte heparan sulphate was associated with profound protein-losing enteropathy in the absence of conventional microscopic abnormalities in the small bowel biopsies of three infants.[315] We investigated the hypothesis that heparin functions as a co-receptor molecule for basic fibroblast growth factor, a role usually performed by heparan sulphate chains on the cell adhesion molecule syndecan-1. A marked reduction of syndecan-1 was found in reparative epithelium from inflammatory bowel disease patients.[316] *In vitro* we were able to demonstrate that removal of heparan sulphate from gastrointestinal epithelial cells reduced the response to basic fibroblast growth factor, and that this could be fully restored by the addition of heparin. We have hypothesized that this is important in the clinical situation.[317]

Basic fibroblast growth factor itself is already known not only to bind heparin, but also to stimulate angiogenesis and promote wound healing in tissues. Its serum concentration has been found to be strongly correlated with disease activity in paediatric Crohn's disease ($r = 0.53$, $P < 0.001$) and somewhat less so in ulcerative colitis ($r = 0.33$, $P = 0.03$);[318] it might be imagined that tissue levels would be more clearly linked still.

We have gone on to demonstrate that the downregulation of syndecan-1 is intimately related to over-expression of TNF-α and a causative association is far from excluded.[319] Our data are supported by an *in vitro* study in which heparin prevented leucocyte adhesion in response to exogenous TNF.[320] This was attributed to the result of induction of the leucocyte adhesion molecules CD11 a and b, and suppression of L-selectin, with no contribution from altered activity of other mediators (P-selectin, ICAM-1 or VCAM-1). There is evidence from Birmingham also for this mechanism[321] and animal model evidence for a specific anti-inflammatory effect of enoxaparin in experimental colitis.[322,323] It certainly appears that heparin has anti-inflammatory actions that have the potential to be important at standard anticoagulant doses. In discussion of a fascinating case report, the Liverpool group[324] postulate that these effects of heparin contributed to its apparent therapeutic role in their patient (with pathergic arthropathy and pyoderma gangrenosum). It is suggested that margination of neutrophils – the degree to which the cells 'roll' along the endothelium – may be of key importance.

HEPARIN IN INFLAMMATORY BOWEL DISEASE THERAPY

Heparin, given for an incidental deep venous thrombosis, was apparently effective in problematic ulcerative colitis.[325] Nine further patients treated by full heparinization have now been reported from the same centre. Nine of the 10 entered remission, rectal bleeding being the first symptom to resolve. Similar uncontrolled data come from other reputable centres,[326] and especially so in Russia. Further small series (in abstract only) record apparent useful effects of therapeutic doses of heparin in Crohn's disease, and extra-intestinal manifestations, indicating that the agent's actions may not necessarily be confined to ulcerative colitis.[327,328]

The clinical response appears to be similar when low molecular weight heparins such as dalteparin[329] and nadroparin[330] are employed, offering advantages in ease of use (controlled data are awaited). However, despite generally low toxicity, there remains a risk of clinically important bleeding associated with unfractionated heparin therapy.[331] As there is evidence that poorly or non-anticoagulant heparins may be even more effective in certain circumstances, and that unusual routes (perhaps oral or by enema?) may be of value,[323] a topically orientated delivery has its attractions.

At last we have the first of several impending reports of controlled trials in ulcerative colitis therapy, from Panes *et al.*[332] Patients with moderately severe ulcerative colitis requiring hospitalization were randomized into a double-blind comparison of placebo tablets plus intravenous unfragmented heparin to bring the activated partial thromboplastin time (APTT) to 1.5–2.0, against methylprednisolone 1 mg/kg with placebo injections, for 14 days. Patients then began a steroid taper over 12 weeks to zero, or heparin continuing at 12 500 units twice daily subcutaneously. In an interim analysis of 25 patients there was no effect from heparin other than a slight fall in CRP and an increased frequency of bleeding (2/12 needing transfusion) with a fairly typical response to prednisolone (69 per cent at 10 days). At 10 days, 90 per cent of the heparin group still had rectal bleeding compared with 31 per cent of the steroid group. The trial was therefore terminated. This was a stiff challenge for heparin and I do not believe that this is the end of the story.

Whatever the conclusions about heparin in specific therapy, this should not be permitted to overshadow the need for anticoagulant precautions to be taken in all patients rendered bedbound by their inflammatory bowel disease (see Chapter 7).

ENDOTHELIAL CELL ADHESION MOLECULES AND THEIR MANIPULATION

Intracellular adhesion molecule-1 (ICAM-1) is closely involved in the binding of leucocytes to vessels in the presence of inflammation. It is known to be upregulated in intestinal mucosa in active Crohn's disease. It is also present on the surface of some antigen-presenting cells, from where it binds to lymphocyte function-associated antigen-1 (LFA-1) on T cells, thus increasing their activation status. An antisense nucleotide to ICAM-1 has been developed, and a dose-ranging study in active Crohn's disease has been completed in Oxford.[333] With alternate-day intravenous administration, 7 of 15 patients receiving active agent were in remission compared with only 1 of 5 given placebo. At 6 months, 5 of the 7 responders were still in remission and had needed a lower cumulative dose of steroids than the controls.

However, in a larger German study (n = 77) of 0.5 mg/kg daily for 2 days to 4 weeks in steroid-refractory Crohn's disease patients, there was no difference from placebo, and the trial was stopped prematurely at planned interim analysis.[334]

The $\alpha4\beta7$ integrin is expressed on blood mononuclear cells (CD4 cells) and is ligand for the mucosal addressin cell adhesion molecule MadCAM-1, which is expressed on gut vascular epithelium. Antibody to $\alpha4\beta7$ should in theory prevent access of T cells to the inflamed gut mucosa (egression of lymphocytes into gut). A series of anti-integrin antibodies are under evaluation in inflammatory bowel disease therapy.

Antibodies to $\alpha4\beta7$ integrin prevent T cells and monocytes from entering the gut in mice models, and there is impressive evidence from treatment of colitis in the cotton-top tamarin.[335] An equivalent antibody for human use now exists: like CDP571, the LDP-02 antibody is humanized. In the first human use, single doses for moderate ulcerative colitis, in a double-blind, dose-ranging, placebo-controlled trial (n = 29) (0.15–2.0 mg/kg i.v.), yielded detectable levels of the antibody in circulation and functional blockade of receptors to more than 2 weeks with the two higher doses.[336] Side effects were mild (19 versus 13 per cent for placebo) and, if representative, the best responses were with 0.5 mg/kg.

There are also promising human data for another humanized antibody – natalizumab – which is active against $\alpha4\beta1$ and $\alpha4\beta7$. In preliminary studies, now being followed by larger-scale controlled trials, there have been indications that there is therapeutic gain associated with a rise in lymphocyte counts and significant alteration of endothelial adhesion molecule expression.[337]

GRANULOCYTE COLONY STIMULATING FACTOR (GCSF)

Noting the similarity of chronic granulomatous disease to Crohn's disease (see Chapter 1) and its response to GCSF,[338] and the similarity of glycogen storage disease type 1b to Crohn's disease (see

Chapter 1) and its response to GCSF,[339] it is not surprising that GSCF has been used in Crohn's disease.[340] This anecdotal report has been followed by two small series with additional support from our own experience (St Mark's and University College London). In a study of five highly resistant patients, there were two probable responses,[341] and in an open study of Neupogen® 300 μg/day for 12 weeks in 17 patients (6 on steroids), 10 improved, including 6 who achieved full remission and 3 with fistulae who seemed to benefit.[342] Three had significant medullary bone pain despite prophylactic analgesia, but there was no other toxicity.

HUMAN GROWTH HORMONE

Employing a rationale based on benefit from nutrition (high-protein supply), its anabolic effects, and data supporting trophic effects of growth hormone in short bowel, 5 mg human growth hormone (Humatrope) was given daily for 1 week, then 1.5 mg/day for 15 weeks, or placebo injections in Crohn's disease. It was evidently difficult to recruit to the study because of injection issues, and only 37 from 597 considered were entered.[343] The CDAI fell and the need for prednisolone fell in actively treated patients, with opposite findings in the placebo group ($P = 0.004$). Immunosuppressant use was static with placebo, and reduced with growth hormone. Side effects of mild oedema and/or headache usually resolved within the first month of treatment. However, despite careful prior selection, two tumours (renal carcinoma and benign schwannoma) came to light during the study period (and also one in the placebo group). This could be a promising agent if the neoplastic potential can be confidently neglected.

Nicotine

Intermittent smokers and those who restart after a period of abstinence often record improvement in ulcerative colitis symptomatology, suggesting that the act of smoking is of continuing direct relevance, and not a marker for other behaviour (or of a genetic predisposition – to both smoking and inflammatory bowel disease phenotype) (see Chapter 1). In the absence of satisfactory explanations for these phenomena, it is suggested that nicotine may be an important mediator of the apparent beneficial effect in ulcerative colitis, perhaps acting via an effect on the neuromotor manifestations of acute inflammation. Nicotine has accordingly been assessed as a potential therapeutic agent.

NICOTINE IN COLITIS THERAPY

A double-blind, placebo-controlled trial of nicotine patches in active ulcerative colitis was reported in 1994.[344] Encouraging results reached significance, but there were irregularities in the study which came in for some criticism, not least in an accompanying editorial.[345] A similar study has now been reported from the Mayo Clinic[346] with comparable results (clinical responses in 39 per cent compared to a mere 9 per cent in the placebo group). These authors included histological assessment, which showed improvement at 4 weeks but of insufficient magnitude to reach significance. There was considerable morbidity, including contact dermatitis and nausea, but also acute pancreatitis. The Mayo group (with colleagues in France) associate the response to nicotine to an effect on IL-8 suppression, and were unable to demonstrate any effect on mucin gene expression.[347]

The Welsh group followed up their original study with a 6-week comparative study using a prednisolone-treated control group.[348] Sixty-one non-smoking patients with mildly to moderately active ulcerative colitis (about 50 per cent of those seen) entered the study, and were randomized to treatment with either oral prednisolone or nicotine patches. Prednisolone was prescribed at

5 mg/day, rising over 9 days to a 15 mg daily dose that then remained static for the remainder of the study period. Nicotine-treated patients received an incremental dose administered by transdermal patch delivering 2.5 mg/day rising 'every 1 to 2 days' to 15 mg, and then to 25 mg daily if remission had not been achieved by 14 days. A reduced dose of nicotine was permitted if side effects occurred. All other therapy was discontinued. Steroid-treated patients received dummy patches, whereas nicotine-treated patients had placebo capsules by mouth. Appropriate effort appears to have been taken to modify the dose/size of placebo patches similarly in the steroid-treated group to ensure maximal preservation of blinding. The rather unorthodox (and arguably suboptimal) steroid regimen is defended on grounds of simplicity and homogeneity, but it seems a pity that a more conventional reducing course was not accommodated within the trial design. The steroid- and nicotine-treated groups proved well matched; the only differences of potential importance were a greater prior use of steroids in the prednisolone group, and somewhat higher global clinical and histological scores in the nicotine group at trial entry. Outcomes were recorded by intention to treat in respect of clinical, sigmoidoscopic and histological scores. There were fewer withdrawals in the steroid-treated group, and it seems probable that many of the withdrawals from the nicotine group were the result of (predictable) pharmacological effects of nicotine; 19 of 30 completed the trial protocol (compared with 24 of 31 with prednisolone). Lowered nicotine doses were required even amongst three of these, to minimize toxicity and retain compliance. Serum studies of nicotine and cotinine indicate that compliance was, however, as stated to the authors. The efficacy of continued blinding (of patients and investigators) is difficult to judge, but has probably not influenced the results of the study. In those who were able to complete the 6-week study period, there was a remission rate of only 32 per cent with nicotine patches, compared with 58 per cent of those completing 6 weeks in the steroid limb of the study. This difference does not reach significance, but when the data are analysed by intention to treat, prednisolone offers clear and significant advantage (e.g. 47 versus 21 per cent for clinical remission; $P = 0.035$). For no criterion does nicotine score more favourably than prednisolone and, although there was clinical improvement with nicotine treatment, this was not accompanied by sigmoidoscopic improvement.

TOPICAL NICOTINE

My impressions have been that colitic patients who smoke consider that they get considerably more benefit from smoking than from nicotine patches, and that non-smoking colitics find the side effects of the nicotine unacceptable. It has therefore been valuable to see promising results from topical administration of nicotine preparations that aim to deliver drug to the site of disease with minimal systemic uptake. Two uncontrolled studies have used nicotine enemas, both of which have proved of value in a good majority of patients with low blood levels of nicotine and its metabolites[349,350] and a Eudragit-coated formulation to be taken by mouth has been examined – so far only in healthy volunteers.[351]

NICOTINE IN COLITIS MAINTENANCE

There is no case for nicotine in maintenance of remission of ulcerative colitis. In a careful study, again performed by the Welsh group, the results from nicotine appeared equivalent to those of placebo.[352] As there is unequivocal benefit from 5-ASA maintenance therapy, it is doubtful whether any further studies in this context could be considered legitimate.

The evidence in favour of smoking (as opposed to nicotine administration alone) is insufficient to warrant its recommendation to ulcerative colitis patients, given its other potentially fatal consequences, despite the comments to the contrary by at least one prominent expert in the ulcerative colitis field! In Crohn's disease, the gastroenterologist has a continuing and unequivocal mandate to direct its cessation.

Miscellaneous therapeutic options

REACTIVE OXYGEN METABOLITES

Oxygen free radical production is increased in inflammatory bowel disease. Neutrophils and granulocytes, both in the peripheral circulation and in the intestinal mucosa, responsible for this almost certainly thereby contribute to the inflammatory process[353] (see Chapter 1). In animal models of colitis, inhibition of free radical production reduces inflammation[354] and Millar et al.[355] indicated that this may prove useful in man also (but in an abstract only despite a 6-year delay), an effect perhaps already in use as one of the mechanisms of action of 5-ASA, and again of relevance to the effects of smoking.

Iron in its ferric state is known to contribute to the generation of reactive oxygen species, prompting a successful trial of chelation with desferrioxamine in pouchitis. This possibility has not yet been assessed in other forms of inflammatory bowel disease, but the addition of allopurinol (a xanthine oxidase inhibitor) or dimethyl sulphoxide (a hydroxyl radical scavenger) to sulphasalazine maintenance has been shown to improve symptoms and prolong remission in ulcerative colitis.[356] Emerit et al.[357] have also reported good long-term results in an open study of refractory Crohn's disease ($n = 34$) using copper zinc superoxide dismutase, an enzyme that accelerates the clearance of O_2^-. Again, controlled trials are awaited.

LOCAL ANAESTHETICS

Evidence for abnormal intestinal innervation[358]

(see Chapter 1) bolsters the same group's good results (all of 21 patients) from topical lignocaine (lidocaine) therapy in distal colitis. There are other reasons for believing that local anaesthetic agents might be of therapeutic value in inflammatory bowel disease, as they can be shown to inhibit leucocyte migration to sites of inflammation,[359] secretion of cytokines from epithelial cell lines[360] and may reduce platelet aggregation and cytokine production.[361] There are, however, still no controlled data for lignocaine use in colitis or support from other centres, there being only a very modest clinical response in this author's patients given the same dose of topical gel. However, Arlander et al. suggest that ropivacaine, a new long-acting local anaesthetic, might usefully be employed.[362] A twice-daily 200 mg dose of ropivacaine gel was given to 12 patients with active distal ulcerative colitis without toxicity, and with indications that endoscopic and histological parameters improved usefully (as did clinical features despite the error in the published abstract that suggests the opposite). Formal comparisons of local anaesthetic agents with established drugs are indicated.

BISMUTH

Following the anecdotal report of efficacy from bismuth salts in microscopic colitis, this has been studied in a small open study of patients with collagenous or lymphocytic colitis in which bismuth subnitrate was compared with budesonide 9 mg.[363] Treated patients received drug in solution at 750 mg thrice daily. Both drugs helped a majority of patients and in retrospective comparison to a similar extent. Formal evaluation would now be reasonable.

ANTIHISTAMINES

Given evidence for involvement of mast cells and therefore of histamine in the Th2 response of ulcerative colitis, it appeared legitimate to examine antihistamines in therapy. Loratadine (an H1 anti-histamine) has been used in addition to steroids and 5-ASA in a small ($n = 16$) controlled trial.[364] At 4- and 6-months follow-up, there had been substantially less cumulative steroid usage in the treated patients (26.0 versus 33.7 mg/kg; 28.5 versus 40.8 mg/kg). This did not apparently reach statistical significance but offers an interesting new angle. If true, it is surprising that this has not previously emerged given the huge use of antihistamines (and, indeed, H2 blockers) in the general population, but a larger study could be informative.

The future?

The selective use of immunomodulators in Crohn's disease is increasingly accepted and the net may soon be spread wider to include ulcerative colitis. However, all currently available therapies have limited efficacy and most have significant clinical toxicity. Incomplete responses and the potential for short- and long-term toxicity leave a continuing need for pharmacological development. Surgical intervention will continue to be necessary for a substantial minority of patients with inflammatory bowel disease for the foreseeable future. Stem cell transplantation and gene therapy for benign disease are already with us, and it cannot be long before they are appropriately assessed in inflammatory bowel disease. In the meantime, there are a few developments nearer to the bedside.

There is no doubt that IL-10 is an active agent in inflammatory bowel disease, but its efficacy has not been sufficiently impressive for it to dominate over infliximab (see above). There are no immediate expectations that it will be made widely available, but its salvation may lie in a fascinating new approach. It has been recognized that lactobacilli can prevent colitis in the IL-10-deficient mouse[365] and a genetically modified strain could prove the beginning of a revolution. *Lactococcus lactis* is a non-pathogenic bacterium used in the dairy industry

that (unusually) is not killed once it releases its cytokines. It has been modified to produce IL-10 at potentially therapeutic levels. When the recombinant bacteria are administered enterally to colitic mice, IL-10 is released (though not readily detected systemically) and the colitis is substantially ameliorated.[366] This is not yet applicable for clinical use as mouse IL-10 is too distinct from the human cytokine but this methodology cannot be far away.

Vaccination may prove to be possible in the therapy of Crohn's disease. Danish workers (in conjunction with Ferring Pharmaceuticals) have inserted a small fragment of ovalbumin into recombinant TNF-α, and then injected this into the same species as the original TNF-α.[367] This TNF-α must itself be inactivated or it is merely destroyed, but in the preliminary mouse experiments it has now been possible to modify circumstances so that these mice produce antibodies to TNF-α. This is relatively sustained but falls with time unless booster doses are given. The position of the ovalbumin in the TNF produces antibodies of different characteristics. In murine models there is already a customizable anti-cachexin and antirheumatoid effect.

More prosaically, but no less relevant to the patient, come the various complementary options. These are frequently sought. No less than 26 per cent of all inflammatory bowel disease patients in the UK have used one or more technique (compared with 17 per cent of general medical patients, although less than the 50 per cent in irritable bowel syndrome); this is especially popular (and pertinent?) in those with adverse social or emotional circumstances and with the less organ-specific symptoms like malaise and tiredness.[368]

It is an exciting time in inflammatory bowel disease therapeutics!

References

1 Ilnyckyj A, Shanahan F, Anton PA, Cheang M, Bernstein CN. Quantification of the placebo

response in ulcerative colitis. *Gastroenterology* 1997; **112**: 1854–8.

2 Brynskov J, Freund L, Norby Rasmussen S, *et al.* A placebo-controlled, double-blind, randomized trial of cyclosporine in active chronic Crohn's disease. *N Engl J Med* 1989; **321**: 845–50.

3 Sutherland L, Singleton J, Sessions J, *et al.* Double blind, placebo controlled trial of metronidazole in Crohn's disease. *Gut* 1991; **32**: 1071–5.

4 Chun A, Chadi RM, Korelitz BI, *et al.* Intravenous corticotrophin vs. hydrocortisone in the treatment of hospitalized patients with Crohn's disease: a randomized double-blind study and follow-up. *Inflamm Bowel Dis* 1998; **4**: 177–81.

5 Marx J. How the glucocorticoids suppress immunity. *Science* 1995; **270**: 232–3.

6 Fahey JV, Guyre PM, Munck A. Mechanisms of anti-inflammatory actions of glucocorticoids. In Weissman G, ed. *Advances in Inflammation Research*, Vol 2. New York: Raven, 1981: 21–51.

7 Reich K, Lingnau F, Williams RM, *et al.* Corticosteroids downregulate BCL2 and induce apoptosis in CD4+ LPL in Crohn's disease. *Gastroenterology* 1996; **110**: A999.

8 Honda M, Orii F, Ayabe T, *et al.* Expression of glucocorticoid receptor β in lymphocytes of patients with glucocorticoid-resistant ulcerative colitis. *Gastroenterology* 2000; **118**: 859–66.

9 Hearing SD, Norman M, Probert CS, Haslam N, Dayan CM. Predicting therapeutic outcome in severe ulcerative colitis by measuring in vitro steroid sensitivity of proliferating peripheral blood lymphocytes. *Gut* 1999; **45**: 382–8.

10 Truelove SC, Witts LJ. Cortisone in ulcerative colitis. Final report on a therapeutic trial. *Br Med J* 1955; **2**: 1041–8.

11 Munkholm P, Langholz E, Davidsen M, Binder V. Frequency of glucocorticoid resistance and dependency in Crohn's disease. *Gut* 1994; **35**: 360–2.

12 Baron JH, Connell AM, Kanaghinis TG, *et al.* Outpatient treatment of ulcerative colitis: comparison between three doses of oral prednisolone. *Br Med J* 1962; **2**: 441–3.

13 Powell-Tuck J, Bown RL, Lennard-Jones JE. A comparison of oral prednisolone given as single or multiple daily doses for active proctocolitis. *Scand J Gastroenterol* 1978; **13**: 833–7.

14 Lai H-C, Fitzsimmons SC, Allen DB, *et al.* Risk of persistent growth impairment after alternate day prednisone treatment in children with cystic fibrosis. *N Engl J Med* 2000; **342**: 851–9.

15 Sinha A, Nightingale JM, West KP. A gradual dose reduction is needed after 2 weeks of oral prednisolone for ulcerative colitis. *Gastroenterology* 2000; **118**(Suppl 2): A782.

16 Malchow H, Ewe K, Brandes JW, *et al.* The European Cooperative Crohn's Disease Study: results of drug treatment. *Gastroenterology* 1984; **86**: 249–66.

17 Modigliani R, Mary JY, Simon JF, *et al.* Clinical, biological, and endoscopic picture of attacks of Crohn's disease. Evolution on prednisolone. Groupe d'Etude Therapeutique des Affections Inflammatoires Digestives. *Gastroenterology* 1990; **98**: 811–18.

18 Franchimont DP, Louis E, Croes F, Belaiche J. Clinical pattern of corticosteroid dependent Crohn's disease. *Eur J Gastroenterol Hepatol* 1998; **10**: 821–5.

19 Nyman-Pantelidis M, Nilsson A, Wagner ZG, Borga O. Pharmacokinetics and retrograde colonic spread of budesonide enemas in patients with distal ulcerative colitis. *Aliment Pharmacol Ther* 1994; **8**: 617–22.

20 Mulder CJJ, Tytgat GNJ. Review article: topical corticosteroids in inflammatory bowel disease. *Aliment Pharmacol Ther* 1993; 7: 125–30.

21 Campieri M, Cottone M, Miglio F, *et al.* Beclomethasone dipropionate enemas versus prednisolone sodium phosphate enemas in the treatment of distal ulcerative colitis. *Aliment Pharmacol Ther* 1998; **12**: 361–6.

22 Anderson FH. The rectal approach to treatment in distal ulcerative colitis. *Lancet* 1995; **346**: 520–1.

23 McIntyre PB, Macrea FA, Berghouse L, English J, Lennard-Jones JE. Therapeutic benefits from a poorly absorbed prednisolone enema in distal colitis. *Gut* 1985; **26**: 822–4.

24 Hanauer SB, Robinson M, Pruitt R, *et al.* Budesonide enema for the treatment of active,

distal ulcerative colitis and proctitis: a dose-ranging study. U.S. Budesonide enema study group. *Gastroenterology* 1998; **115**: 525–32.

25 Tarpila S, Turunen U, Sepäälä K, *et al.* Budesonide enema in active haemorrhagic proctitis: a controlled trial against hydrocortisone foam enema. *Aliment Pharmacol Ther* 1994; **8**: 591–5.

26 Löfberg R, Thomsen OØ, Langholz E, *et al.* Budesonide versus prednisolone retention enemas in active distal ulcerative colitis. *Aliment Pharmacol Ther* 1994; **8**: 623–9.

27 Pruitt, R, Katz S, Bayless T, Levine J. Repeated use of budesonide enema is safe and effective for the treatment of acute flares of distal ulcerative colitis. *Gastroenterology* 1996; **110**: A995.

28 Greenberg GR, Feagon BG, Martin F, *et al.* Oral budesonide for active Crohn's disease. *N Engl J Med* 1994; **331**: 836–41.

29 Rutgeerts P, Löfberg R, Malchow H, *et al.* A comparison of budesonide with prednisolone for active Crohn's disease. *N Engl J Med* 1994; **331**: 842–5.

30 Gross V, Andus T, Caesar I, *et al.* Oral pH-modified release budesonide versus 6-methylprednisolone in active Crohn's disease. German/Austrian Budesonide Study Group. *Eur J Gastroenterol Hepatol* 1996; **8**: 905–9.

31 Campieri M, Ferguson A, Doe W, Persson T, Nilsson LG. Oral budesonide is as effective as oral prednisolone in active Crohn's disease. The Global Budesonide Study Group. *Gut* 1997; **41**: 209–14.

32 Papi C, Luchetti R, Gili L, Montanti S, Koch M, Capurso L. Budesonide in the treatment of Crohn's disease. A meta-analysis. *Gastroenterology* 2000; **118**(Suppl 2): A781.

33 Löfberg R, Danielsson A, Suhr O, *et al.* Oral budesonide versus prednisolone in patients with active extensive and left-sided ulcerative colitis. *Gastroenterology* 1996; **110**: 1713–18.

34 Kolkman JJ, Molmann HW, Mollmann AC, *et al.* Beneficial effect of oral budesonide for distal ulcerative colitis: a comparative study of Budenofalk® 3 mg TID vs 9 mg OD. *Gastroenterology* 2000; **118**(Suppl 2): A779.

35 Hawthorne AB, Record CO, Holdsworth CD, *et al.* Double blind trial of oral fluticasone propi-

onate v prednisolone in the treatment of active ulcerative colitis. *Gut* 1993; **34**: 125–8.

36 Greenberg GR, Feagan BG, Martin F, *et al.* Oral budesonide as maintenance treatment for Crohn's disease: a placebo-controlled, dose ranging study. *Gastroenterology* 1996; **110**: 45–51.

37 Löfberg R, Rutgeerts P, Malchow H, *et al.* Budesonide prolongs time to relapse in ileal and ileocaecal Crohn's disease. A placebo controlled one year study. *Gut* 1996; **39**: 82–6.

38 D'Haens G, Verstraete A, Cheyns K, Aerden I, Bouillon R, Rutgeerts P. Bone turnover during short-term therapy with methylprednisolone or budesonide in Crohn's disease. *Aliment Pharmacol Ther* 1998; **12**: 419–24.

39 Baron JH, Connell AM, Lennard-Jones JE, Avery-Jones F. Sulphasalazine and salcylazosulphanilamide in ulcerative colitis. *Lancet* 1962; **1**: 1094–6.

40 Misiewicz JJ, Lennard-Jones JE, Connell AM, Baron JH, Avery Jones F. Controlled trial of sulphasalazine in maintenance therapy for ulcerative colitis. *Lancet* 1965; **1**: 185–8.

41 Khan AZ, Piris J, Truelove SC. An experiment to determine the active therapeutic moiety of sulphasalazine. *Lancet* 1977; **2**: 892–5.

42 Greenfield SM, Punchard NA, Teare JP, Thompson RPH. Review article: the mode of action of aminosalicylates in inflammatory bowel disease. *Aliment Pharmacol Ther* 1993; 7: 369–83.

43 Hartley MG, Hudson MJ, Swarbrick ET, Grace RH, Gent AE, Hellier MD. Sulphasalazine treatment and the colorectal mucosa-associated flora in ulcerative colitis. *Aliment Pharmacol Ther* 1996; **10**: 157–63.

44 Nielsen OH, Bondesen S. Kinetics of 5-aminosalicylic acid after jejunal installation in man. *Br J Pharmacol* 1983; **16**: 738–40.

45 Fallingborg J, Christensen LA, Ingeman-Nielsen M, Jacobsen BA, Abildgaard K, Rasmussen HH. pH-profile and regional transit times of the normal gut measured by a radiotelemetry device. *Aliment Pharmacol Ther* 1989; **3**: 605–13.

46 Sasaki Y, Hada R, Nakajima H, Fukuda S, Munakata A. Improved localizing method of radiopill in measurement of entire gastrointestinal

pH profiles: colonic luminal pH in normal subjects and patients with Crohn's disease. *Am J Gastroenterol* 1997; **92**: 114–18.

47 Christensen LA, Slot O, Sanchez G, *et al.* Release of 5-aminosalicylic acid from Pentasa during normal and accelerated intestinal transit time. *Br J Clin Pharmacol* 1987; **23**: 365–9.

48 Rijk MC, van Schaik A, van Tongeren JH. Disposition of mesalazine from mesalazine-delivering drugs in patients with inflammatory bowel disease, with and without diarrhoea. *Scand J Gastroenterol* 1992; **27**: 863–8.

49 Nugent SG, Kumar D, Yazaki ET, Evans SF, Rampton DS. Gut pH and transit time in ulcerative colitis appear sufficient for complete dissolution of pH-dependent 5-ASA-containing capsules. *Gastroenterology* 2000; **118**(Suppl 2): A781.

50 McIntyre PB, Rodrigues CA, Lennard-Jones JE, *et al.* Balsalazide in the maintenance treatment of patients with ulcerative colitis, a double-blind comparison with sulphasalazine. *Aliment Pharmacol Ther* 1988; **2**: 237–43.

51 Schroeder KW, Tremaine WJ, Ilstrup DM. Coated oral 5-aminosalicylic acid therapy for mildly to moderately active ulcerative colitis. A randomized study. *N Engl J Med* 1987; **317**: 1625–9.

52 Järnerot G. Withdrawal rates because of diarrhea in Dipentum treated patients with ulcerative colitis are low when Dipentum is taken with food and dose-titrated. *Gastroenterology* 1996; **110**: A932.

53 Kruis W, Brandes JW, Schreiber S, *et al.* Olsalazine versus mesalazine in the treatment of mild to moderate ulcerative colitis. *Aliment Pharmacol Ther* 1998; **12**: 707–15.

54 Green JR, Lobo AJ, Holdsworth CD, *et al.* Balsalazide is more effective and better tolerated than mesalamine in the treatment of acute ulcerative colitis. *Gastroenterology* 1998; **114**: 15–22.

55 Pruitt R, Hanson J, Safdi M, *et al.* Balsalazide is superior to mesalamine in the time to improvement of signs and symptoms of acute ulcerative colitis. *Gastroenterology* 2000; **118**(Suppl 2): A120–1.

56 Abenhaim L, Sutherland LR, Field LG, *et al.* Has the introduction of a new mesalamine containing compound altered the clinical course of ulcerative colitis patients? *Gastroenterology* 1996; **110**: A850.

57 Courtney M, Nunes D, Bergin C, *et al.* Randomised comparison of olsalazine and mesalazine in prevention of relapses in ulcerative colitis. *Lancet* 1992; **339**: 1279–81.

58 Laursen LS, Stokholm M, Bukhave K, Rask-Madsen J, Lauritsen K. Disposition of 5-aminosalicylic acid by olsalazine and three mesalazine preparations in patients with ulcerative colitis: comparison of intraluminal colonic concentrations, serum values, and urinary excretion. *Gut* 1990; **31**: 1271–6.

59 Green JR, Gibson JA, Kerr GD, *et al.* Maintenance of remission of ulcerative colitis: a comparison between balsalazide 3 g daily and mesalazine 1.2 g daily over 12 months. *Aliment Pharmacol Ther* 1998; **12**: 1207–16.

60 Fockens P, Mulder CJJ, Tytgat GNJ, *et al.* Comparison of the efficacy and safety of 1.5 vs 3.0 g oral slow-release mesalazine (Pentasa) in the maintenance treatment of ulcerative colitis. *Eur J Gastroenterol Hepatol* 1995; **7**: 1025–30.

61 Schroeder KW, Tremaine WJ, Ilstrup DM. Coated oral 5-aminosalicylic acid therapy for mildly to moderately active ulcerative colitis. A randomized study. *N Engl J Med* 1987; **317**: 1625–9.

62 Ardizzone S, Petrillo M, Imbesi V, Cerutti R, Bollani S, Bianchi-Porro G. Is maintenance therapy always necessary for patients with ulcerative colitis in remission? *Aliment Pharmacol Ther* 1999; **13**: 373–9.

63 Messori A, Brignola C, Trallori G, *et al.* Effectiveness of 5-aminosalicylic acid for maintaining remission in patients with Crohn's disease: a meta-analysis. *Am J Gastroenterol* 1994; **89**: 692–8.

64 Singleton JW, Hanauer SB, Gitnick GL, *et al.* Mesalamine capsules for the treatment of active Crohn's disease: results of a 16-week trial. *Gastroenterology* 1993; **104**: 1293–301.

65 Prantera C, Cottone M, Pallone F. Mesalamine in the treatment of mild to moderate active Crohn's ileitis: results of a randomized, multicenter trial. *Gastroenterology* 1999; **116**: 521–6.

66 Tromm A, Griga T, May B. Oral mesalazine for the treatment of Crohn's disease: clinical efficacy with respect to pharmacokinetic properties. *Hepatogastroenterology* 1999; **46**: 3124–35.

67 Steinhart AH, Hemphill D, Greenberg GR. Sulfasalazine and mesalazine for the maintenance therapy of Crohn's disease: a meta-analysis. *Am J Gastroenterol* 1994; **89**: 2116–24.

68 Sutherland LR, Martin F, Bailey RJ, *et al.* A randomized, placebo-controlled, double-blind trial of mesalamine in the maintenance of remission of Crohn's disease. *Gastroenterology* 1997; **112**: 1069–77.

69 de Franchis R, Omodei P, Ranzi T, *et al.* Controlled trial of oral 5-aminosalicylic acid for the prevention of early relapse in Crohn's disease. *Aliment Pharmacol Ther* 1997; **11**: 845–52.

70 Camma C, Giunta M, Rosselli M, Cottone M. Mesalamine in the maintenance treatment of Crohn's disease: a meta-analysis adjusted for confounding variables. *Gastroenterology* 1997; **113**: 1465–73.

71 Caprilli R, Andreoli A, Capurso L, *et al.* Oral mesalazine (5-aminosalicylic acid; Asacol) for the prevention of post-operative recurrence of Crohn's disease. *Aliment Pharmacol Ther* 1994; **8**: 35–43.

72 McLeod RS, Wolff BG, Steinhart AH, *et al.* Prophylactic mesalamine treatment decreases postoperative recurrence of Crohn's disease. *Gastroenterology* 1995; **109**: 404–13.

73 Florent C, Cortot A, Quandale P, *et al.* Placebo-controlled clinical trial of mesalazine in the prevention of early endoscopic recurrences after resection for Crohn's disease. *Eur J Gastroenterol Hepatol* 1996; **8**: 229–34.

74 Lochs H, Mayer M, Fleig WE, *et al.* Prophylaxis of postoperative relapse in Crohn's disease with mesalamine. *Gastroenterology* 2000; **118**: 264–73.

75 Frieri G, Pimpo MT, Andreoli A, *et al.* Prevention of post-operative recurrence of Crohn's disease requires adequate mucosal concentration of mesalazine. *Aliment Pharmacol Ther* 1999; **13**: 577–82.

76 Sturgeon JB, Bhatia P, Hermens D, Miner PB Jr. Exacerbation of chronic ulcerative colitis with mesalamine. *Gastroenterology* 1995; **108**: 1889–93.

77 Kapur KC, Williams GT, Allison MC. Mesalazine induced exacerbation of ulcerative colitis. *Gut* 1995; **37**: 838–9.

78 *British National Formulary*, 39th edition. London: British Medical Association and Royal Pharmaceutical Society of Great Britain, 2000.

79 Wang KK, Bowyer BA, Fleming CR, Schroeder KW. Pulmonary infiltrates and eosinophilia associated with sulfasalazine. *Mayo Clin Proc* 1984; **59**: 343–6.

80 Jordan A, Cowan RE. Reversible pulmonary disease and eosinophilia associated with sulphasalazine. *J Roy Soc Med* 1988; **81**: 233–5.

81 Anonymous. Nephrotoxicity associated with mesalazine. Committee on Safety of Medicines. *Current Problems* 1990; **30**: 2.

82 Thuluvath PJ, Ninkovic M, Calam J, Anderson M. Mesalazine induced interstitial nephritis. *Gut* 1994; **35**: 1493–6.

83 Stoa-Birketveldt G, Florholmen J. The systemic load and efficient delivery of active 5-aminosalicylic acid in patients with ulcerative colitis on treatment with olsalazine or mesalazine. *Aliment Pharmacol Ther* 1999; **13**: 357–61.

84 Asacol Study Group. Sensitive markers of renal dysfunction are elevated in chronic ulcerative colitis. *Gastroenterology* 1995; **108**: A919.

85 Bonnet J. Nephropathy and 5-aminosalicylic acid. *Gastroenterol Clin Biol* 1998; **22**: 663–4.

86 Hussain F, Ajjan R, Weir N, Trudgill N, Riley S. Single and divided dose delayed-release mesalazine: are traditional dosing regimens outmoded? *Gastroenterology* 1996; **110**: A928.

87 Farthing MJG, Rutland MD, Clark ML. Retrograde spread of hydrocortisone containing foam given intrarectally in ulcerative colitis. *Br Med J* 1979; **287**: 822–4.

88 Van Bodegraven AA, Boer RO, Lourens J, Tuynman HARE, Sindram JW. Distribution of mesalazine enemas in active and quiescent ulcerative colitis. *Aliment Pharmacol Ther* 1996; **10**: 327–32.

89 Campieri M, Corbelli C, Gionchetti P, *et al.* Spread and distribution of 5-ASA colonic foam and 5-ASA enema in patients with ulcerative colitis. *Dig Dis Sci* 1992; **37**: 1890–7.

90 Gionchetti P, Ardizzonne S, Benvenuti ME, *et al.* A new mesalazine gel enema in the treatment of left-sided ulcerative colitis: a randomised controlled multicentre trial. *Aliment Pharmacol Ther* 1999; **13**: 381–8.

91 Lee FI, Jewell DP, Mani V, *et al.* A randomised trial comparing mesalazine and prednisolone foam enemas in patients with acute distal ulcerative colitis. *Gut* 1996; **38**: 229–33.

92 Marshall JK, Irvine EJ. Rectal corticosteroids versus alternative treatments in ulcerative colitis: a meta-analysis. *Gut* 1997; **40**: 775–81.

93 Mulder CJJ, Fockens P, Meijer JWR, Van der Heide H, Wiltink EHH, Tytgat GNJ. Beclomethasone diproprionate (3mg) versus 5-aminosalicylic acid (2g) versus the combination of both (3mg/2g) as retention enemas in active ulcerative proctitis. *Eur J Gastroenterol Hepatol* 1996; **8**: 549–54.

94 Safdi M, DeMicco M, Sninsky C, *et al.* A double-blind comparison of oral versus rectal mesalamine versus combination therapy in the treatment of distal ulcerative colitis. *Am J Gastroenterol* 1997; **92**: 1867–71.

95 Gionchetti P, Rizzello F, Venturi A, *et al.* Comparison of oral with rectal mesalazine in the treatment of ulcerative proctitis. *Dis Colon Rectum* 1998; **41**: 93–7.

96 d'Albasio G, Pacini F, Camarri E, *et al.* Combined therapy with 5-aminosalicylic acid tablets and enemas for maintaining remission in ulcerative colitis: a randomized double-blind study. *Am J Gastroenterol* 1997; **92**: 1143–7.

97 Hinojosa J, Agueda A, Panes J, *et al.* Multicenter randomized trial comparing oral topical and oral plus topical mesalazine treatment in active distal ulcerative colitis. *Gastroenterology* 2000; **118**(Suppl 2): A778–9.

98 Vecchi M, Meucci G, Gionchetti P, *et al.* Comparison of oral versus combination mesalazine therapy in active ulcerative colitis: a double-blind, double dummy, randomized, multicenter Italian study. *Gastroenterology* 2000; **118**(Suppl 2): A783.

99 Campieri M, Gionchetti P, Belluzi A, *et al.* Optimum dosage of 5-aminosalicylic acid as rectal enemas in patients with active ulcerative colitis. *Gut* 1991; **32**: 929–31.

100 Gionchetti P, Rizzello F, Venturi A, *et al.* Comparison of mesalazine suppositories in proctitis and distal proctosigmoiditis. *Aliment Pharmacol Ther* 1997; **11**: 1053–7.

101 Mantzaris GJ, Hatzis A, Petraki K, Spiliadi C, Triantaphyllou G. Intermittent therapy with high-dose 5-aminosalicylic acid enemas maintains remission in ulcerative proctitis and proctosigmoiditis. *Dis Colon Rectum* 1994; **37**: 58–62.

102 Marteau P, Crand J, Foucault M, Rambaud JC. Use of mesalazine slow release suppositories 1 g three times per week to maintain remission of ulcerative proctitis: a randomised double blind placebo controlled multicentre study. *Gut* 1998; **42**: 195–9.

103 Ardizzone S, Doldo P, Ranzi T, *et al.* Mesalazine foam (Salofalk foam) in the treatment of active distal ulcerative colitis. A comparative trial vs Salofalk enema. *Ital J Gastroenterol Hepatol* 1999; **31**: 677–84.

104 O'Donnell LJ, Arvind AS, Hoang P, *et al.* Double blind, controlled trial of 4-aminosalicylic acid and prednisolone enemas in distal ulcerative colitis. *Gut* 1992; **33**: 947–9.

105 Marteau P, Halphen M. Etude comparative ouverte randomisée de l'efficacité et de la tolérance de lavements de 2g d'acide 4-amino-salicylique (4-ASA) et de 1g d'acide 5-amino-salicylique (5-ASA) dans les formes basses de rectocolite hémorragique. *Gastroenterol Clin Biol* 1995; **19**: 31–5.

106 Kozarek RA. Review article: immunosuppressive therapy for inflammatory bowel disease. *Aliment Pharmacol Ther* 1993; **7**: 117–23.

107 Hassan C, Marinaki A, Ansari A, Duley J, Shobowale-Bakre E, Sanderson JD. Thiopurine methyl transferase genotype in patients with inflammatory bowel disease treated with azathioprine. *Gut* 1999; **45**(Suppl V): A15.

108 Colonna T, Korelitz BI. The role of leukopenia in the 6-mercaptopurine induced remission of refractory Crohn's disease. *Am J Gastroenterol* 1994; **89**: 362–6.

109 Berg PS, George J, Present DH, Bodian C, Rubin PH. 6MP – is leukopenia required to induce

remission in the treatment of ulcerative colitis? *Gastroenterology* 1996; **110**: A863.

110 Campbell SS, Ghosh S. Maintenance of remission in inflammatory bowel disease by azathioprine: is neutropenia necessary? *Gastroenterology* 2000; **118**(Suppl 2): A785.

111 Yates CR, Krynetski EY, Loennechen T, *et al.* Molecular diagnosis of thiopurine S-methyltransferase deficiency: genetic basis for azathioprine and mercaptopurine intolerance. *Ann Intern Med.* 1997; **126**: 608–14.

112 Belaiche J, Desager JP, Horsmans Y, Louis E. Is the dosage of red blood cell 6-thioguanine concentration useful in the management of Crohn's disease treated with azathioprine and 6-mercaptopurine? *Gastroenterology* 2000; **118**(Suppl 2): A784.

113 Dubinsky MC, Hassard PV, Kam LY, *et al.* Serial 6-mercaptopurine metabolite measurements in combination with dose escalation unmasks an important biochemical explanation for '6-mercaptopurine resistance'. *Gastroenterology* 2000; **118**(Suppl 2): A890.

114 Cuffari C, Hunt S, Harris M, Bayless T. Erythrocyte 6-thioguanine metabolite levels predict clinical responsiveness to therapy in inflammatory bowel disease. *Gastroenterology* 2000; **118**(Suppl 2): A785.

115 Gupta P, Gokhale R, Kirschner BS. 6-mercaptopurine metabolite levels in children with inflammatory bowel disease: lack of correlation of 6-thioguanine levels with clinical response. *Gastroenterology* 2000; **118**(Suppl 2): A787.

116 Lowry PW, Franklin CL, Weaver AL, *et al.* Cross-sectional study of inflammatory bowel disease patients taking azathioprine or 6-mercaptopurine: lack of correlation between disease activity and 6-thioguanine nucleotide concentration. *Gastroenterology* 2000; **118**(Suppl 2): A788.

117 McGovern DPB, Hussaini SH, Reynolds NJ, Dalton HR. Can thiopurine methyl transferase levels predict efficacy and side effects of azathioprine in patients with inflammatory bowel disease? *Gut* 1999; **45**(Suppl V): A204.

118 Connell WR, Kamm MA, Ritchie JK, Lennard-Jones JE. Bone marrow toxicity caused by azathioprine in inflammatory bowel disease: 27 years of experience. *Gut* 1993; **34**: 1081–5.

119 Present DH, Meltzer ST, Krumholz MP, Wolke A, Korelitz BI. 6-Mercaptopurine in the management of inflammatory bowel disease: short- and long-term toxicity. *Ann Intern Med* 1989; **111**: 641–9.

120 Fraser AG, Jewell DP. Side effects of azathioprine treatment given for inflammatory bowel disease – a 30 year audit. *Gastroenterology* 2000; **118**(Suppl 2): A787.

121 McGovern DP, Shobowale-Bakre E-M, Duley J, Travis SP. Early azathioprine intolerance in inflammatory bowel disease patients is imidazole-related and independent of thiopurine methyl transferase activity. *Gastroenterology* 2000; **118**(Suppl 2): A890.

122 Present DH, Korelitz BI, Wisch N, Glass JL, Sachar DB, Pasternack BS. Treatment of Crohn's disease with 6-mercaptopurine. A long-term randomized double-blind study. *N Engl J Med* 1980; **402**: 981–7.

123 Candy S, Wright J, Gerber M, Adams G, Gerig M, Goodman R. A controlled double blind study of azathioprine in the management of Crohn's disease. *Gut* 1995; **37**: 674–8.

124 D'Haens G, Geboes K, Ponette E, Penninckx F, Rutgeerts P. Healing of severe recurrent ileitis with azathioprine therapy in patients with Crohn's disease. *Gastroenterology* 1997; **112**: 1475–81.

125 Pearson DC, May GR, Fick GH, Sutherland L. Azathioprine and 6-mercaptopurine in Crohn disease. A meta-analysis. *Ann Intern Med* 1995; **123**: 132–42.

126 Sandborn WJ, Tremaine WJ, Wolf DC, *et al.* Lack of effect of intravenous administration on time to respond to azathioprine for steroid-treated Crohn's disease. North American Azathioprine Study Group. *Gastroenterology* 1999; **117**: 527–35.

127 Kader HA, Theoret Y, Tolia V, *et al.* A prospective randomized double blind placebo controlled study to assess the efficacy of intravenous loading of azathioprine in children and adolescents with inflammatory bowel disease. *Gastroenterology* 2000; **118**(Suppl 2): A118.

128 Korelitz BI, Present DH. Favorable effect of 6-mercaptopurine on fistulae of Crohn's disease. *Dig Dis Sci* 1985; **30**: 58–64.

129 Lecomte T, Contou J-F, Carbonnel F, *et al.* Effect of azathioprine or 6-mercaptopurine on perianal lesions of Crohn's disease. *Gastroenterology* 2000; **118**(Suppl 2): A785.

130 O'Donoghue DP, Dawson AM, Powell-Tuck J, Brown RL, Lennard-Jones JE. Double blind withdrawal trial of azathioprine as maintenance treatment for Crohn's disease. *Lancet* 1978; **2**: 955–7.

131 Markowitz J, Rosa J, Grancher K, Aiges H, Daum F. Long term 6-mercaptopurine treatment in adolescents with Crohn's disease. *Gastroenterology* 1990; **99**: 1347–51.

132 Lémann M, Cuillerier E, Bouhnik Y, *et al.* Azathioprine for prevention of Crohn's recurrence after ileal or colonic resection. *Gastroenterology* 1996; **110**: A948.

133 Kirk AP, Lennard-Jones JE. Controlled trial of azathioprine in chronic ulcerative colitis. *Br Med J* 1982; **284**: 1291–2.

134 Present DH. 6-Mercaptopurine and other immunosuppressive agents in the treatment of Crohn's disease and ulcerative colitis. *Gastroenterol Clin North Am* 1989; **18**: 57–71.

135 Adler DJ, Korelitz BI. The therapeutic efficacy of 6-mercaptopurine in refractory ulcerative colitis. *Am J Gastroenterol* 1990; **85**: 717–22.

136 Hawthorne AB, Logan RFA, Hawkey CJ, *et al.* Randomised controlled trial of azathioprine withdrawal in ulcerative colitis. *Br Med J* 1992; **305**: 20–2.

137 George J, Present DH, Pou R, Bodian C, Rubin PH. The long-term outcome of ulcerative colitis treated with 6-mercaptopurine. *Am J Gastroenterol* 1996; **91**: 1711–14.

138 Kim PS, Zlatanic J, Korelitz BI, Gleim GW. Optimum duration of treatment with 6-mercaptopurine for Crohn's disease. *Am J Gastroenterol* 1999; **94**: 3254–7.

139 Bouhnik Y, Lémann M, Mary J-Y, *et al.* Long-term follow-up of patients with Crohn's disease treated with azathioprine or 6-mercaptopurine. *Lancet* 1996; **347**: 215–19.

140 Flanagan WM, Corthesy B, Bram RJ, Crabtree GR. Nuclear association of a T-cell transcription factor blocked by FK-506 and cyclosporin A. *Nature* 1991; **352**: 803–7.

141 Hodgson H. Cyclosporin in inflammatory bowel disease. *Aliment Pharmacol Ther* 1991; **5**: 343–50.

142 Lichtiger S, Present DH, Kornbluth A, *et al.* Cyclosporine in severe ulcerative colitis refractory to steroid therapy. *N Engl J Med* 1994; **330**: 1841–5.

143 Jewell DP, Lennard-Jones JE and the Cyclosporin Study Group of Great Britain and Ireland. Oral cyclosporin for chronic active Crohn's disease. *Eur J Gastroenterol Hepatol* 1994; **6**: 499–505.

144 Feagan BG, McDonald JWD, Rochon J, *et al.* Low-dose cyclosporine for the treatment of Crohn's disease. *N Engl J Med* 1994; **330**: 1846–51.

145 Stange EF, Modigliani R, Pena AS, *et al.* European trial of cyclosporine in chronic active Crohn's disease: a 12 month study. *Gastroenterology* 1995; **109**: 774–82.

146 Feagan B. Cyclosporine in Crohn's disease: a meta-analysis. *Inflamm Bowel Dis* 1995; **1**: 335–6.

147 Present DH, Lichtiger S. Efficacy of cyclosporine in treatment of fistula of Crohn's disease. *Dig Dis Sci* 1994; **39**: 374–80.

148 Chapman RW, Selby WS, Jewell DP. Controlled trial of intravenous metronidazole as an adjunct to corticosteroids in severe ulcerative colitis. *Gut* 1986; **27**: 1210–12.

149 Cohen RD, Stein R, Hanauer SB. Intravenous cyclosporin in ulcerative colitis: a five-year experience. *Am J Gastroenterol* 1999; **94**: 1587–92.

150 Cohen RD, Brodsky AL, Hanauer SB. A comparison of the quality of life in patients with severe ulcerative colitis after total colectomy versus medical treatment with intravenous cyclosporin. *Inflamm Bowel Dis* 1999; **5**: 1–10.

151 Hyde GM, Thillainayagam AV, Jewell DP. Intravenous cyclosporin as rescue therapy in severe ulcerative colitis: time for a reappraisal? *Eur J Gastroenterol Hepatol* 1998; **10**: 411–13.

152 Gurudu SR, Griffel LH, Gialanella RJ, Das KM Cyclosporine therapy in inflammatory bowel disease: short-term and long-term results. *J Clin Gastroenterol* 1999; **29**: 151–4.

153 Sandborn WJ, Tremaine WJ, Schroeder KW, *et al.* A placebo-controlled trial of cyclosporine enemas for mildly to moderately active left-sided ulcerative colitis. *Gastroenterology* 1994; **106**: 1429–35.

154 Taylor AC, Connell WR, Elliott R, d'Apice AJ. Oral cyclosporin in refractory inflammatory bowel disease. *Aust N Z J Med* 1998; **28**: 179–83.

155 Kornbluth A, Present DH, Lichtiger S, Hanauer S. Cyclosporin for severe ulcerative colitis: a user's guide. *Am J Gastroenterol* 1997; **92**: 1424–8.

156 Abreu-Martin MT, Vasiliauskas EA, Gaiennie J, Voigt B, Targan SR. Continuous infusion cyclosporine is effective for severe acute Crohn's disease . . . but for how long? *Gastroenterology* 1996; **110**: A851.

157 Vega R, Bertran X, Menacho M, *et al.* Cytomegalovirus infection in patients with inflammatory bowel disease. *Am J Gastroenterol* 1999; **94**: 1053–6.

158 Sternthal M, George J, Kornbluth A, Lichtiger S, Present D. Toxicity associated with the use of cyclosporin in patients with inflammatory bowel disease. *Gastroenterology* 1996; **110**: A1019.

159 Hermida-Rodriguez C, Cantero-Perona J, Garcia-Valriberas R, Pajares-Garcia JM, Mate-Jimenez J. High-dose intravenous cyclosporine in steroid refractory attacks of inflammatory bowel disease. *Hepatogastroenterology* 1999; **46**: 2265–8.

160 Quan VA, Saunders BP, Hicks BH, Sladen GE. Cyclosporin treatment for ulcerative colitis complicated by fatal *Pneumocystis carinii* pneumonia. *Br Med J* 1997; **314**: 363–4.

161 Van Gossum A, Schmit A, Adler M, *et al.* Short- and long-term efficacy of cyclosporin administration in patients with acute severe ulcerative colitis. Belgian IBD Group. *Acta Gastroenterol Belg* 1997; **60**: 197–200.

162 Yee GC, Stanley DL, Pessa LJ. Effect of grapefruit juice on blood cyclosporin concentration. *Lancet* 1995; **345**: 955–6.

163 D'Haens G, Bourgeois S, Hiele M, *et al.* Two and four mg/kg/day of intravenous cyclosporine are equally effective in severe attacks of ulcerative colitis. *Gastroenterology* 2000; **118**(Suppl 2): A786.

164 Kozarek R, Patterson D, Gelfand M, Botoman V, Ball T, Wilske K. Methotrexate induces clinical and histologic remission in patients with refractory inflammatory bowel disease. *Ann Intern Med* 1989; **110**: 353–6.

165 Lémann M, Chamiot-Prieur C, Mesnard B, *et al.* Methotrexate for the treatment of refractory Crohn's disease. *Aliment Pharmacol Ther* 1996; **10**: 309–14.

166 Zenjari T, Lémann M, Mesnard B, *et al.* Methotrexate in Crohn's disease: long-term efficacy and toxicity. *Gastroenterology* 1996; **110**: A1053.

167 Feagan BG, Rochon J, Fedorak RN, Irvine EJ. Methotrexate for the treatment of Crohn's disease. *N Engl J Med* 1995; **332**: 292–7.

168 Egan LJ, Sandborn WJ, Tremaine WJ, *et al.* A randomized dose-response and pharmacokinetic study of methotrexate for refractory inflammatory Crohn's disease and ulcerative colitis. *Aliment Pharmacol Ther* 1999; **13**: 1597–604.

169 Feagan BG, Fedorak RN, Irvine EJ, *et al.* A comparison of methotrexate with placebo for the maintenance of remission in Crohn's disease. *N Engl J Med* 2000; **342**: 1627–32.

170 Hermida C, Cantero J, Moreno-Otero R, Mate-Jimenez J. Methotrexate and 6-mercaptopurine in steroid-dependent inflammatory bowel disease patients: a randomized controlled clinical trial. *Gut* 1999; **45**(Suppl V): A132.

171 Oren R, Arber N, Odes S, *et al.* Methotrexate in chronic active ulcerative colitis: a double-blind, randomized, Israeli multicenter trial. *Gastroenterology* 1996; **110**: 1416–21.

172 Whiting-O'Keefe QE, Fye KH, Sack KD. Methotrexate and histologic hepatic abnormalities: a meta-analysis. *Am J Med* 1991; **90**: 711–16.

173 Reynolds J, Trellis D, Abu-Elmagd K, Fung J. The rationale for FK506 in inflammatory bowel disease. *Can J Gastroenterol* 1993; 7: 208–10.

174 Lowry PW, Weaver AL, Tremaine WJ, Sandborn WJ. Combination therapy with oral tacrolimus (FK506) and azathioprine or 6-mercaptopurine for treatment-refractory Crohn's disease perianal fistulae. *Inflamm Bowel Dis* 1999; 5: 239–45.

175 Ierardi E, Principi M, Rendina A, *et al.* Oral tacrolimus long term therapy in Crohn's disease with steroid resistance or dependence. *Gut* 1999; **45**(Suppl V): A287.

176 Fellermann K, Herrlinger KR, Witthoeft T, Holmann N, Ludwig D, Stange EF. Tacrolimus (FK506): a new immunosuppressant for steroid refractory inflammatory bowel disease. *Gastroenterology* 2000; **118**(Suppl 2): A786.

177 Fickert P, Hinterleitner TA, Wenzl HH, *et al.* Mycophenolate mofetil in patients with Crohn's disease. *Am J Gastroenterol* 1998; **93**: 2529–32.

178 Neurath MF, Wanitschke R, Peters M, Krummenauer F, Meyer-zum-Buschenfelde KH, Schlaak JF. Randomised trial of mycophenolate mofetil versus azathioprine for treatment of chronic active Crohn's disease. *Gut* 1999; **44**: 625–8.

179 Wenzl HH, Hinterleitner TA, Fickert P, Aichbichler BW, Metzler O, Petritsch W. Low efficacy of long-term mycophenolate mofetil in patients with Crohn's disease. *Gastroenterology* 2000; **118**(Suppl 2): A790.

180 Skelly MM, Curtis H, Jenkins D, Hawkey CJ. Toxicity of mycophenolate mofetil in patients with inflammatory bowel disease. *Gastroenterology* 2000; **118**(Suppl 2): A789.

181 Lopez-Cubero SO, Sullivan KM, McDonald GB. Course of Crohn's disease after allogeneic marrow transplantation. *Gastroenterology* 1998; **114**: 433–40.

182 Kashyap A, Forman SJ. Autologous bone marrow transplantation for non-Hodgkin's lymphoma resulting in long-term remission of coincidental Crohn's disease. *Br J Haematol* 1998; **103**: 651–2.

183 Soderholm JD, Juliusson G, Sjodahl R. Long-term endoscopic remission in a case of Crohn's disease after autologous bone marrow transplantation. *Gastroenterology* 2000; **118**(Suppl 2): A789.

184 Sartor RB. Antimicrobial therapy of inflammatory bowel disease: implications for pathogenesis and management. *Can J Gastroenterol* 1993; 7: 132–8.

185 Ambrose NS, Allan RN, Keighley MR, *et al.* Antibiotic therapy for treatment in relapse of intestinal Crohn's disease. A prospective randomized study. *Dis Colon Rectum* 1985; **28**: 81–5.

186 Brandt LJ, Bernstein LH, Boley SJ, *et al.* Metronidazole therapy for perineal Crohn's disease: a follow-up study. *Gastroenterology* 1982; **83**: 383–5.

187 Rutgeerts P, Hiele M, Geboes K, *et al.* Controlled trial of metronidazole treatment for prevention of Crohn's recurrence after ileal resection. *Gastroenterology* 1995; **108**: 1617–21.

188 Duffy LF, Daum F, Fisher SE, *et al.* Peripheral neuropathy in Crohn's disease patients treated with metronidazole. *Gastroenterology* 1985; **88**: 681–4.

189 Colombel JF, Lémann M, Cassagnou M, *et al.* A controlled trial comparing ciprofloxacin with mesalazine for treatment of active Crohn's disease. *Am J Gastroenterol* 1999; **94**: 674–8.

190 Turunen UM, Farkkila MA, Hakala K, *et al.* Long-term treatment of ulcerative colitis with ciprofloxacin: a prospective double-blind, placebo-controlled study. *Gastroenterology* 1998; **115**: 1072–8.

191 Mantzaris GJ, Archavlis E, Christoforidis P, *et al.* A prospective randomized controlled trial of oral ciprofloxacin in acute ulcerative colitis. *Am J Gastroenterol* 1997; **92**: 454–6.

192 Burke DA, Axon AT, Clayden SA, Dixon MF, Johnston D, Lacey RW. The efficacy of tobramycin in the treatment of ulcerative colitis. *Aliment Pharmacol Ther* 1990; 4: 123–9.

193 Casellas F, Borruel N, Papo M, *et al.* Antiinflammatory effects of enterically coated amoxicillin-clavulanic acid in active ulcerative colitis. *Inflamm Bowel Dis* 1998; 4: 1–5.

194 Vega R, Bertran X, Menacho M, *et al.* Cytomegalovirus infection in patients with inflammatory bowel disease. *Am J Gastroenterol* 1999; **94**: 1053–6.

195 Moonka D, Furth EE, MacDermott RP, Lichtenstein GR. Pouchitis associated with primary cytomegalovirus infection. *Am J Gastroenterol* 1998; **93**: 264–6.

196 Moss A, Carbone J, Kressel H. Radiologic and clinical assessment of broad-spectrum antibiotic therapy in Crohn's disease. *Am J Roentgenol* 1978; **131**:787–90.

197 Lichtenstein G. Medical therapies for inflammatory bowel disease. *Curr Opin Gastroenterol* 1993; 9: 588–99.

198 Thayer WR, Reinert SE, Natarajan R, Szaro J. Rifabutin/streptomycin in the treatment of

Crohn's disease. A double-blind controlled trial. *Gastroenterology* 1996; **110**: A1027.

199 Rutgeerts P, Geboes K, Vantrappen G, *et al*. Rifabutin and ethambutol do not help recurrent Crohn's disease in the neoterminal ileum. *J Clin Gastroenterol* 1992; **15**: 24–8.

200 Douglass A, Cann PA, Bramble MG. An open pilot study of antimicrobial therapy in patients with unresponsive Crohn's disease. *Gut* 1999; **45**(Suppl V): A127.

201 Gui GP, Thomas PR, Tizard ML, Lake J, Sanderson JD, Hermon-Taylor J. Two-year-outcomes analysis of Crohn's disease treated with rifabutin and macrolide antibiotics. *J Antimicrob Chemother* 1997; **39**: 393–400.

202 Gibson GR, Fuller R. Aspects of in vitro and in vivo research approaches directed toward identifying probiotics and prebiotics for human use. *J Nutr* 2000; **130**(2S Suppl): 391S–5S.

203 Favier C, Neut C, Mizon C, Cortot A, Colombel JF, Mizon J. Fecal beta-D-galactosidase production and bifidobacteria are decreased in Crohn's disease. *Dig Dis Sci* 1997; **42**: 817–22.

204 Giaffer MH, Holdsworth CD, Duerden BI. The assessment of faecal flora in patients with inflammatory bowel disease by a simplified bacteriological technique. *J Med Microbiol* 1991; **35**: 238–43.

205 Kruis W, Schutz E, Fric P, Fixa B, Judmaier G, Stolte M. Double-blind comparison of an oral *Escherichia coli* preparation and mesalazine in maintaining remission of ulcerative colitis. *Aliment Pharmacol Ther* 1997; **11**: 853–8.

206 Rembacken BJ, Snelling AM, Hawkey PM, Chalmers DM, Axon AT. Non-pathogenic *Escherichia coli* versus mesalazine for the treatment of ulcerative colitis: a randomised trial. *Lancet* 1999; **354**: 635–9.

207 Guslandi M. Flare-up of Crohn's disease is prevented by *Saccharomyces boulardii*. *Gastroenterology* 2000; **118**(Suppl 2): A779.

208 Ishikawa H, Imaoka A, Umesaki Y, Tanaka R, Ohtani T. Randomized controlled trial of the effect of bifidobacterium-fermented milk on ulcerative colitis. *Gastroenterology* 2000; **118**(Suppl 2): A779.

209 Venturi A, Gionchetti P, Rizzello F, *et al*. Impact on the composition of the faecal flora by a new probiotic preparation: preliminary data on maintenance treatment of patients with ulcerative colitis. *Aliment Pharmacol Ther* 1999; **13**: 1103–8.

210 Campieri M, Rizzello F, Venturi A, *et al*. Combination of antibiotic and probiotic treatment is efficacious in prophylaxis of post-operative recurrence of Crohn's disease: a randomized controlled study vs mesalamine. *Gastroenterology* 2000; **118**(Suppl 2): A781.

211 Hennequin C, Kauffmann-Lacroix C, Jobert A, *et al*. Possible role of catheters in *Saccharomyces boulardii* fungemia. *Eur J Clin Microbiol Infect Dis* 2000; **19**: 16–20.

212 Fernandez-Banares F, Hinojosa J, Sanchea-Lombrana JL, *et al*. Randomized clinical trial of *Plantago ovata* seeds (dietary fiber) as compared with mesalamine in maintaining remission in ulcerative colitis. *Am J Gastroenterol* 1999; **94**: 427–33.

213 Bouhnik Y, Riottot M, Telotte A, Attar A, Dyard F, Flourié B. Lactulose ingestion increases fecal bifidobacterial counts. A randomised double blind study in healthy humans. *Gut* 1999; **45**(Suppl V): A288.

214 Tragnone A, Valpiani D, Miglio F, *et al*. Dietary habits as risk factors for inflammatory bowel disease. *Eur J Gastroenterol Hepatol* 1995; **7**: 47–51.

215 Ballegaard M, Bjergstrom A, Brondum S, Hylander E, Jensen L, Ladefoged K. Self-reported food intolerance in chronic inflammatory bowel disease. *Scand J Gastroenterol* 1997; **32**: 569–71.

216 Samuelsson SM, Ekbom A, Zack M, Helmick CG, Adami HO. Risk factors for extensive ulcerative colitis and ulcerative proctitis: a population based case-control study. *Gut* 1991; **32**: 1526–30.

217 Varghese TJ, Coomansingh D, Richardson S, *et al*. Clinical effect on ulcerative colitis with dietary supplementation by omega-3 fatty acids: a double blind randomised study. *Gastroenterology* 2000; **118**(Suppl 2): A588.

218 Bjørck S, Bosaeus I, Ek E, *et al*. Food induced stimulation of the antisecretory factor can improve symptoms in human inflammatory bowel disease: a study of a concept. *Gut* 2000; **46**: 824–9.

219 Riordan AM, Ruxton CH, Hunter JO. A review of associations between Crohn's disease and consumption of sugars. *Eur J Clin Nutr* 1998; **52**: 229–38.

220 Pearson M, Teahon K, Levi AJ, Bjarnason I. Food intolerance and Crohn's disease. *Gut* 1993; **34**: 783–7.

221 Griffiths AM, Ohlsson A, Sherman PM, Sutherland LR. Meta-analysis of enteral nutrition as a primary treatment of active Crohn's disease. *Gastroenterology* 1995; **108**: 1056–67.

222 Silk DB. Medical management of severe inflammatory disease of the rectum: nutritional aspects. *Baillières Clin Gastroenterol* 1992; **6**: 27–41.

223 O'Morain CA. Nutritional therapy in ambulatory patients. *Dig Dis Sci* 1987; **32**: 95S–9S.

224 Giaffer MH, Cann P, Holdsworth CD. Long-term effects of elemental and exclusion diets for Crohn's disease. *Aliment Pharmacol Ther* 1991; **5**: 115–25.

225 Teahon K, Bjarnason I, Pearson M, Levi AJ. Ten years' experience with an elemental diet in the management of Crohn's disease. *Gut* 1990; **31**: 1133–7.

226 O'Morain C, Segal AW, Levi AJ. Elemental diet as primary treatment of acute Crohn's disease: a controlled trial. *Br Med J* 1984; **288**: 1859–62.

227 Saverymuttu S, Hodgson HJF, Chadwick VS. Controlled trial comparing prednisolone with an elemental diet plus non-absorbable antibiotics in active Crohn's disease. *Gut* 1985; **26**: 994–8.

228 Sanderson IR, Udeen S, Davies PSW, Savage MO, Walker-Smith JA. Remission induced by an elemental diet in small bowel Crohn's disease. *Arch Dis Child* 1987; **61**: 123–7.

229 Malchow H, Steinhardt HJ, Lorenz-Meyer H, *et al.* Feasibility and effectiveness of a defined-formula diet regimen in treating active Crohn's disease. European Co-operative Crohn's Disease Study III. *Scand J Gastroenterol* 1990; **25**: 235–44.

230 Thomas AG, Taylor F, Miller V. Dietary intake and nutritional treatment in childhood Crohn's disease. *J Pediatr Gastroenterol Nutr* 1993; **17**: 75–81.

231 González-Huix F, De León R, Fernández-Bañares F, *et al.* Polymeric enteral diets as primary treatment of active Crohn's disease: a prospective steroid controlled trial. *Gut* 1993; **34**: 778–82.

232 Ruemmele FM, Roy CC, Levy E, Seidman EG. Nutrition as primary therapy in pediatric Crohn's disease: fact or fantasy? *J Pediatr* 2000; **136**: 285–9.

233 Gorard DA, Hunt JB, Payne-James JJ, *et al.* Initial response and subsequent course of Crohn's disease treated with elemental diet or prednisolone. *Gut* 1993; **34**: 1198–202.

234 Lochs H, Steinhardt HJ, Klaus-Wentz B, *et al.* Comparison of enteral nutrition and drug treatment in active Crohn's disease. Results of European Co-operative Crohn's Disease Study IV. *Gastroenterology* 1991; **101**: 881–8.

235 Riordan AM, Hunter JO, Cowan RE, *et al.* Treatment of active Crohn's disease by exclusion diet: East Anglian multicentre controlled trial. *Lancet* 1993; **342**: 1131–4.

236 Davison SM, Johnson T, Chapman S, Booth IW, Murphy MS. Disease localisation in elemental diet therapy for Crohn's disease: a study of response using 99mTc-HMPAO leukocyte scintigraphy. *Gastroenterology* 1996; **110**: A797.

237 Leiper K, Woolner JT, Parker TJ, *et al.* A randomised double blind controlled trial of high versus low long chain triglyceride whole protein feed in active Crohn's disease. *Gastroenterology* 2000; **118**(Suppl 2): A583.

238 Gassull MA, Fernandez-Banares F, Cabre E, *et al.* Fat composition is the differential factor to explain the primary therapeutic effect of enteral nutrition in Crohn's disease. Results of a double-blind randomized multicenter European trial. *Gastroenterology* 2000; **118**(Suppl 2): A117.

239 Lomer MC, Harvey RC, Evans SM, Thompson RP, Powell JJ. A low microparticle diet in Crohn's disease. *Gastroenterology* 2000; **118**(Suppl 2): A584.

240 Alun Jones V, Dickinson RJ, Workman E, *et al.* Crohn's disease: maintenance of remission by diet. *Lancet* 1985; **2**: 177–80.

241 Wilschanski M, Sherman P, Pencharz P, Davis L, Corey M, Griffiths A. Supplementary enteral nutrition maintains remission in paediatric Crohn's disease. *Gut* 1996; **38**: 543–8.

242 Verma S, Giaffer MH. Maintenance of remission in Crohn's disease using oral nutritional

supplementation. A comparative study with normal food. *Gut* 1999; **45**(Suppl V): A285.

243 Greenberg G. Nutritional support in inflammatory bowel disease: current status and future directions. *Scand J Gastroenterol* 1992; **27**(Suppl 192): 117–22.

244 Norday A. Is there a rational role for N-3 fatty acids (fish oil) in clinical medicine? *Drugs* 1991; **42**: 331.

245 Eliakim R, Karmeli F, Chorev M, Okon E, Rachmilewitz D. Effect of drugs on colonic eicosanoid accumulation in active ulcerative colitis. *Scand J Gastroenterol* 1992; **27**: 968–72.

246 Stenson W, Cort D, Rodgers J, *et al.* Dietary supplementation with fish oil in ulcerative colitis. *Ann Intern Med* 1992; **87**: 609–14.

247 Hawthorne AB, Daneshmend TK, Hawkey CJ, *et al.* Treatment of ulcerative colitis with fish oil supplementation: a prospective 12 month randomised controlled trial. *Gut* 1992; **33**: 922–8.

248 Belluzzi A, Brignola C, Campieri M, Pera A, Boschi S, Miglioli M. Effect of an enteric-coated fish-oil preparation on relapses in Crohn's disease. *N Engl J Med* 1996; **334**: 1557–60.

249 Roediger WEW. The colonic epithelium in ulcerative colitis: an energy deficiency disease? *Lancet* 1980; **2**: 712–15.

250 Harig JM, Soergel KH, Komorowski RA, Wood CM. Treatment of diversion colitis with short chain fatty acid irrigation. *N Engl J Med* 1989; **320**: 23–8.

251 Briel JW, Zimmerman DD, De Boer LM, Van der Kwast TH, Schouten WR. Short-chain fatty acid irrigation in the treatment of diversion colitis. A prospective double-blind randomized study. *Gastroenterology* 2000; **118**(Suppl 2): A580.

252 Pitcher MCL, Cummings JH. Hydrogen sulphide: a bacterial toxin in ulcerative colitis? *Gut* 1996; **39**: 1–4.

253 Senagore A, MacKeigan J, Scheider M, Ebrom S. Short chain fatty acid enemas: a cost effective alternative in the treatment of nonspecific proctosigmoiditis. *Dis Colon Rectum* 1992; **35**: 923–7.

254 Vernia P, Villotti G, Annese V, *et al.* Combined topical butyrate/5-ASA therapy is more effective than 5-ASA alone in refractory distal ulcerative colitis. A double-blind placebo-controlled study. *Gut* 1999; **45**(Suppl V): A23.

255 Nightingale JMD, Rathbone BJ, West KP, Mayberry JF, Wicks ACW. Butyrate enemas are less effective than prednisolone enemas in treating distal or left sided ulcerative colitis. *Gut* 1995; **37**(Suppl 2): A41.

256 Steinhart AH, Hiruki T, Brzezinski A, Baker JP. Treatment of left-sided ulcerative colitis with butyrate enemas: a controlled trial. *Aliment Pharmacol Ther* 1996; **10**: 729–36.

257 Scheppach W, Christl SU, Bartram HP, Richter F, Kasper H. Effects of short-chain fatty acids on the inflamed colonic mucosa. *Scand J Gastroenterol Suppl* 1997; **222**: 53–7.

258 Connell AM, Lennard-Jones JE, Misiewicz JJ, Baron JH, Avery Jones F. Comparison of acetarsol and prednisolone-21-phosphate suppositories in the treatment of idiopathic proctitis. *Lancet* 1965; **1**: 238–9.

259 Forbes A, Britton TC, House IM, Gazzard BG. Safety and efficacy of acetarsol suppositories in unresponsive proctitis. *Aliment Pharmacol Ther* 1989; **3**: 553–6.

260 Wardle TD, Hall L, Turnberg LA. Inter-relationships between inflammatory mediators released from colonic mucosa in ulcerative colitis and their effects on colonic secretion. *Gut* 1993; **34**: 503–8.

261 Hawthorne AB, Boughton-Smith NK, Whittle BJ, Hawkey CJ. Colorectal leukotriene B4 synthesis *in vitro* in inflammatory bowel disease: inhibition by the selective 5-lipoxygenase inhibitor BWA4C. *Gut* 1992; **33**: 513–17.

262 Collawn C, Rubin P, Perez N, *et al.* Phase II study of the safety and efficacy of a 5-lipoxygenase inhibitor in patients with ulcerative colitis. *Am J Gastroenterol* 1992; **87**: 342–6.

263 Peppercorn M, Das K, Elson C, *et al.* Zileuton, a 5-lipoxygenase inhibitor, in the treatment of active ulcerative colitis: a double blind placebo controlled trial. *Gastroenterology* 1994; **106**: A751.

264 Hawkey CJ, Dube LM, Rountree LV, Linnen PJ, Lancaster JF. A trial of zileuton versus mesalazine or placebo in the maintenance of remission of ulcerative colitis. The European Zileuton Study

Group For Ulcerative Colitis. *Gastroenterology* 1997; **112**: 718–24.

265 Gertner D, Rampton D, Stevens T, Lennard-Jones J. Verapamil inhibits in-vitro leukotriene B4 release by rectal mucosa in active ulcerative colitis. *Aliment Pharmacol Ther* 1992; **6**: 163–8.

266 Widomski D, Fretland DJ, Gasiecki AF, Collins PW. The prostaglandin analogs, misoprostol and SC-46275, potently inhibit cytokine release from activated human monocytes. *Immunopharmacol Immunotoxicol* 1997; **19**: 165–74.

267 Ratnaike RN, Jones TE. Mechanisms of drug-induced diarrhoea in the elderly. *Drugs Aging* 1998; **13**: 245–53.

268 Hawkey C, Rampton D. Prostaglandins and the gastrointestinal mucosa: are they important in its function, disease or treatment? *Gastroenterology* 1985; **89**: 1462–88.

269 Rampton D, Collins C. Review article: thromboxanes in inflammatory bowel disease – pathogenic and therapeutic implications. *Aliment Pharmacol Ther* 1993; 7: 357–67.

270 Collins CE, Benson MJ, Burnham WR, Rampton DS. Picotamide inhibition of excess *in vitro* thromboxane B2 release by colorectal mucosa in inflammatory bowel disease. *Aliment Pharmacol Ther* 1996; **10**: 315–20.

271 Casellas F, Papo M, Guarner F, *et al.* Effects of thromboxane synthase inhibition on *in vivo* release of inflammatory mediators in chronic ulcerative colitis. *Eur J Gastroenterol Hepatol* 1995; 7: 221–6.

272 Schreiber S, Heinig T, Thiele HG, Raedler A. Immunoregulatory role of interleukin 10 in patients with inflammatory bowel disease. *Gastroenterology* 1995; **108**: 1434–44.

273 Van Deventer SJH, Elson CO, Fedorak RN, *et al.* Multiple doses of intravenous interleukin-10 in steroid-refractory Crohn's disease. *Gastroenterology* 1997; **113**: 383–9.

274 Fedorak RN, Gangl A, Elson CO, *et al.* Safety, tolerance, and efficacy of multiple doses of subcutaneous interleukin-10 in mild to moderate active Crohn's disease. *Gastroenterology* 1998; **114**: A974.

275 Vincenti F, Kirkman R, Light S, *et al.* Interleukin-2-receptor blockade with daclizumab to prevent acute rejection in renal transplantation. *N Engl J Med* 1998; **338**: 161–5.

276 Sands BE, Bank S, Sninsk CA, *et al.* Preliminary evaluation of safety and activity of recombinant human interleukin 11 in patients with active Crohn's disease. *Gastroenterology* 1999; **117**: 58–64.

277 Fuss IJ, Marth T, Neurath MF, Pearlstein GR, Jain A, Strober W. Anti-interleukin 12 treatment regulates apoptosis of Th1 T cells in experimental colitis in mice. *Gastroenterology* 1999; **117**: 1078–88.

278 Madsen SM, Schlichting P, Davidsen B, *et al.* An open, randomized study comparing systemic interferon-alpha-2a and prednisolone enemas in the treatment of left-sided ulcerative colitis. *Gut* 1999; **45**(Suppl V): A286.

279 Debinski H, Forbes A, Kamm MA. Low dose interferon gamma for refractory Crohn's disease. *Ital J Gastroenterol Hepatol* 1997; **29**: 403–6.

280 Neurath MF, Pettersson S, Meyer zum Buschenfelde K-H, Strober W. Local administration of antisense phosphorothioate oligonucleotides to the p65 subunit of NF-κB abrogates established experimental colitis in mice. *Nat Med* 1996; **2**: 998–1004.

281 Powrie F, Leach MW, Mauze S, Caddle LB, Coffman RL. Phenotypically distinct subtypes of CD4+ T cells induce or protect from chronic intestinal inflammation in C.B-17 SCID mice. *Int Immunol* 1993; **5**: 1461–71.

282 Powrie F, Lesch MW, Mauze S, Menon S, Caddle LB, Coffman RL. Inhibition of Th1 responses prevents inflammatory bowel disease in SCID mice reconstituted with CD45Rbhi CD4+ T cells. *Immunity* 1994; **1**: 553–62.

283 Baert FJ, D'Haens GR, Peeters M, *et al.* Tumor necrosis factor alpha antibody (infliximab) therapy profoundly down-regulates the inflammation in Crohn's ileocolitis. *Gastroenterology* 1999; **116**: 22–8.

284 Van Dullemen HM, Van Deventer SJH, Hommes DW, *et al.* Treatment of Crohn's disease with anti-tumor necrosis factor chimeric monoclonal antibody (cA2). *Gastroenterology* 1995; **109**: 129–35.

285 Targan SR, Hanauer SB, Van Deventer S, *et al.* A short-term study of chimeric monoclonal

antibody cA2 to tumor necrosis factor α for Crohn's disease. *N Engl J Med* 1997; **337**: 1029–35.

286 Rutgeerts P, D'Haens G, Targan S, *et al.* Efficacy and safety of retreatment with anti-tumor necrosis factor (infliximab) to maintain remission in Crohn's disease. *Gastroenterology* 1999; **117**: 761–9.

287 D'Haens G, Van Deventer S, Van Hogezand R, *et al.* Endoscopic and histological healing with infliximab anti-tumor necrosis factor antibodies in Crohn's disease: a European multicenter trial. *Gastroenterology* 1999; **116**: 1029–34.

288 Nikolaus S, Fölsch UR, Raedler A, Schreiber S. Increased peripheral production of TNFα and mucosal levels of activated NFκb predict relapse after treatment with infliximab in patients with Crohn's disease. *Gut* 1999; **45**(Suppl V): A2.

289 Vermeire S, Monsuur F, Groenen P, *et al.* Response to anti-TNFα treatment is associated with the TNFα-308*1 allele. *Gastroenterology* 2000; **118**: A654.

290 Marion JF, Bodian C, Lisa T, *et al.* TNF microsatellite polymorphism does not predict response to infliximab in patients with Crohn's disease. *Gastroenterology* 2000; **118**: A655.

291 Wong JB, Loftus EV, Sandborn WJ, Feagon BG. Estimating the cost-effectiveness of infliximab for Crohn's disease. *Gastroenterology* 1999; **116**: A105–6.

292 Toy LS, Scherl EJ, Kornbluth A, *et al.* Complete bowel obstruction following initial response to infliximab therapy for Crohn's disease: a series of a newly described complication. *Gastroenterology* 2000; **118**(Suppl 2): A569.

293 Pittman R, Toy LS, Kornbluth A, Present DH. Pretreatment with 6-mercaptopurine/azathioprine prolongs clinical response time in Crohn's disease patients with fistulizing disease treated with infliximab. *Gastroenterology* 2000; **118**(Suppl 2): A788.

294 Stack WA, Mann SD, Roy AJ, *et al.* Randomised controlled trial of CDP571 antibody to tumour necrosis factor-α in Crohn's disease. *Lancet* 1997; **349**: 521–4.

295 Sandborn WJ, Targan SR, Hanauer SB, *et al.* A randomized controlled trial of CDP571, a humanized antibody to TNFα, in moderately to severely active Crohn's disease. *Gastroenterology* 2000; **118**: A655.

296 Feagan BG, Sandborn WJ, Baker JP, *et al.* A randomized double-blind placebo-controlled multi-center trial of the engineered human antibody to TNF (CDP571) for steroid sparing and maintenance of remission in patients with steroid-dependent Crohn's disease. *Gastroenterology* 2000; **118**: A655.

297 Moreland LW, Schiff MH, Baumgartner SW, *et al.* Etanercept therapy in rheumatoid arthritis: a randomized controlled trial. *Ann Intern Med* 1999; **130**: 478–86.

298 D'Haens G, Swijsen C, Noman M, Lemmens L, Geboes K, Rutgeerts P. Etanercept (TNF receptor fusion protein, Enbrel®) is effective and well tolerated in active refractory Crohn's disease: results of a single center pilot study. *Gastroenterology* 2000; **118**(Suppl 2): A656.

299 Moreria A, Sampaio E, Zmuidzinas A, Frindt P, Smith K, Kaplan G. Thalidomide exerts its inhibitory action on tumor necrosis factor alpha by enhancing mRNA degradation. *J Exp Med* 1993; **177**: 1675–80.

300 Vasiliauskas EA, Kam LY, Abreu-Martin MT, *et al.* An open-label pilot study of low-dose thalidomide in chronically active, steroid-dependent Crohn's disease. *Gastroenterology* 1999; **117**: 1278–87.

301 Ehrenpreis ED, Kane SV, Cohen LB, Cohen RD, Hanauer SB. Thalidomide therapy for patients with refractory Crohn's disease: an open-label trial. *Gastroenterology* 1999; **117**: 1271–7.

302 Wedel S, Bauditz J, Suk A, Lochs H. Efficacy of thalidomide in Crohn's disease. *Gut* 1999; **45**(Suppl V): A133.

303 Kam LY, Vasiliauskas EA, Abreu MT, Hassard PV, Zeldis J, Targan SR. Open labeled pilot study of thalidomide as a novel therapy for medically resistant ulcerative colitis. *Gastroenterology* 2000; **118**(Suppl 2): A582.

304 Bauditz J, Haemling J, Ortner M, Lochs H, Raedler A, Schreiber S. Treatment with tumour necrosis factor inhibitor oxpentifylline does not improve corticosteroid dependent chronic active Crohn's disease. *Gut* 1997; **40**: 470–4.

305 Watkins PE, Warren BF, Stephens S, Ward P, Foulkes R. Treatment of ulcerative colitis in the cottontop tamarin using antibody to tumour necrosis factor alpha. *Gut* 1997; **40**: 628–33.

306 Evans RC, Clarke L, Heath P, Stephens S, Morris AI, Rhodes JM. Treatment of ulcerative colitis with an engineered human anti-TNFalpha antibody CDP571. *Aliment Pharmacol Ther* 1997; **11**: 1031–5.

307 Sands BE, Podolsky DK, Tremaine WJ, *et al.* Chimeric monoclonal anti-tumor necrosis factor antibody (cA2) in the treatment of severe, steroid-refractory ulcerative colitis. *Gastroenterology* 1996; **110**: A1008.

308 Levin S, Fischer S, Christie D, Haggitt R, Ochs H. Intravenous immunoglobulin therapy for active extensive and medically refractory idiopathic ulcerative or Crohn's colitis. *Am J Gastroenterol* 1992; **87**: 91–100.

309 Bicks RO, Groshart KD. The current status of T-lymphocyte apheresis (TLA) treatment of Crohn's disease. *J Clin Gastroenterol* 1989; **11**: 136–8.

310 Lerebours E, Bussel A, Modigliani R, *et al.* Treatment of Crohn's disease by lymphocyte apheresis: a randomized controlled trial. *Gastroenterology* 1994; **107**: 357–61.

311 Sawada K, Ohnishi K, Kosaka T, *et al.* Leukocytapheresis with leukocyte removal filter as new therapy for ulcerative colitis. *Ther Apher* 1997; **1**: 207–11.

312 Emmrich J, Seyfarth M, Fleig W, Emmrich F. Treatment of inflammatory bowel disease with anti-CD4 monoclonal antibody. *Lancet* 1991; **338**: 570–1.

313 Canva-Delcambre V, Jacquot S, Robinet E, *et al.* Treatment of severe Crohn's disease with anti-CD4 monoclonal antibody. *Aliment Pharmacol Ther* 1996; **10**: 721–7.

314 Stronkhorst A, Radema S, Yon SL, *et al.* CD4 antibody treatment in patients with active Crohn's disease, a phase 1 dose finding study. *Gut* 1997; **40**: 320–7.

315 Murch SH, Winyard PJD, Koletzko S, *et al.* Congenital enterocyte heparan sulphate deficiency with massive albumin loss, secretory diarrhoea, and malnutrition. *Lancet* 1996; **347**: 1299–301.

316 Day R, Ilyas M, Daszak P, Talbot I, Forbes A. Expression of syndecan-1 in inflammatory bowel disease and a possible mechanism of heparin therapy. *Dig Dis Sci* 1999; **44**: 2508–15.

317 Day R, Forbes A. Heparin, cell adhesion, and pathogenesis of inflammatory bowel disease. *Lancet* 1999; **354**: 62–5.

318 Bousvaros A, Zurakowski D, Fishman SJ, *et al.* Serum basic fibroblast growth factor in pediatric Crohn's disease. Implications for wound healing. *Dig Dis Sci* 1997; **42**: 378–86.

319 Day R, Rowlands D, Knight S, Forbes A. Epithelial syndecan-1 expression is reduced by tumour necrosis factor-α *in vitro*. *Gut* 1999; **45**(Suppl V): A125.

320 Salas A, Sans M, Soriano A, *et al.* Heparin attenuates TNF-α induced inflammatory response through a CD11b dependent mechanism. *Gut* 2000; **47**: 88–96.

321 Lalor P, Adams DH, Langman MJS, Michell NP. Inhibition of neutrophil recruitment: how heparin ameliorates ulcerative colitis? *Gut* 2000; **46**(Suppl II): A2.

322 Dotan I, Hershkoviz R, Karmeli F, Rachmilewitz D. Low molecular weight heparin (clexane) significantly ameliorates experimental colitis. *Gastroenterology* 1999; **116**: A702.

323 Tyrrell DJ, Horne AP, Holme KR, Preuss JM, Page CP. Heparin in inflammation: potential therapeutic applications beyond anticoagulation. *Adv Pharmacol* 1999; **46**: 151–208.

324 Dwarakanath AD, Yu LG, Brookes C, *et al.* 'Sticky' neutrophils pathergic arthritis and response to heparin in pyoderma gangrenosum complicating ulcerative colitis. *Gut* 1995; **37**: 585–8.

325 Gaffney PR, Doyle CT, Gaffney A, Hogan J, Hayes DP, Annis P. Paradoxical response to heparin in 10 patients with ulcerative colitis. *Am J Gastroenterol* 1995; **90**: 220–3.

326 Evans RC, Wong VS, Morris AI, Rhodes JM. Treatment of corticosteroid-resistant ulcerative colitis with heparin – a report of 16 cases. *Aliment Pharmacol Ther* 1997; **11**: 1037–40.

327 Dupas JL, Brazier F, Yzet T, Roussel B, Duchmann JC, Iglicki F. Treatment of active Crohn's disease with heparin. *Gastroenterology* 1996; **110**: A900.

328 Brazier F, Yzet T, Duchmann JC, Iglicki F, Dupas JL. Effect of heparin treatment on extra-intestinal manifestations associated with inflammatory bowel disease. *Gastroenterology* 1996; **110**: A872.

329 Torkvist L, Thorlacius H, Sjoqvist U, *et al.* Low molecular weight heparin as adjuvant therapy in active ulcerative colitis. *Aliment Pharmacol Ther* 1999; **13**: 1323–8.

330 Vrij AA, Schoon EJ, Hemker HC, Stockbrugger RW. Low molecular weight heparin treatment in steroid refractory ulcerative colitis. *Gastroenterology* 1999; **116**: A841.

331 Folwaczny C, Wiebecke B, Loeschke K. Unfractioned heparin in the therapy of patients with highly active inflammatory bowel disease. *Am J Gastroenterol* 1999; **94**: 1551–5.

332 Panes J, Esteve M, Cabre E, *et al.* Comparison of heparin and steroids in the treatment of moderate and severe ulcerative colitis. *Gastroenterology* 2000; **118**: A874.

333 Yacyshyn BR, Bowen-Yacyshyn MB, Jewell L, *et al.* A placebo controlled trial of ICAM-1 antisense oligonucleotide in the treatment of Crohn's disease. *Gastroenterology* 98; **114**: 1133–42.

334 Schreiber S, Malchow H, Kruis W, *et al.* Antisense ICAM-1 (ISIS-2302) for subcutaneous treatment of chronic active Crohn's disease: lack of efficacy in a prospective double-blind multicenter randomized trial. *Gastroenterology* 2000; **118**(Suppl 2): A568–9.

335 Hesterberg PE, Winsor-Hines D, Briskin MJ, *et al.* Rapid resolution of chronic colitis in the cotton-top tamarin with an antibody to a gut-homing integrin $\alpha 4\beta 7$. *Gastroenterology* 1996; **111**: 1373–80.

336 Feagan BG, McDonald JWD, Greenberg G, *et al.* An ascending dose trial of a humanized $\alpha 4\beta 7$ antibody in ulcerative colitis. *Gastroenterology* 2000; **118**: A874.

337 Gordon FH, Rana S, Tahami F, Khan K, Amlot PL, Pounder RE. Adhesion molecule expression in inflammatory bowel disease patients treated with natalizumab (Antegren®), a humanized antibody to A4 integrin. *Gastroenterology* 2000; **118**: A344.

338 Myrup B, Valerius NH, Mortensen PB. Treatment of enteritis in CGD with granulocyte colony stimulating factor. *Gut* 1998; **42**: 127–30.

339 Roe TF, Coates TD, Thomas DW, Miler JH, Gilsanz V. Treatment of chronic inflammatory bowel disease in glycogen storage disease type 1b with colony stimulating factors. *N Engl J Med* 1992; **326**: 1666–9.

340 Vaughan D, Drumm B. Treatment of fistulas with granulocyte colony stimulating factor in a patient with Crohn's disease. *N Engl J Med* 1999; **340**: 239–40.

341 Dejaco C, Gasche C, Poetze R, *et al.* Safety and efficacy of granulocyte colony stimulating factor for treatment of severe endoscopic postoperative recurrence in Crohn's disease. *Gastroenterology* 2000; **118**(Suppl 2): A566.

342 Korzenik JR, Dieckgraefe BK. Immuno-stimulation in Crohn's disease: results of a pilot study of G-CSF in mucosal and fistulizing Crohn's disease. *Gastroenterology* 2000; **118**: A874–5.

343 Slonim AE, Bulone L, Damore MB, *et al.* A preliminary study of growth hormone therapy for Crohn's disease. *N Engl J Med* 2000; **342**: 1633–7.

344 Pullan, RD, Rhodes J, Ganesh S, *et al.* Transdermal nicotine for active ulcerative colitis. *N Engl J Med* 1994; **330**: 811–15.

345 Hanauer SB. Nicotine for colitis – the smoke has not yet cleared. *N Engl J Med* 1994; **330**: 856–7.

346 Sandborn WJ, Tremaine WJ, Offord KP, *et al.* Transdermal nicotine for mildly to moderately active ulcerative colitis. A randomized, double-blind, placebo-controlled trial. *Ann Intern Med* 1997; **126**: 364–71.

347 Louvet B, Buisine MP, Desreumaux P, *et al.* Transdermal nicotine decreases mucosal IL-8 expression but has no effect on mucin gene expression in ulcerative colitis. *Inflamm Bowel Dis* 1999; **5**: 174–81.

348 Thomas GAO, Rhodes J, Ragunath K, *et al.* Transdermal nicotine compared with oral prednisolone therapy for active ulcerative colitis. *Eur J Gastroenterol Hepatol* 1996; **8**: 769–76.

349 Sandborn WJ, Tremaine WJ, Leighton JA, *et al.* Nicotine tartrate liquid enemas for mildly to moderately active left-sided ulcerative colitis

unresponsive to first-line therapy: a pilot study. *Aliment Pharmacol Ther* 1997; **11**: 663–71.

350 Green JT, Thomas GA, Rhodes J, *et al.* Nicotine enemas for active ulcerative colitis – a pilot study. *Aliment Pharmacol Ther* 1997; **11**: 859–63.

351 Compton RF, Sandborn WJ, Lawson GM, *et al.* A dose-ranging pharmacokinetic study of nicotine tartrate following single-dose delayed-release oral and intravenous administration. *Aliment Pharmacol Ther* 1997; **11**: 865–74.

352 Thomas GAO, Rhodes J, Mani V, *et al.* Transdermal nicotine as maintenance therapy for ulcerative colitis. *N Engl J Med* 1995; **332**: 988–92.

353 Verspaget H, Mulder T, Van der Sluys Veer A, Pena A, Lamers C. Reactive oxygen metabolites and colitis: a disturbed balance between damage and protection: a selective review. *Scand J Gastroenterol* 1991; **26**: 44–51.

354 Kesharvarzian A, Haydeck J, Zabihi R, Doria M, D'Astice M, Sorenson JR. Agents capable of eliminating reactive oxygen species. Catalase, WR-2721, or $Cu(II)_2(2,5\text{-DIPS})_4$ decrease experimental colitis. *Dig Dis Sci* 1992; **37**: 1866–73.

355 Millar AD, Blake DR, Rampton DS. An open trial of antioxidant nutrient therapy in active ulcerative colitis. *Gut* 1994; **35**(Suppl 5): S29.

356 Salim A. Role of oxygen derived free radical scavengers in the management of recurrent attacks of ulcerative colitis: a new approach. *J Lab Clin Med* 1992; **119**: 710–17.

357 Emerit J, Pelletier S, Likforman J, *et al.* Phase II trial of copper zinc superoxide dismutase in the treatment of Crohn's disease. *Free Radic Res Commun* 1991; **12–13**: 563–9.

358 Bjørck S, Dahlstrom A, Ahlman H. Topical treatment of ulcerative proctitis with lidocaine. *Scand J Gastroenterol* 1989; **24**: 1061–72.

359 MacGregor RR, Thorner RE, Wright DM. Lidocaine inhibits granulocyte adherence and prevents granulocyte delivery to inflammatory sites. *Blood* 1980; **56**: 203–9.

360 Lahav M, Bar-Meir S, Tal R, Chowers Y. Lidocaine inhibits secretion of pro-inflamamtory mediators from HT29 intestinal epithelial cells. *Gastroenterology* 2000; **118**: A97.

361 Feinstein MB, Fiekers J, Fraser C. An analysis of the mechanism of local anesthetic inhibition of platelet aggregation and secretion. *J Pharmacol Exp Ther* 1976; **197**: 215–28.

362 Arlander E, Ost A, Ståhlberg, Löfberg R. Ropivacaine gel in active distal ulcerative colitis and proctitis – a pharmacokinetic and exploratory clinical study. *Aliment Pharmacol Ther* 1996; **10**: 73–81.

363 Bohr J, Olesen M, Tysk C, Järnerot G. Budesonide and bismuth in microscopic colitis. *Gut* 1999; **45**(Suppl V): A202.

364 Raithel M, Schwab D, Winterkamp S, Weidenhiller M, Ottmann B, Hahn EG. Double-blind placebo-controlled randomized pilot trial of additional H1-receptor antagonist treatment in active ulcerative colitis. *Gastroenterology* 2000; **118**(Suppl 2): A587.

365 Madsen KL, Doyle JS, Jewell LD, *et al. Lactobacillus* species prevents colitis in interleukin 10 gene-deficient mice. *Gastroenterology* 1999; **116**: 1107–14.

366 Steidler L, Hans W, Schotte L, *et al.* Treatment of murine colitis by *Lactococcus lactis* secreting interleukin-10. *Science* 2000; **289**: 1352–5.

367 Jensen MR, Dalum I, Steinaa L, *et al.* Immunization against TNFα – a new approach for the treatment of inflammatory bowel disease. *Gastroenterology* 2000; **118**: A873.

368 Langmead L, Chitnis M, Rampton DS. Complementary therapy in inflammatory bowel disease patients: who uses it and why? *Gastroenterology* 2000; **118**(Suppl 2): A119.

Problematic ulcerative colitis, and surgery for inflammatory bowel disease

Acute severe or fulminant colitis

Acute severe or fulminant colitis remains an important clinical problem and is still responsible for major morbidity and occasional mortality. In many respects the medical management is simple, but the necessity for and timing of surgery remain difficult to judge. Much of this section is therefore taken up with consideration of prognostic indicators early in the clinical course, and the related indications for timely surgical intervention. Fulminant colitis was defined in the 1950s by Truelove and Witts, from the combination of frequent bloody diarrhoea with evidence of systemic illness. No better definition has emerged, other than in the form of minor modifications of the original description, such as that from the Oxford group in the 1980s (Table 4.1).[1]

Table 4.1 Definition of fulminant colitis

In a patient with established ulcerative colitis, the presence of:

more than 5 bloody stools per 24 hours
and at least one of
fever (> 37°C)
tachycardia (> 90/min)
ESR > 30 mm/h
haemoglobin < 100 g/L
albumin < 35 g/L

Most patients with very active disease have many of the signs of systemic disease, and any patient with a complication of aggressive colitis (such as toxic megacolon) would be considered to have fulminant colitis even in the unlikely event of their absence.

The mortality of fulminant colitis has fallen substantially since the middle of the twentieth century, from around 50 per cent before the introduction of steroids in the early 1950s,[2] to around 1.5 per cent in most centres now. This reduction has not, however, been the result of single critical changes in practice, as even steroids brought the mortality down only to around 30 per cent in the early 1960s. The improvement almost certainly reflects earlier diagnosis, better medical and perioperative care (including safer anaesthesia), but possibly most importantly, the greater sharing of management between physicians and surgeons. Unfortunately this cooperation appears to function least well in centres with the least experience of life-threatening colitis. Any patient sick enough to warrant admission for ulcerative colitis also warrants referral to both medical and surgical gastroenterologists. This practice makes joint planning easier and eliminates the surgeons' concerns that some patients are referred too late, as well as the physicians' frustrations when, having managed the patient actively for some days and reached the conclusion that surgery is inevitable, the surgeon chooses to observe for a further period whilst becoming familiar with the patient!

There is rarely a substantial differential diagnosis when the patient is already known to have ulcerative colitis, but the occasional patient with Crohn's disease presents in this way, and the largest group of patients with a final diagnosis of indeterminate colitis are those in whom an initial fulminant presentation led to early resection. However, in the known colitic as well as in the new case, it is essential to exclude infective causes, and perhaps especially, superimposed *Clostridium difficile* infection (see Chapter 2).

The immediate management of fulminant colitis includes bed rest, and intravenous steroids, with parenteral fluids and blood if necessary. There are few data favouring a particular steroid, although adrenocorticotropic hormone (ACTH) may offer minor advantage if the patient has not previously been exposed to steroid therapy. It may not even be necessary to give the steroid parenterally as (for example) in Denmark similar results are obtained from high-dose oral therapy. A daily regimen based on prednisolone or methylprednisolone 1 mg/kg or hydrocortisone 4 mg/kg is appropriate, whichever route is chosen. Some centres consider that the addition of topical steroids is also helpful. Response to steroid therapy can be anticipated in about two-thirds of these patients.[3] There is no evidence that the routine addition of antibiotics is helpful, and a small deleterious difference between treated and untreated groups has been documented from the development of antibiotic-related pseudomembranous colitis. There is no place for nutritional intervention as specific therapy (although it will clearly be an important part of adjunctive management and especially so in the malnourished patient). Bowel rest does not appear to offer any advantage, with evidence that normal eating produces similar results to fasting, with or without parenteral nutrition.[4]

Urgent surgery is almost always indicated in fulminant colitis if complications arise. It is mandatory in the event of perforation, and virtually so in massive haemorrhage (which can be considered to be the case in any patient requiring a transfusion of more than 6 units or daily administration of blood). Surgery should naturally follow full resuscitative measures and should be performed by an experienced colorectal surgeon.

Toxic megacolon complicates no more than 10 per cent of cases with fulminant colitis, but is the major indication for surgery in around 25 per cent of the most urgent cases. The condition is readily defined from the diameter of the colon or caecum on a plain abdominal radiograph (Figure 4.1). It is usually easiest to identify in the transverse colon, where a diameter in excess of 5.5 cm is considered diagnostic in the context of acute colitis. The predominance of this site simply reflects the colonic anatomy, as this is generally the least dependent part of the colon when the patient lies supine, and is therefore gas-filled and most easily

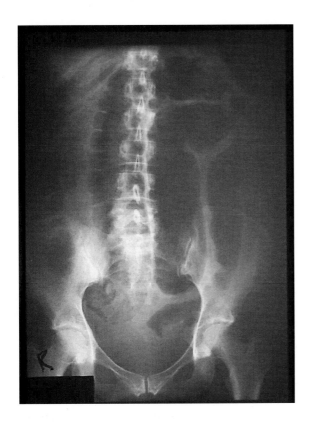

Figure 4.1 Toxic megacolon clearly demonstrated on plain abdominal film. This case was of interest because megacolon developed in the absence of pan-colitis, and the well-preserved pattern of taeniae in the right colon even in the presence of distal dilatation testifies to this. There was no response to brief intensive medical therapy; surgery confirmed the severity of the condition but also its persistent limited extent.

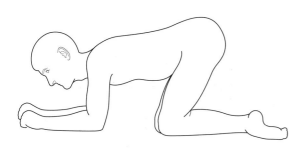

Figure 4.2 The knee–elbow position as advocated for relief of megacolon; when achieved, the rectosigmoid becomes the most superior part of the gastrointestinal tract, facilitating spontaneous passage of flatus.

visualized. A caecal diameter of more than 9 cm has identical significance. Many gastroenterologists and most surgeons consider megacolon to be an absolute indication for colectomy. This is a safe but perhaps unnecessarily aggressive strategy. It is probably reasonable to permit 24 hours of medical therapy in a patient who presents untreated with megacolon, but megacolon developing during therapy or persisting for more than 24 hours despite therapy should lead to colectomy. In this context the value of rolling the patient or encouraging the taking up of certain postures may be valuable (as also in the patient distressed by air insufflation at colonoscopy). The British technique[5] (Figure 4.2) places the patient in the knee–elbow position, whereas the North American method implies more rolling of the patient (to the prone position every few hours), often combined with the use of a rectal tube to help in deflation of the distal bowel.[6] Both techniques are reported to resolve megacolon without subsequent need for surgery. All forms of medical therapy for megacolon may, however, be considered to be temporizing manoeuvres, as around 50 per cent of patients so treated come to colectomy within a year. Equally, some of these are able to have elective surgery with its obvious advantages relative to emergency resection.

It should be remembered that evidence even for such serious complications as perforation and frank faecal peritonitis can be masked by the high doses of steroids being used. A low threshold for surgical intervention should be maintained.

Predictors for failure of medical therapy once the major complications have been sought and excluded reflect evidence of disease severity and involvement of the full thickness of the colon. A detailed review of patients presenting to St Mark's Hospital with fulminant colitis identified a number of criteria for poor outcome (Table 4.2).[7] More recent data[8,9] led to similar conclusions, adding a short history, extensive colitis, anaemia, and high erythrocyte sedimentation rate (ESR). The Oxford data were derived from study of the 49 patients seen there on 51 occasions over an 18-month period in which cyclosporin was available but not uniformly used (14/51 cases; see Chapter 3).[8] Outcomes were

defined as: complete response (fewer than four stools per day with no blood by day 7); partial response (more than three stools or blood on day 7 but colectomy not performed that admission); or colectomy. As is typical in studies of fulminant colitis, 29 per cent required colectomy during the acute admission. The stool frequency and the C-reactive protein (CRP) on days 1–5 were associated with the final outcomes, such that on day 3, 85 per cent of patients with more than eight stools on that day, or between three and eight stools and a CRP >45, would require colectomy. The authors comment appropriately that these patients should be identified and managed carefully, but there is an element of circular reasoning. Although surgery clearly will not have been decided upon because of continuing bloody diarrhoea and a high CRP alone, this combination is a very powerful one, as it includes a verifiable and distressing symptom, and one of the more objective markers of disease. It is most unlikely therefore that the Oxford authors were uninfluenced in their decisions about surgery by the very markers that they now propose as predictors. Of arguably greater value is the observation that the partial responders at 7 days had a 60 per cent chance of continuing symptoms, an 82 per cent risk of needing continuing immunosuppression, and a 40 per cent chance of colectomy during the follow-up period (median 12 months).

Table 4.2 Adverse prognostic factors in fulminant colitis

Criterion	Failure rate
> 8 stools/day	33%
Pulse rate > 100/min	36%
Maximum temperature > 38°C	56%
Serum albumin < 30 g/L	42%
Presence of mucosal islands on plain abdominal radiograph	75%
Small bowel dilatation	73%

The CRP is probably more informative than the sedimentation rate in inflammatory bowel disease, and elevated levels have similar adverse significance. The failure of the CRP to fall with medical therapy is particularly important. As corticosteroids suppress all the acute phase proteins even in the absence of reduced inflammation at the site of most interest, their failure to decrease the CRP indicates progressive and uncontrolled disease.[10]

Severe diarrhoea is accompanied by a loss of sodium and hydrogen ions, and an abnormally acid stool. This can lead in turn to a systemic metabolic alkalosis. Given that most sick patients develop a metabolic acidosis, the presence of alkalosis should be taken seriously, and Caprilli et al.[11] consider this a useful adverse prognostic feature.

In addition to toxic megacolon itself, there are two other key abnormalities discernible from the plain film. The presence of mucosal islands along the length of the colon indicates a virtually complete loss of the mucosal surface, the beginnings of full-thickness damage to the bowel and a very high risk of later perforation if colectomy is not undertaken (Table 4.2). The islands – raised areas protruding into the lumen – are in fact the last remaining regions of relatively preserved mucosa. Similarly, the presence of (three or more) dilated loops of small bowel is predictive of a poorer outcome (Table 4.2) and, indeed, of the development of toxic megacolon itself,[12,13] the Oxford group finding this sign in 73 per cent of those who subsequently required surgery, compared with in only 43 per cent of those responding to medical therapy. When there were five or more distended loops, all patients required surgery. Again there is some difficulty in interpretation given that earlier data[7] predicted these outcomes and presumably had some bearing on the decision to embark on surgical intervention.

Almer et al.[14] have, in effect, expanded on the plain abdominal film with their study of 'air enema radiography' in 35 (of 49) patients with acute severe colitis who went on to surgery, and in whom they felt that the plain film was not adequate. Air was 'gently insufflated' under fluoroscopic control, with patients on their left sides, aiming to reach the caecum. A 'sufficient volume' of air was judged as that at which the mucosal outline was easily seen and in most cases was between 500 and 800 mL. There was excellent agreement between radiological assessment of depth of mucosal ulceration and that demonstrable histologically in the resected colon – overall accuracy was 86 per cent. It is not clear whether the technique was useful in those who did not need surgery, and the paper does not entirely exclude a relationship between the procedure and a subsequent adverse event (such as perforation). It is likely, but unproven, that the technique is as safe as instant barium enema, which has a very impressive safety record.[15] It is almost certainly safer than colonoscopy in this setting. Colonoscopy was responsible for a major complication in one of only 46 patients with severe disease in a report from the principal protagonists of the technique.[16] It is nevertheless surprising that air enema was necessary in such a high proportion of patients, since the required information would be expected from the unenhanced plain film much more often than in the 22 per cent of cases (11 of 49) reported.

A suggested framework of clinical and investigatory monitoring is given in Table 4.3. Most of the elements are standard observations, but it is surprisingly informative to collect the various items onto a single 'colitis observations proforma'. Although there is implicit benefit in a daily assessment of the fulminant colitic by a senior clinician, who will often be able to provide a reliable overall assessment from clinical review alone, the global assessments made by the well-supported junior using the proforma are rarely different. Measurement of abdominal girth is notoriously irreproducible and is not recommended.

Table 4.3 Fulminant colitis: suggested framework for clinical and investigatory monitoring

Pulse	6 hourly
Temperature	6 hourly
Stool frequency	Recorded on daily basis
Stool consistency	Recorded on daily basis
Presence of blood?	Recorded on daily basis
Abdominal tenderness?	Recorded on daily basis
Nature of bowel sounds	Recorded on daily basis
Serum electrolytes	Daily
Full blood count	Daily
Plain abdominal radiograph	Daily
Serum CRP (or ESR)	Thrice weekly
Serum albumin	Thrice weekly
'Global assessment'	Daily – recorded as better, same, or worse

Early surgery should be considered for fulminant colitis if any complication develops, or if there is an overall deterioration despite appropriate medical therapy. Surgery should also be planned if there has been no improvement by around 5 days from the initiation of aggressive steroid therapy. Surgery is probably indicated in all patients in whom any monitoring criterion worsens, even if the overall status appears quite reasonable, and particularly so when the CRP fails to fall, or if one of the key radiological signs emerges. A useful aphorism runs as follows: 'When the patient feels well but the signs are bad, the colon is usually a mess and should be removed', or more simply: 'If in doubt, operate'.

There is probably only one operation to be considered in this context – the subtotal colectomy with ileostomy formation (and probably a mucous fistula to vent the rectosigmoid). This aborts the emergency, avoids the dangers of extensive pelvic dissection in the acute situation, and permits elective pouch surgery to be considered at leisure. Even with this approach, colectomy for fulminant colitis has a mortality in the region of 5 per cent (compared with less than 1 per cent for taxing, pouch-creating, elective surgery – see below).

The place of ciclosporin in the management of the fulminant colitic is dealt with in detail in Chapter 3, but neither its use nor that of other medical therapies should be permitted to delay laparotomy in the unresponsive patient if we are to retain the improved prognosis that has come from the earlier and safer surgery practised through the past 25 years.

It should be recognized that a single episode of fulminant colitis – however catastrophic – once survived without surgery, ceases to have any direct bearing on surgical planning for that patient. Although such patients do not escape future severe exacerbations, their risk thereof and of needing surgery is no greater than for other individuals with similar disease extent (and may be less)[17] (see Chapter 2).

Problematic distal ulcerative colitis

In most cases, distal ulcerative colitis will respond well to the simple measures outlined in Chapter 3, the northern European emphasis on topical steroids for acute disease gradually being eroded by increasing use of topical 5-ASA, with probable greater efficacy if also greater cost. Unfortunately, there are patients in whom the disease is manifestly limited to a short segment of distal bowel, but in whom symptom control is not achieved. In many cases, this is because the problem is a functional one akin to irritable bowel syndrome rather than predominantly the result of uncontrolled inflammation. In this event, endoscopic examination reveals unremarkable macroscopic features, although care should be taken to ensure that active disease does not exist proximal to the lowermost zone within range of the rigid sigmoidoscope where disease has been controlled by topical therapy. If symptoms do appear out of proportion to objective criteria, it is reasonable to consider symptomatic measures in addition to continuing topical 5-ASA (or steroid) therapy. Loperamide or another opioid may be sufficient, but many patients obtain greater benefit from increased fibre (for example as ispaghula) or lactulose, as proximal constipation is just as often the cause of distress (see Chapter 2). There is also some evidence that lactulose, by virtue of its intraluminal metabolism to short-chain fatty acids, may have a therapeutic effect on colitis in its own right[18] (unpublished observations). Other strategies used for irritable bowel syndrome can also be valuable.

When the distal disease is macroscopically active, the combination of topical steroid and 5-ASA is worth trying (see Chapter 3), and patience can also be rewarded, many patients coming into remission over 6–8 weeks simply by continuing a regimen that was not initially helpful. Alternative topical regimens based on the various agents outlined in Chapter 3 have their advocates, and it will often be appropriate to conduct therapeutic trials. Reliable data are lacking, especially in this context of resistant disease. When a selection of such measures have failed, and especially if there are indicators of systemic disease such as an elevated platelet count or CRP, I am comfortable managing the patient as if the colitis was more extensive and am accordingly happy to consider

systemic steroids and azathioprine. Azathioprine has not been subjected to controlled trial in this context but appears to yield a response rate comparable to that in patients with more extensive disease.

Surgery is obviously a less attractive proposition when much of the colon is felt to be normal, but will be appropriate in some resistant patients. The correct operation is total colectomy, since more limited resection is almost always followed by aggressive relapse in the previously normal bowel (see below). Between 10 and 15 per cent of the colectomies performed for ulcerative colitis at St Mark's are currently in patients with intractable limited disease, and at least 5 per cent might be expected for this indication in a more general colorectal surgical practice.

Surgery

Surgery is rarely the first therapy considered in inflammatory bowel disease but often proves an important component of overall management in affected patients. The indications for early and occasionally emergency surgery for fulminant colitis have been enumerated above, but in other circumstances the decision should be more of an elective one with contributions to the decision-making process from each of the three key parties: physician, surgeon and patient.

ULCERATIVE COLITIS

Surgery is required in ulcerative colitis for one of three main indications:

- uncontrolled severe acute disease and especially so if there are complications;
- uncontrolled chronic disease, with either a lack of adequate response to medical therapy, or steroid dependence;
- the development of long-term complications such as dysplasia or frank malignancy (see Chapter 8).

At least 70 per cent of procedures are performed for the second indication in all the major centres. This is also the most patient-dependent indication, and careful analysis of the severity of symptoms and realistic expectations of surgery are essential in management planning.

Surgery for ulcerative colitis should be almost synonymous with total colectomy, because partial colectomy is usually followed by problematic relapse in the retained colon, and because the patient is otherwise left at risk of colorectal carcinoma. In a typical series of seven elderly patients in whom deliberately conservative surgery with segmental resection was performed, even limited follow-up revealed troublesome recurrence in all.[19] This recurrence of colitis is a problem even when documented distal disease has been fully resected, leaving apparently healthy proximal colon. A report from Varma and colleagues lends support to the numerous anecdotes to this effect.[20] All four patients treated by segmental resection had a major relapse in the neoterminal colon within 11 months (median 6 months), and no fewer than three required early completion colectomy and proctectomy. The complex course also reduced the eligibility for pouch surgery, further emphasizing the poor final outcome.

Total proctocolectomy with formation of an end ileostomy remains a viable option with relatively low (but significant) immediate complication rates, and a short period of perioperative morbidity; the cancer risk is eliminated and colitic symptoms are abolished. However, the presence of a permanent ileostomy is unacceptable to many, and the lifetime complication rate is well in excess of 50 per cent. In a detailed actuarial analysis of 150 patients with an end ileostomy, the 20-year frequency of stomal complications reached 75 per cent in ulcerative colitis (and 56 per cent in Crohn's disease).[21] There were a variety of skin problems, retraction and/or herniation of the stoma, and overt intestinal obstruction in 23 per cent. Revisional surgery had been necessary in 28 per cent of those where the stoma had been created for ulcerative colitis (and 16 per cent in Crohn's disease).

Good though the results of proctocolectomy and ileostomy generally are, it is understandable that patients seek more normal continence. Kock devised a continent ileostomy by fashioning a pouch from the terminal ileum, which was then secured to the abdominal wall. Parks took this idea a step further in the 1970s by anastomosing a similar pouch to the anal canal, thus creating the pelvic ileoanal pouch and a more truly restorative procedure, which has changed surgical practice. This has become the most frequently performed surgical procedure for ulcerative colitis in specialist centres – 75 of 145 operations at St Mark's through 1986–90,[22] and 57 of 79 first definitive procedures in 1998.[23] This is not the place for a detailed analysis of the surgical techniques, but an awareness of the principal options is worthwhile. The first decision is whether the surgery should be performed in a single operation or spread over two or more sessions. The patient with fulminant colitis should almost certainly have a simple (and safe) colectomy and ileostomy, with the later option of pouch creation when in remission. A consensus had been forming that a single-stage procedure in which the colectomy, proctectomy, and pouch creation were done together (with no defunctioning ileostomy) was appropriate for the majority of patients undergoing elective surgery. All defunctioning ileostomies need to be closed at some stage and are not themselves without complications. However, the consequences of pouch leakage are greatly reduced by a protecting up-stream stoma and many experienced surgeons have reverted to a two-stage procedure. Only in the more insistent patient in whom there is no technical difficulty with the pouch formation or greater than average anxieties about pelvic sepsis is a single-stage procedure undertaken.

The pouch may be made from a single loop or from multiple loops of ileum – the so-called 'J', 'S'

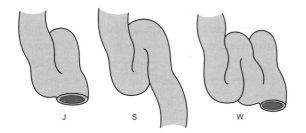

J   S   W

Figure 4.3 Three formats used in creation of the ileoanal pouch. The more 'folds' made in the terminal ileum, the greater the volume of the pouch and the less the need for frequent evacuation. The efferent limb of the 'S' pouch has been associated with a higher incidence of outlet obstruction and is now less favoured.

or 'W' pouch (Figure 4.3), may be stapled or hand sewn, and may be secured to the anal canal with a varying degree of stripping of the distal rectal and transitional mucosa. Stapling devices lend some degree of technical simplicity and speed in pouch creation, and aid the creation of a very distal anastomosis without damage to the anal sphincters, but leave a small 'cuff' of rectal mucosa which may pose a small but real risk of future neoplasia.

There is a tendency for the healthy pouch to take on a number of characteristics of normal colon (Plate 8). The normal villous pattern of the terminal ileum becomes somewhat blunted with shortening and broadening of the villi. It is unclear to what extent this represents an appropriate accommodation to the new reservoir function and the altered bacterial flora and to what degree it may be considered pathological. The magnitude of this colonic metaplasia does not appear to predict short- or long-term complications, however.

The different configurations of pouch anatomy have been compared frequently, but rarely in a controlled fashion. Most centres have moved firmly away from the 'S' pouch because of outflow problems (see below) and it has been felt that the decision between the 'J' and the 'W' was a compromise between the larger volume and assumed better final functional capacity of the latter, and the simpler surgery and shorter length of small bowel sacrificed in the former. A well-constructed, randomized, controlled trial done in Leeds has therefore been most helpful.[24] Sixty

patients received either a 'J' or a 'W' pouch constructed with 30 or 40 cm of ileum, respectively. At 1 year all were continent, although eight had minor leakage of mucus, and all were able to defer defecation for at least 15 minutes. The median bowel frequency was 5/24 hours in both groups of patients and there were no apparent differences in clinical outcome. The authors felt there was no longer any justification for the more complex procedure, and recommend a 30 cm 'J' pouch created with linear stapling instruments.

The commonest reasons for pouch failure are perianal and/or pelvic sepsis and unknowing pouch creation in Crohn's disease (but see below), with some patients falling prey to intractable inflammation within the pouch – pouchitis (see Chapter 1 and below). Pelvic sepsis affects around 15 per cent of patients to some extent, and although it rarely leads to loss of the pouch, it is responsible for considerable distress and protracted hospital stays. Early postoperative intestinal obstruction is seen in around 10 per cent and may also substantially delay discharge, up to half of affected patients needing further laparotomy;[25] the longer-term outcome of this complication is, however, good. Even including early cases at St Mark's (when the institution was still on the 'learning curve'), the cumulative rate of pouch failure was only 12 per cent at 5 years.[26] The magnitude of the undertaking from the patient's perspective should not, however, be underestimated, as 68 per cent of patients had required readmission during those 5 years for reasons other than for ileostomy closure, and roughly half of those had required further laparotomy. Typically, 3 months' morbidity can be expected even when things go well. It should be recognized that defecatory function is not normal in patients with a satisfactory pouch, as the frequency of evacuation is usually three to six times daily. This is not, however, associated with urgency or with much night-time waking, and patients can usually adapt well to this constraint, which is so much more predictable than their prior experiences with colitis. Comparisons with patients' own assessments of outcomes from proctocolectomy and ileostomy are heavily in favour of the reconstructive operation.[27] Even those patients unlucky enough to be troubled by some degree of incontinence report a preference for their new state compared with the prior colitis (and tend to wish that their surgery had been performed sooner).[28] A nice contrast is posed by patients having a restorative proctocolectomy for polyposis coli (for cancer prevention) in whom there were no previous colonic symptoms and in whom these failings are perceived less favourably.

Very few units now recommend colectomy with ileorectal anastomosis because rectal symptoms may still be a problem (to the extent of compromising continence) and because of the continuing concern about neoplasia. This may, however, be an appropriate option in the young patient who is very keen to avoid an ileostomy but who is not ready to invest the time required for pouch creation (or to run the remote risk of neuronal damage compromising sexual function). In this circumstance, a relatively generous portion of distal bowel should be left in continuity to avoid the need for two pelvic procedures. These patients need careful follow-up with attention to neoplastic risk as if total colitis still persisted until the rectum is finally removed (see Chapter 8).

Pouchitis

Inflammation within the newly created ileoanal pouch may be the result of gastrointestinal infection,

surrounding sepsis in the pelvis, or of mechanical deficiencies such as outlet obstruction, but also occurs when these factors are absent. This 'pouchitis' must be defined carefully and requires histological as well as clinical and endoscopic evidence for its confirmation. Publications and clinical decisions on pouchitis in the absence of these criteria should be treated with great reserve. Pouchitis is recognized in the Kock pouch as well as in the pelvic pouch at a comparable frequency[29] and is presumed to have little or nothing to do with the location of the pouch, but more to do with the underlying disease, as it hardly ever occurs in patients having pouch surgery for familial polyposis coli. It remains poorly understood, but several strands of evidence favour the idea that to some extent it represents ulcerative colitis of the ileal cells transformed by colonic metaplasia (see Chapter 1). It is possible that an imbalance in the intestinal flora is aetiologically important in the pathogenesis of pouchitis and the microflora of the ileal reservoir have accordingly been analysed.[30] Patients with pouchitis proved to have an increased number of aerobes and clostridia, with fungal species that were not found in controls, and relatively fewer anaerobes and lactobacilli. The prevailing pH also was more alkaline in those with pouchitis (6.5 versus 5.4). Unfortunately, these authors do not make the crucial distinction between the effects of pouchitis and the situation prior to its onset; these findings may all be secondary to pouchitis that has arisen for an unconnected reason. Serial estimations and challenge studies with the patients' own faecal stream prior to ileostomy closure in progress at St Mark's will hopefully clarify this. Pouchitis is probably not more common in those with pANCA (see Chapter 1).[31,32]

A frequency of pouchitis (at some time) in the region of 20 per cent is to be expected, but problematic disease is much less common, and leads to pouch excision in well under 5 per cent of patients in most series. There do not appear to be any reliable clinical pointers to a higher risk of pouchitis in ulcerative colitis patients apart from a slightly higher risk in males[33] and in those with initially the most extensive colitis.[34]

Pouchitis most commonly presents acutely with proctitis-like symptoms that settle rapidly with or without intervention, but in about half of those affected there are recurrent relapsing or continual symptoms. It leads to a loss of the normal vascular pattern at endoscopy, with a variable degree of inflammation, contact bleeding and occasionally frank ulceration. None of these features is sufficiently specific for the diagnosis to be made without supportive histology. Given the uncertainties of symptom-based diagnosis of pouchitis, it should now be expected that all patients in whom pouchitis is considered will have endoscopic and histological verification. The scoring system devised by the Mayo Clinic is helpful in the research context and not unduly complex for routine use[35] (see Appendix A). The microscopic changes include a prominent polymorphonuclear cell infiltrate in the acute phase, with a greater involvement of lymphocytes and other mononuclear inflammatory cells with developing chronicity (Plate 9). The histological features may be patchy and tend to affect the most distal part of the pouch preferentially.[36] Infective causes should be excluded by appropriate investigation. Cytomegalovirus has been especially implicated in patients with chronic pouchitis who show no response to steroids; the Mayo Clinic group have elicited good clinical and histological results from ganciclovir therapy in two such patients.[37]

Pouchitis therapy is still at a relatively immature stage. Metronidazole (400 mg thrice daily) has been shown in a small, blinded crossover study of relatively intractable pouchitis to offer a significant advantage in terms of a reduced frequency of evacuation but without histological or other objective improvements.[38] This remains, nevertheless, the first intervention of most clinicians and often appears valuable; it is unclear whether its apparent

effect is primarily an antimicrobial one, but the anecdotal support for the use of ciprofloxacin and other antibiotics suggests that this is a correct interpretation. Uncontrolled data favour the combination of ciprofloxacin and rifaximin (which has a broad spectrum and is not absorbed from the gut), with up to 88 per cent of those with chronic inflammation showing a response.[39] Careful trials with controlled data are seriously needed, and a good start has been made by Campieri's group with a well-designed and innovative study of a probiotic mixture comprising four strains of lactobacilli, three of bifidobacteria and a streptococcus. All the patients had documented chronic pouchitis (clinical, endoscopic and histological criteria) and were pretreated with antibiotics[39] to bring them into remission, prior to randomization to treatment with the probiotic cocktail or placebo for 9 months. Three of 20 treated patients relapsed during the 9 months compared with all 20 of those on placebo ($P < 0.001$).[40] There are some reservations about the methodology, with regrets that the microbiological surveillance was incomplete, but the blinding appears to have been secure and the outcome measures were verifiable. Sadly all the treated patients relapsed once the probiotic cocktail was withdrawn, as tends to be the case with this form of intervention (see Chapter 3). Campieri's group have also used probiotics in attempts at preventing pouchitis. In a 12-month postoperative study they demonstrated a difference in the incidence of pouchitis (8 of 20 in the control group and 2 of 20 of those treated; $P < 0.05$).[41]

Preliminary data from a small pouchitis study indicate similar efficacy from budesonide enemas to that of oral metronidazole.[42] By intention to treat, there were 7 responses (and 6 remissions) in 12 patients treated with 2 mg budesonide daily for 6 weeks, compared with 7 (and 6) of 14 patients given metronidazole. There were more adverse events with metronidazole. The results do not have statistical power but lend some support to the common clinical practice of employing steroid enemas when metronidazole has failed. Various alternatives and variations on these themes have been utilized, including systemic steroids, topical and oral 5-ASA preparations, and a range of topical agents otherwise thought valuable in the management of proctitis. Fortunately, despite this therapeutic uncertainty, most patients finally do well and excision of a pouch for intractable pouchitis is a rare event.

Functional disorders of the pouch also exist and deserve brief comment, not least because the affected patient is perhaps the most likely to be referred from the specialist pouch surgeon to the physician with an interest in inflammatory bowel disease. The commonest functional disorder is the early postoperative intestinal obstruction for which no mechanical cause can be demonstrated. Although laparotomy may occasionally be necessary to prove this, the prognosis is generally good and continuing action unnecessary. Frequency of pouch action is greatest in the first weeks after surgery and usually settles to the three to six times daily alluded to above. Higher frequency in the absence of pouchitis is usually relatively readily overcome by incremental therapy with loperamide or other opioids. Occasionally patients behave as if the small bowel were a great deal shorter than it is known to be, exhibiting 'short bowel syndrome'. Although this tends to be a transient phenomenon, it may last for some weeks and require intensive fluid and nutritional support during this time (see Chapter 7).

Difficulty in pouch evacuation was a much commoner problem in the early days of pouch surgery, and particularly in the case of the 'S' pouch with its efferent limb (Figure 4.3), an operation now avoided by most surgeons for this reason. There remain a few (< 5 per cent) patients who need to intubate with a soft catheter to achieve defecation, and others who continue to have a major problem with unpredictable evacuation. Postoperative problems are not predicted by preoperative physiological or other assessments, with the proviso only that preoperative sphincter function must be reasonably normal; however successful the pouch, the reservoir contents will never have the solidity of a normal stool. Investigation of the problematic pouch by contrast pouchography (analogous to the defecating proctogram) will usually permit the exclusion of pouch outlet obstruction, and may demonstrate oddities of pouch configuration (such as a floppy pouch that twists on itself), that help to determine the place, if any, for revisional surgery. When no structural abnormality can be identified, the patient can at least be reassured that the pouch is viable, itself a cause of great relief to many who fear pouch excision and ileostomy more even than substantial difficulties with the pouch. Continuing management is then symptom orientated, and may include the careful use of enemas or behavioural techniques such as biofeedback. More authoritative advice will no doubt become available with time.

One of the main justifications for pouch surgery in ulcerative colitis, as opposed to ileorectal anastomosis, is to avoid the risk of rectal carcinoma. Theoretically the pouch eliminates this risk, but there are two notes of caution. Since the mucosa of the pouch usually takes on a number of colonic characteristics, it is possible that it may also become at risk of colonic-type neoplasia with the passing of time (or, indeed, independently of colonic metaplasia, given the stasis and altered flora which are alien to the normal distal small bowel). Second, there remains the possibility of rectal mucosal cells being retained (accidentally from inadequate mucosal stripping, or unavoidably in the transitional zone above the anal canal). Although the literature contains a small collection of case reports of so-called pouch cancers, careful reading indicates that these generally (if not exclusively) reflect incomplete rectal excision. It is too soon to be sure, however, that the first risk is only hypothetical, especially in the light of the two following reports. The clearest case for invasive adenocarcinoma arising in true ileal mucosa within a pouch is a single patient in whom a J pouch created for ulcerative colitis transformed into a site of malignancy 14 years later.[43] However, this was a special case, in as much as the pouch was defunctioned for most of this time. Dysplasia was found in a subgroup of Swedish pouch patients in whom the postoperative course was complicated by continuing severe pouchitis associated with permanent subtotal or total villous atrophy, which constituted 9 per cent of the series.[44] Dysplasia was low grade and affected three patients (3.4 per cent of all pouch patients) at a mean follow-up of 6.3 years. It affected mucosa of apparently small bowel origin, and was present at numerous sites (on eight occasions, in 63 biopsies in the three patients). The prognostic significance of this observation is not yet known, and clearly there is also a low background rate of spontaneous adenocarcinoma in ileal tissue. Continued clinical surveillance and regular pouch biopsy are evidently warranted.

Pre-anastomotic ileitis after colectomy for ulcerative colitis

In addition to the well-recognized pouchitis described above, there is also an increasing awareness of post-colectomy ileitis. It is rare but occurs after all forms of colectomy and re-anastomosis for ulcerative colitis, and maybe particularly so in the neoterminal ileum immediately proximal to an ileoanal pouch. An Israeli group examined nine cases of their own and the scant previous literature to try to identify potential risk factors and valuable therapeutic strategies.[45] Careful re-evaluation for Crohn's disease was a necessary exclusion criterion. There was no apparent common feature in terms of surgical technique, the condition occurring after ileorectal anastomosis and with Kock and ileoanal pouches. There was independence from proctitis and from pouchitis (which was absent in most cases). Potential specific microbial agents

were not demonstrable. The magnitude of symptoms ranged from none to those of a severe ileitis with stricturing and ulceration demonstrable at ileoscopy. As the condition is also described after colectomy for colorectal carcinoma,[45] it is probable that it has an explanation separate from prior ulcerative colitis. Treatment is a problem, there being a poor response to steroids and 5-ASA, but azathioprine may have a place in the resistant case.

CROHN'S DISEASE

There are important differences in approach when surgery for Crohn's disease is considered. Key amongst these are the high lifetime frequency of surgery in this disease (>50 per cent), involvement of the small bowel, the potential for permanent nutritional dependency if a major proportion of the intestine is removed, the absence of any confident expectation of 'cure' of the underlying condition, and the possibilities pre- and postoperatively of other complications. Emergency surgery is less often required for colonic Crohn's than for ulcerative colitis, as fulminant colitis and its complications are much less common (see above). Urgent surgical intervention may, however, be required for intestinal obstruction from stenotic disease, or for the effects of sepsis and abscess formation (see Chapter 7). Fistula surgery is rarely best embarked upon on an emergency footing (see Chapter 7). Unfortunately, more than 50 per cent of all patients operated on for Crohn's disease will have postoperative relapse and most of these will need further surgery.[46] Figures as high as 75 per cent lifetime reoperation rates are readily found in the literature.[47]

The high postoperative relapse rates in all forms of Crohn's disease (see also Chapter 3) should not be allowed to detract from the excellent surgical results that can be obtained, and especially in the first-time patient with localized ileocaecal disease failing to respond to standard medical measures. At least 40 per cent of such patients will have uncomplicated surgery and prolonged remission, which will be lifelong in a sizeable minority. Representative data include those of the Cleveland Clinic, where resection led to prolonged surgery-free survival in 47 per cent to 56 per cent depending on the site of the original disease,[48] of the Leuven group, who record 66 per cent of patients symptom-free at 3 years postoperatively,[49] and the Leiden group where 44 per cent remained free of further surgery at 20 years.[50] Patients who have already had surgery, those with fistulae, and those with other complications cannot be given such a good prognosis. Although good results are certainly still achieved, the proportion decreases with each additional procedure and complication.

There is a curious phenomenon influencing the nature of postoperative recurrence which has been clearly documented by the Chicago group.[51] For reasons yet to be explained, when Crohn's disease recurs after resection, it affects a similar length of intestine with a remarkable degree of consistency (26 cm versus 24 cm; correlation coefficient: 0.70), but is not then progressive with time.

It is probable that technical considerations have a generalizable impact on surgical results. Apart from the obvious justifications for careful case selection and an experienced inflammatory bowel disease surgeon, there are arguments in favour of stapled rather than sutured anastomoses, and of side-to-side rather than end-to-end anastomosis. The complication rate (17 versus 8 per cent) and reoperation rate (43 versus 2 per cent) were much higher with end-to-end suturing than with equivalent stapling in one uncontrolled series.[52] The Birmingham group reached similar conclusions from their own retrospective analysis (complication rate: 23 versus 7 per cent; reoperation rate: 33 versus 2 per cent),[53] but acknowledged important biases of recruitment date and shorter flow-up in the stapled cohort, and commendably went on to a controlled trial.[54] The trial compared the outcome after conventional sutured closure of a loop ileostomy closure with stapled ileostomy closure. There was good balancing of patients between the two groups for all the standard independent risk factors, and their perioperative course was not obviously different, apart from a higher frequency of postoperative obstruction in the sutured group (14 versus 3 per cent), which just failed to reach statistical significance (probably through underpowering of the study). In short-term follow-up there had not been a difference in relapse rate. Whilst it is probable that the stapled patients achieve advantage, this is at some financial cost and without useful reduction in operating time (median 4 minutes less). As it is postulated that the side-to-side anastomosis may give better results by virtue of providing a wider anastomotic lumen, the Birmingham group have unfortunately muddied the waters somewhat by their comparison of a side-to-side stapled anastomosis with a sutured end-to-end join.

The risk of relapse has much to do with the continuity of small and large bowel. When a terminal ileostomy is created, the frequency of relapse is relatively low, the Leuven group quoting a typical relapse rate of 29 per cent,[49] which unfortunately reverts to the general risk of relapse if the ileostomy is subsequently closed. Some possible mechanisms for this phenomenon are discussed in Chapter 1. In practice, patient management is not greatly influenced by this knowledge, as there is a natural tendency of patients and surgeons alike to avoid stoma formation if at all possible, reserving it for the patient with pan-colitis, especially when there is intractable perianal disease implicating the sphincter zone, and when continence has been prejudiced or entirely lost. A stoma may be created with the intention that it will be temporary (to be closed when the perineum or distal colorectum has recovered), but it is my experience that in almost 50 per cent of such cases, closure never becomes feasible. Patients undergoing surgery for difficult Crohn's disease should always be aware that a stoma may be a necessary intervention, and that even an intentionally temporary stoma may become permanent.

Conservative surgery in small bowel Crohn's disease has an important place, nevertheless, and is generally to be preferred precisely because of the high risk of recurrence (despite improving postoperative maintenance with pharmacological agents – see Chapter 3) and the concern that future surgery will lead to borderline or actual short bowel syndrome. Most surgeons will therefore choose to perform reparative stricturoplasty unless there is a very well defined (and relatively short) section of diseased small bowel. This procedure entails a longitudinal division of the stricture with a transverse anastomosis of the enterotomy created (Figures 4.4 and 4.5). Sites for surgical attention can be identified by the peroperative passage of a 2.5 cm balloon along the small bowel with stricturoplasty (or resection) performed at each site that the balloon will not pass. There is a low immediate morbidity from stricturoplasty with a postoperative dehiscence rate of around 5 per cent, which is more impressive when one considers that a single patient may have upwards of 10 stricturoplasties at one operative session, but depressing when this so often means an enterocutaneous fistula.[55,56] The postoperative recurrence rate is unsurprisingly substantial; at 12 months, over 96 per cent of Tjandra's patients were without obstructive symptoms, but in

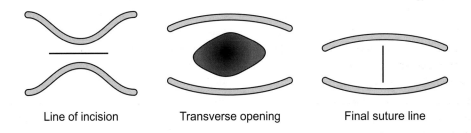

Line of incision   Transverse opening   Final suture line

Figure 4.4 The Heineke–Mikulicz stricturoplasty for conservational ileal stricture surgery.

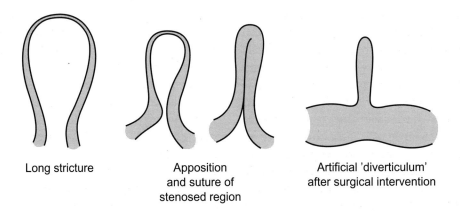

Long stricture   Apposition and suture of stenosed region   Artificial 'diverticulum' after surgical intervention

Figure 4.5 The Finney stricturoplasty for the more lengthy ileal stricture.

continuing follow-up, 13 per cent required further stricture surgery.[55] Although one might expect the best results for stricturoplasty to be confined to patients in whom the predominant problem is fibrous stricturing with little current inflammation, this does not seem universally to be the case. Not only do some stenoses with an active inflammatory component do well, but the inflammation may also settle with apparent recovery of the bowel at the site of the surgical incision, with future relapses just as, or more, likely to affect previously unaffected parts of the small bowel.[55] It may be for similar reasons that endoscopically detected but surgically inapparent lesions do not appear to impart a worse prognosis if left undisturbed.[57] As it has been known for many years that residual microscopic disease left at conventional resection has no impact on the relapse rate, we should perhaps be unsurprised at these observations.[58]

The situation in respect of the lower bowel is a little different. Scandinavian data indicate, first of all, that the patient with isolated colonic Crohn's disease is less likely to need surgery in the first few years after diagnosis than the patient with small bowel involvement,[46] but surgery is nonetheless indicated in more than 50 per cent.[59] Because the colon, despite its role in fluid and electrolyte balance, is nutritionally less essential, and because of concerns of colonic recurrence if partial colectomy is performed, there has been a feeling that total colectomy should be favoured whenever colectomy is indicated. Segmental colonic resection has been thought to predispose not only to recurrence in the residual colon, but to a more aggressive, less controllable disease that leads to completion colectomy soon afterwards. There are no controlled data to help us, although a trial between segmental resection and ileorectal anastomosis would be entirely legitimate. A controlled trial comparing segmental resection to colectomy and ileostomy would also be of interest but this would be most unlikely to be acceptable to

patients or ethical committees. Personal experience indicates that some patients do well with segmental resection and some do badly, but it is rarely at all clear preoperatively which outcome is to be expected.

A German group have tried to help with a long-term analysis of 142 patients with segmental resections performed at a single centre,[59] comparing this with 28 patients who had an initial colectomy (often with retention of the rectum). The initial distribution of disease was typical of those for other centres with the exception perhaps of a rather high rate of rectal involvement (40 per cent). Based on a mean of well over 7 years of follow-up from the time of first surgery, they constructed actuarial statistics for the first 10 years. Clinical recurrence occurred in 63 per cent, and 33 per cent needed further surgery by 10 years. The presence of a colocolic anastomosis did increase the risk of relapse (but only by about 32 per cent), as did the presence of perianal disease (which doubled the relapse rate). However, the risk of progression to completion colectomy was only 11 per cent at 10 years after segmental resection, with 8 per cent needing a terminal ileostomy, compared with a 25 per cent stoma rate in those treated initially by resection and ileorectal anastomosis. The authors advocate a more liberal policy towards segmental colectomy, but it must be accepted that there has been a high degree of selection leading to the initial surgical decision. Contemporary French data (still only available in abstract form) on the place of ileorectal anastomosis in Crohn's surgery reach a less encouraging conclusion, with a high failure rate, leading to proctectomy in 50 per cent of their patients during as little as 2 years of follow-up.[60] Again, patients with anorectal disease were least likely to do well, and poorer outcomes were recorded in those with extra-intestinal manifestations of their disease. British data specifically comparing subtotal colectomy (with ileorectal anastomosis) and initial proctocolectomy (clearly not comparable patients or controlled data) indicate high rates of complications for both operations (32 versus 53 per cent respectively).[61] The symptomatic recurrence rate thereafter was, however, significantly lower in the group with an initial ileostomy (29 versus 68 per cent; $P < 0.0001$). As perianal disease generally predicts a worse prognosis (see, for example, reference 59), data such as these should help the clinician to guide the patient in need of colonic surgery as to the relative merits of creation of a definitive stoma. The state of the rectum and the perianal region clearly has a major influence on surgical planning and, as in all inflammatory bowel disease surgery, the informed patient will (and should) often be the final arbiter.

Appendicectomy in unsuspected Crohn's disease presenting as acute appendicitis?

As preoperative ultrasound and laparoscopic evaluation and intervention become more common, the surprise finding of terminal ileal or ileocaecal Crohn's disease at grid-iron incision for suspected appendicitis is less frequent than in the past, but the question remains as to what should be done when it is found. Teaching has been to remove the appendix, on the basis that this is what the scar will be taken to indicate in future, but this introduces a risk of postoperative fistula (and other complications) and is arguably unethical if the appendix itself is healthy. No less than 2.5 per cent ($n = 36$) of all Crohn's disease surgery was performed in this context over 9 years at the Lahey Clinic.[62] Ten patients had ileocolic resection, 23 had appendicectomy (one with ileocaecal bypass) and only three had a simple diagnostic laparotomy. Fifty per cent of those having 'a Crohn's operation' needed further surgery within a mean of 18 years, whereas 92 per cent of those having an appendicectomy required surgery for Crohn's disease within a mean of 3 years (four for fistula and two for perforation). The authors are inclined to advocate ileocolic resection. However, the initial operating surgeon

will have decided on a course of action influenced by the state of the ileum and caecum as well as by the (presumably healthy) appendix, and these data may just as logically provide support for a strategy of non-intervention. Had the appendicectomy not been performed, the patient may not have run into trouble. The modern, well-informed patient can probably be trusted to remember whether or not the organ has been removed so long as he or she is told.

Pouch surgery in Crohn's disease

Ileoanal pouch construction in Crohn's has been vetoed by most inflammatory bowel disease practitioners because of the anxieties in respect of pelvic sepsis, pouch breakdown, and the potentially catastrophic effects of disease recurrence. However, for reasons alluded to elsewhere (Chapter 2), it is not always possible to exclude Crohn's disease as a cause of colitis, and sometimes a previously confident diagnosis of ulcerative colitis proves incorrect. Some of these patients have had 'accidental' pouch surgery and the results are perhaps not as bad as might be expected.

The Mayo Clinic have reviewed the long-term outcome in patients with pouches created inadvertently in Crohn's disease ($n = 37$).[63] In six, the diagnosis became apparent early on from the histology of the resection specimen, and nine had an initial diagnosis of indeterminate colitis. Eleven patients developed complex fistulae (pouch-cutaneous, $n = 6$; pouch-vaginal, $n = 4$; or pouch-vesical, $n = 1$), 20 developed active Crohn's disease in the pouch (10 of whom also had anal involvement, 4 had isolated anal canal disease and 3 had Crohn's elsewhere). At 10 years (range, 3–14), the pouch remained in functional continuity in 20 patients with a median frequency of seven times daily, but had been defunctioned in 7 patients, and excised in 10 (failure rate 45 per cent). The Paris group have been heavily criticized for their paper which recorded respectable results in 13 such patients, criticism being levelled not for their inclusion of these patients, but for the use of pouch surgery in a further 18 patients in whom the diagnosis was known to be Crohn's disease and in whom the operation was a deliberate 'high-risk' strategy.[64] There has also been some surprise that so many patients could be found to fulfil the stated criteria of colonic Crohn's without either ileal or anorectal disease. Follow-up is still relatively short (mean 59 months) and caution is certainly required, but the 6 per cent relapse rate (Crohn's disease affecting the pouch in two patients) and the 19 per cent complication rate are remarkably good. As the authors note, the complication rate is neither statistically nor numerically different from their own results in ulcerative colitis, and is comparable to that for ulcerative colitis series at other centres. When it is remembered that the appropriate comparator is not pouch surgery in ulcerative colitis but alternative surgery in Crohn's disease with generally higher overall relapse and complication rates even for terminal ileostomy (the surgical 'best option'), the possibility of pouch construction for the Crohn's patient with severe but isolated colonic disease should no longer be dismissed out of hand.

When a pouch has been created inadvertently in Crohn's disease and active disease recurs, there may prove to be value from infliximab. In retrospective review there appeared to have been remission in six of seven treated patients, all of whom had some benefit.[65] In four patients, the indication was pre-pouch ileitis, one of whom also had a perianal fistula, and in three it was for pouch-vaginal fistula, but up to four infusions were administered and there are no controlled data.

Non-surgical predictive factors for relapse after surgery for Crohn's disease

It is probable that the underlying disease phenotype is of key importance in governing the risk of postoperative relapse (see Chapter 1), some patients having an 'innate' higher risk, perhaps genetically determined. Nonetheless, there are factors that are amenable to intervention. Most authors find a strong link between continued smoking and risk of relapse after surgery for Crohn's disease[66–68] and, although this is not a universal finding,[46] there are sufficient grounds arguing against smoking that cessation should be the strong advice to all patients in the preoperative and postoperative periods. Postoperative medical prophylaxis has been disappointing (the need for meta-analysis to show clear benefit indicates a low magnitude of gain) (see Chapter 3), but this may reflect a failure of stratification. If all patients (whether of high or low innate relapse risk) are considered together, the value of modest but selective influences may be obscured. Potentially helpful data have emerged from a study of postoperative tissue cytokine levels in which interleukin-10 concentrations were substantially lower in those who went on to early (endoscopically determined) relapse than in those who retained healthy postoperative appearances.[69] The particulars of the study are unlikely to be clinically applicable but the concept that cytokine status in the immediate postoperative period is predictive of those at greater or lesser risk could help to select patients for secondary prophylactic intervention.

DIVERSION COLITIS

When the rectum has been defunctioned but not resected there is a frequency of relapse divided uncertainly between defunction/diversion proctitis and reactivated Crohn's, which together affect around half the patients so treated. It may be difficult to distinguish accurately between the two forms of proctitis clinically or histologically (see Chapter 2). The recognition and diagnosis of diversion colitis are plagued by inconsistencies, but histological abnormalities are almost always to be found on biopsy. In a well-documented series in which the final conclusions were drawn from resection specimens, 14 of the 15 cases (helpfully) had many features in common.[70] There was diffuse, mild, chronic inflammation, with a variable extent of mild architectural abnormality of the crypts, minor crypt abscesses and follicular lymphoid hyperplasia. In other words, the changes are those of mild ulcerative colitis rather than ones suggestive of Crohn's disease. A French series of 48 patients indicates that, over 8 years of follow-up, one-third of these patients can be expected to come to proctectomy – most of whom will have had preoperative proctitis – and that prolonged rectal remission is the fortunate outcome in only about 30 per cent. Again, the results of this study are as yet available only in abstract form.[71]

LAPAROSCOPY IN INFLAMMATORY BOWEL DISEASE SURGERY

A section on surgery in inflammatory bowel disease can no longer stand without comment on the role of laparoscopy. Colorectal surgeons were late to enter the laparoscopic arena, but are now doing so with a highly variable degree of enthusiasm. Fazio's group have been publishing on laparoscopically assisted resections for Crohn's disease for several years[72] and techniques for ileostomy creation have also been developed.[73] At present it remains reasonable to conclude that laparoscopic methodology is technically possible in some patients and may permit an easier convalescence,[74,75] but with the proviso that it will rarely be suitable for those with extensive previous surgery, adhesions and complex fistulae, and has yet to prove itself in formal comparison with the more established methods employed at open surgery.

ENDOSCOPIC STRICTURE DILATATION

Anorectal strictures have been dilated by surgeons and patients since mythological times with good results. There is always concern that strictures of the large bowel complicating inflammatory bowel disease have neoplastic potential (see Chapter 8), but with initial and periodic histological assessment their dilatation can also be routinely undertaken with the expectation of good results.[76] More proximal strictures can now be reached endoscopically and with reliable, modern, through-the-scope balloons, endoscopic therapy became a technical possibility. The problem with earlier balloons was not so much their small calibre but their short length, which led to them slipping proximally or distally as the balloon was inflated. Now that balloons of 5 cm or more in length and up to 25 mm in diameter are routinely available, this is much less of a problem. Virtually all colonic and anastomotic strictures are theoretically accessible. There is still a technical failure rate (stricture too tight or its distal opening too angled for access), and a perforation rate, both in the region of 5–10 per cent depending on selection criteria. There are no clear comparative data for long-term results from dilatation. My clinical impression has been that patients with inactive disease and entirely or mainly fibrous stricturing can achieve good and long-lasting results, but those with any degree of inflammatory activity get little benefit, apart perhaps from a placebo response which is lost after 2 or 3 weeks. I tend to reserve this approach for patients with negative inflammatory markers and negative white cell scans. The literature is a little more positive but inclusion criteria are not uniform and there has been no controlled trial. Papers inevitably come from endoscopy enthusiasts, and there may be a publication bias towards better results. The Leuven group probably have most experience and reported on their technical success in dilating 16 of 18 strictures in 1992.[77] Their more recent review includes 55 patients with 59 strictures (average length 40 mm) treated on 78 occasions.[78] All these patients were considered resistant to medical therapy and would otherwise have been treated surgically. Dilatation, with a water-filled balloon, was to 18 mm, and to

25 mm in the more recent patients. It was possible to pass a colonoscope through 73 per cent of the strictures after dilatation, and a further 17 per cent of procedures were considered technical successes. There were six perforations, only two of which necessitated laparotomy and resection; there was no mortality. Kaplan–Meier estimation of recurrence-free survival time indicated that around 40 per cent of patients remained well to 3 years, and that surgery had been avoided in more than 60 per cent at 3 years. The results compare favourably with those to be expected from surgical stricturoplasty,[55] but there are important identifiable differences between the patients included in surgical and endoscopic series, not least the higher frequency of multiple strictures in the former. There is a continuing case for both forms of intervention in appropriately selected patients.

ENDOSCOPIC STENTING FOR BENIGN DISEASE

Stenotic Crohn's disease can, nonetheless, be difficult to manage. Surgical resection is often inappropriate in the patient who has received substantial previous resection, and, despite many successes, balloon and surgical stricturoplasty may fail. A small group of patients remains, therefore, for whom a more permanent endoscopic solution is sought in the form of stenting. There is a convincing literature for the use of metal stents in malignant colonic obstruction, which is either for lifelong palliation in the patient with disseminated disease, or as a short-term measure to allow full resuscitation in the patient who is unfit for surgery at the time of presentation and who goes on to a potentially curative resection (complete with the stent) once stable. Neither scenario is naturally applicable in Crohn's disease or ulcerative colitis as the conditions are not fatal, and a major reason for considering non-resectional techniques is to avoid compromising an already short bowel. It is not surprising, therefore, that the literature is scant.

Matsuhashi *et al.* have reported their short-and medium-term happiness with the procedure[79] and it is legitimate to consider it a technical option for a small number of carefully selected patients in whom a dominant stricture is within endoscopic range and in whom there is acceptance that the risk of permanent foreign body placement is outweighed by the expected benefits. These anxieties may diminish with the further development of biodegradable stent materials, currently under evaluation in cardiological practice, and for other gastrointestinal purposes.

References

1 Chapman RW, Selby WS, Jewell DP. Controlled trial of intravenous metronidazole as an adjunct to corticosteroids in severe ulcerative colitis. *Gut* 1986; **27**: 1210–12.

2 Truelove SC, Witts LJ. Cortisone in ulcerative colitis. Final report on a therapeutic trial. *Br Med J* 1955; **2**: 1041–8.

3 Truelove SC, Willoughby CP, Lee EG, Kettlewell MGW. Further experience in the treatment of severe attacks of ulcerative colitis. *Lancet* 1978; **2**: 1086–8.

4 McIntyre PB, Powell-Tuck J, Wood SR, *et al.* Controlled trial of bowel rest in the treatment of severe acute colitis. *Gut* 1986; **27**: 481–5.

5 Panos MZ, Wood MJ, Asquith P. Toxic megacolon: the knee–elbow position relieves bowel distension. *Gut* 1993; **34**: 1726–7.

6 Present DH, Wolfson D, Gelernt IM, Rubin PH, Bauer J, Chapman ML. Medical decompression of toxic megacolon by rolling. A new technique of decompression with favorable long-term follow-up. *J Clin Gastroenterol* 1988; **10**: 485–90.

7 Lennard-Jones JE, Ritchie JK, Hilder W, Spicer CC. Assessment of severity in colitis: a preliminary study. *Gut* 1975; **16**: 579–84.

8 Travis SPL, Farrant JM, Ricketts C, *et al.* Predicting outcome in severe ulcerative colitis. *Gut* 1996; **38**: 905–10.

9 Meyers S, Lerer PK, Feuer EJ, Johnson JW, Janowitz HD. Predicting the outcome of corticoid

therapy for acute ulcerative colitis. Results of a prospective, randomized, double-blind clinical trial. *J Clin Gastroenterol* 1987; **9**: 50–4.

10 Oshitani N, Kitano A, Fukushima R, *et al.* Predictive factors for the response of ulcerative colitis patients during the acute phase treatment. *Digestion* 1990; **46**: 107–13.

11 Caprilli R, Frieri G, Latella G, Vernia P, Santoro ML. Faecal excretion of bicarbonate in ulcerative colitis. *Digestion* 1986; **35**: 136–42.

12 Chew CN, Nolan DJ, Jewell DP. Small bowel gas in severe ulcerative colitis. *Gut* 1991; **32**: 1535–7.

13 Caprilli R, Vernia P, Latella G, Torsoli A. Early recognition of toxic megacolon. *J Clin Gastroenterol* 1987; **9**: 160–4.

14 Almer S, Bodemar G, Franzen L, Lindström E, Nyström P-O, Ström M. Use of air enema radiography to assess depth of ulceration during acute attacks of ulcerative colitis. *Lancet* 1996; **347**: 1731–5.

15 Bartram CI. Barium radiology. *Scand J Gastroenterol Suppl* 1994; **203**: 20–3.

16 Carbonnel F, Laver GNEA, Lémann M, *et al.* Colonoscopy of acute colitis: a safe and reliable tool for assessment of severity. *Dig Dis Sci* 1994; **39**: 1550–7.

17 Järnerot G, Rolny P, Sandberg-Gertzen H. Intensive intravenous treatment of ulcerative colitis. *Gastroenterology* 1985; **89**: 1005–13.

18 Mortensen PB, Clausen MR. Short-chain fatty acids in the human colon: relation to gastrointestinal health and disease. *Scand J Gastroenterol Suppl* 1996; **216**: 132–48.

19 Condie JD Jr, Leslie KO, Smiley DF. Surgical treatment for inflammatory bowel disease in the older patient. *Surg Gynecol Obstet* 1987; **165**: 135–42.

20 Varma JS, Browning GGP, Smith AN, Small WP, Sircus W. Mucosal proctectomy and coloanal anastomosis for distal ulcerative proctocolitis. *Br J Surg* 1987; **74**: 381–3.

21 Leong AP, Londono-Schimmer EE, Phillips RK. Life-table analysis of stomal complications following ileostomy. *Br J Surg* 1994; **81**: 727–9.

22 Melville DM, Ritchie JK, Nicholls RJ, Hawley PR. Surgery for ulcerative colitis in the era of the pouch: the St Mark's Hospital experience. *Gut* 1994; **35**: 1076–80.

23 Wilkinson K. Research records. In Forbes A, Power E, eds. *St. Mark's Hospital Annual Report 1998*. London: St Mark's Academic Institute, 1998, 131–3.

24 Johnston D, Williamson ME, Lewis WG, Miller AS, Sagar PM, Holdsworth PJ. Prospective controlled trial of duplicated (J) versus quadruplicated (W) pelvic ileal reservoirs in restorative proctocolectomy for ulcerative colitis. *Gut* 1996; **39**: 242–7.

25 Wexner SD, Jagerman D, Lavery D, Fazio V. Ileoanal reservoir. *Am J Surg* 1990; **159**: 178–85.

26 Setti-Carraro P, Ritchie JK, Wilkinson KH, Nicholls RJ, Hawley PR. The first 10 years' experience of restorative proctocolectomy for ulcerative colitis. *Gut* 1994; **35**: 1070–5.

27 Kohler L, Pemberton JH, Zinsmeister AR, Kelly KA. Quality of life after proctocolectomy: a comparison of Brooke ileostomy, Kock pouch and ileal pouch–anal anastomosis. *Gastroenterology* 1991; **101**: 679–84.

28 Keighley MRB. Review article: the management of pouchitis. *Aliment Pharmacol Ther* 1996; **10**: 449–57.

29 Svaninger G, Nordgren S, Oresland T, Hulten L. Incidence and characteristics of pouchitis in the Kock continent ileostomy and the pelvic pouch. *Scand J Gastroenterol* 1993; **28**: 695–700.

30 Ruseler-Van Embdem JG, Schouten WR, Van Lieshout LM. Pouchitis: result of microbial imbalance? *Gut* 1994; **35**: 658–64.

31 Esteve M, Mallolas J, Klaasen J, *et al.* Antineutrophil cytoplasmic antibodies in sera from colectomised ulcerative colitis patients and its relation to the presence of pouchitis. *Gut* 1996; **38**: 894–8.

32 Aisenberg J, Wagreich J, Shim J, *et al.* Perinuclear anti-neutrophil cytoplasmic antibody and refractory pouchitis. A case-control study. *Dig Dis Sci* 1995; **40**: 1866–72.

33 Setti-Carraro P, Talbot IC, Nicholls RJ. Long-term appraisal of the histological appearances of the ileal reservoir mucosa after restorative proctocolectomy for ulcerative colitis. *Gut* 1994; **35**: 1721–7.

34 Luukkonen P, Jarvinen H, Tanskanen M, Kahri A. Pouchitis – recurrence of the inflammatory bowel disease? *Gut* 1994; **35**: 243–6.

35 Sandborn WJ, Tremaine WJ, Batts KP, Pemberton JH, Phillips SF. Pouchitis after ileal pouch–anal anastomosis: a Pouchitis Disease Activity Index. *Mayo Clin Proc* 1994; **69**: 409–15.

36 Moskowitz RL, Shepherd NA, Nicholls RJ. An assessment of inflammation in the reservoir after restorative proctocolectomy with ileoanal ileal reservoir. *Int J Colorect Dis* 1986; **1**: 167–74.

37 Munoz-Juarez M, Pemberton JH, Sandborn WJ, Tremaine WJ, Dozois RR. Misdiagnosis of specific cytomegalovirus infection of the ileoanal pouch as refractory idiopathic chronic pouchitis. *Dis Colon Rectum* 1999; **42**: 117–20.

38 Madden MV, McIntyre AS, Nicholls RJ. Double-blind crossover trial of metronidazole versus placebo in chronic unremitting pouchitis. *Dig Dis Sci* 1994; **39**: 1193–6.

39 Gionchetti P, Rizzello F, Venturi A, *et al.* Antiobiotic combination therapy in patients with chronic, treatment resistant pouchitis. *Aliment Pharmacol Ther* 1999; **13**: 713–18.

40 Gionchetti P, Rizzello F, Venturi A, *et al.* Oral bacteriotherapy as maintenance treatment in patients with chronic pouchitis: a double-blind, placebo-controlled trial. *Gastroenterology* 2000; **119**: 305–9.

41 Gionchetti P, Rizzello F, Venturi A, *et al.* Prophylaxis of pouchitis onset with probiotic therapy: a double-blind placebo controlled trial. *Gastroenterology* 2000; **118**: A190.

42 Sambuella A, Boerr L, Negreira S, *et al.* Budesonide enemas versus oral metronidazole in pouchitis: a double-blind, double-dummy controlled trial. *Gastroenterology* 2000; **118**: A874.

43 Iwama T, Kamikawa J, Higuchi T, *et al.* Development of invasive adenocarcinoma in a long-standing diverted ileal J-pouch for ulcerative colitis: report of a case. *Dis Colon Rectum* 2000; **43**: 101–4.

44 Veress B, Reinholt FP, Lindquist K, Löfberg R, Liljeqvist L. Long-term histomorphological surveillance of the pelvic pouch: dysplasia develops in a subgroup of patients. *Gastroenterology* 1995; **109**: 1090–7.

45 Hallak A, Baratz M, Santo M, *et al.* Ileitis after colectomy for ulcerative colitis or carcinoma. *Gut* 1994; **35**: 373–6.

46 Moum B, Ekbom A, Vatn MH, *et al.* Clinical course during the 1st year after diagnosis in ulcerative colitis and Crohn's disease. Results of a large, prospective population-based study in southeastern Norway, 1990–93. *Scand J Gastroenterol* 1997; **32**: 1005–12.

47 Williams JG, Wong WD, Rothenberger DA, Goldberg SM. Recurrence of Crohn's disease after resection. *Br J Surg* 1991; **78**: 10–19.

48 Whelan G, Farmer RG, Fazio VW, Goormastic M. Recurrence after surgery in Crohn's disease. Relationship to location of disease (clinical pattern) and surgical indication. *Gastroenterology* 1985; **88**: 1826–33.

49 Rutgeerts P, Geboes K, Vantrappen G, Beyls J, Kerremans R, Hiele M. Predictability of the postoperative course of Crohn's disease. *Gastroenterology* 1990; **99**: 956–63.

50 Shivananda S, Hordijk ML, Pena AS, Mayberry JF. Crohn's disease: risk of recurrence and reoperation in a defined population. *Gut* 1989; **30**: 990–5.

51 D'Haens GR, Gasparaitis AE, Hanauer SB. Duration of recurrent ileitis after ileocolonic resection correlates with presurgical extent of Crohn's disease. *Gut* 1995; **36**: 715–17.

52 Hashemi M, Novell JR, Lewis AA. Side-to-side stapled anastomosis may delay recurrence in Crohn's disease. *Dis Colon Rectum* 1998; **41**: 1293–6.

53 Yamamoto T, Bain IM, Mylonakis E, Allan RN, Keighley MR. Stapled functional end-to-end anastomosis versus sutured end-to-end anastomosis after ileocolonic resection in Crohn disease. *Scand J Gastroenterol* 1999; **34**: 708–13.

54 Hasegawa H, Radley S, Morton DG, Keighley MR. Stapled versus sutured closure of loop ileostomy: a randomized controlled trial. *Ann Surg* 2000; **231**: 202–4.

55 Tjandra JJ, Fazio VW. Stricturoplasty without concomitant resection for small bowel obstruction in Crohn's disease. *Br J Surg* 1994; **81**: 561–3.

56 Spencer MP, Nelson H, Wolff BG, Dozois RR. Strictureplasty for obstructive Crohn's disease: the Mayo experience. *Mayo Clin Proc* 1994; **69**: 33–6.

57 Klein O, Colombel JF, Lescut D, *et al.* Remaining small bowel endoscopic lesions at surgery have no influence on early anastomotic recurrences in Crohn's disease. *Am J Gastroenterol* 1995; **90**: 1949–52.

58 Heuman R, Boeryd B, Bolin T, Sjodahl R. The influence of disease at the margin of resection on the outcome of Crohn's disease. *Br J Surg* 1983; **70**: 519–21.

59 Makowiec F, Paczulla D, Schmidtke C, Starlinger M. Long-term follow-up after resectional surgery in patients with Crohn's disease involving the colon. *Z Gastroenterol* 1998; **36**: 619–24.

60 Cattan P, Lémann M, Fritsch S, *et al.* Criteria predicting rectal conservation failure after subtotal colectomy in Crohn's disease. *Gastroenterology* 1996; **110**: A880.

61 Yamamoto T, Keighley MR. Proctocolectomy is associated with a higher complication rate but carries a lower recurrence rate than total colectomy and ileorectal anastomosis in Crohn colitis. *Scand J Gastroenterol* 1999; **34**: 1212–15.

62 Weston LA, Roberts PL, Schoetz DJ Jr, Coller JA, Murray JJ, Rusin LC. Ileocolic resection for acute presentation of Crohn's disease of the ileum. *Dis Colon Rectum* 1996; **39**: 841–6.

63 Sagar PM, Dozois RR, Wolff BG. Long-term results of ileal pouch–anal anastomosis in patients with Crohn's disease. *Dis Colon Rectum* 1996; **39**: 893–8.

64 Panis Y, Poupard B, Nemeth J, Lavergne A, Hautefeuille P, Valleur P. Ileal pouch/anal anastomosis for Crohn's disease. *Lancet* 1996; **347**: 854–7.

65 Ricart E, Panaccione R, Loftus EV, Tremaine WJ, Sandborn WJ. Successful management of Crohn's disease of the ileoanal pouch with infliximab. *Gastroenterology* 1999; **117**; 429–32.

66 Holdstock G, Savage D, Harman M, Wright R. Should patients with inflammatory bowel disease smoke? *Br Med J* 1984; **288**: 362.

67 Cosnes J, Carbonnel F, Beaugerie L, Le Quintrec Y, Gendre JP. Effects of cigarette smoking on the long-term course of Crohn's disease. *Gastroenterology* 1996; **110**: 424–31.

68 Breuer-Katschinski BD, Hollander N, Goebell H. Effect of smoking on the course of Crohn's disease. *Eur J Gastroenterol Hepatol* 1996; **8**: 225–8.

69 Meresse B, Desreumaux P, Rutgeerts P, *et al.* Low ileal IL-10 mRNA levels is predictive of endoscopic recurrence after surgery in patients with Crohn's disease. *Gut* 1999; **45**(Suppl V): A195.

70 Geraghty JM, Talbot IC. Diversion colitis: histological feature in the colon and rectum after defunctioning colostomy. *Gut* 1991; **32**: 1020–3.

71 Quandalle P, Tryohen F, Gambiez L, Paris JC, Colombel JF, Cortot A. Long term follow up of patients with excluded rectum in Crohn's disease. *Gastroenterology* 1996; **110**: A996.

72 Milsom JW, Lavery IC, Böhm M, Fazio VW. Laparoscopically assisted ileocolectomy in Crohn's disease. *Surg Laparosc Endosc* 1993; **3**: 77–80.

73 Roe AM, Barlow AP, Durdey P, Eltringham WK, Espiner HJ. Indications for laparoscopic formation of intestinal stomas. *Surg Laparosc Endosc* 1994; **4**: 345–7.

74 Bauer JJ, Harris MT, Grumbach NM, Gortine SR. Laparoscopic-assisted intestinal resection for Crohn's disease. *Dis Colon Rectum* 1995; **38**: 712–15.

75 Canin-Endres J, Salky B, Gattorno F, Edye M. Laparoscopically assisted intestinal resection in 88 patients with Crohn's disease. *Surg Endosc* 1999; **13**: 595–9.

76 Linares L, Moreira LF, Andrews H, *et al.* Natural history and treatment of anorectal strictures complicating Crohn's disease. *Br J Surg* 1988; **75**: 653–6.

77 Breysem Y, Janssens JF, Coremans G, Vantrappen G, Hendrickx G, Rutgeerts P. Endoscopic balloon dilation of colonic and ileo-colonic Crohn's strictures: long-term results. *Gastrointest Endosc* 1992; **38**: 142–7.

78 Couckuyt H, Gevers AM, Coremans G, Hiele M, Rutgeerts P. Efficacy and safety of hydrostatic balloon dilatation of ileocolonic Crohn's strictures: a prospective longterm analysis. *Gut* 1995; **36**: 577–80.

79 Matsuhashi N, Nakajima A, Suzuki A, Yazaki Y, Takazoe M. Long-term outcome of non-surgical strictureplasty using metallic stents for intestinal strictures in Crohn's disease. *Gastrointest Endosc* 2000; **51**: 343–5.

Obstetrics and paediatrics

Fertility and pregnancy in inflammatory bowel disease

MALE FERTILITY AND DRUG SAFETY

In males, there appear to be few problems aside from the temporarily reduced fertility in the obviously sick individual requiring in-patient care. Overall male fertility in inflammatory bowel disease has not been shown to be different from the general population.[1] Sulphasalazine is, however, responsible for reversible oligospermia.[2,3] The remaining spermatozoa are probably normal, and many normal pregnancies have occurred in the partners of men taking the drug. It is no longer acceptable to continue this drug in a man planning a family given that the available alternative aminosalicylate (5-ASA) drugs are without this side effect.

There are hypothetical dangers to the fetus from preconception exposure of the father to immunosuppressive drugs such as azathioprine. These dangers have not been demonstrated in any reported series and it is likely that any adverse effect is negligible or extremely rare.[4] An Austrian group have now examined the influence of azathioprine on some aspects of male fertility in inflammatory bowel disease.[2] Semen was examined and compared with international standards in respect of sperm density, motility and morphology in 21 treated patients aged between 18 and 57 (median 32). Most semen parameters were within

the World Health Organization standard, and five patients became fathers of healthy children whilst on azathioprine. No significant changes were noted (in 15 patients with multiple estimations) from pretreatment measurements or during drug use.

It is a reasonable practice to inform prospective parents of the potential hazard and, whenever possible, to withdraw these drugs in the pre-conception period. There is especial concern, but no reliable data, in respect of the use of thalidomide and methotrexate, given their catastrophic effects when taken by pregnant women; best advice is that prospective fathers should suspend their use in the pre-conception period.

The risk of inflammatory bowel disease affecting the offspring is similar whether the father or mother is affected (around 10 per cent) (see also Chapter 1), but this has been estimated to rise to about one in three if both parents have inflammatory bowel disease.[5]

FEMALE FERTILITY

The fertility of women with inflammatory bowel disease is probably nearly normal, but slightly fewer children are born to such women than to their peers without disease, and it is difficult to be sure whether this reflects social choices (obviously influenced by having to cope with a chronic disease), medical advice, or a failure of desired conception. The mean of 0.4 further infants born after a diagnosis of Crohn's disease was made (despite less use of contraception) compared with 0.7 born to controls in the same time interval in one survey suggests a true inhibiting effect of the disease.[6] Women with ulcerative colitis and Crohn's disease had normal fertility when compared with the general population of north-east Scotland,[7] but infertility problems were more frequent in women who had undergone IBD surgery than in those who had not (12 versus 5 per cent for Crohn's; 25 versus 7 per cent for ulcerative colitis). Infertility occurs for all the reasons that may affect other women, with a small additional group of those with Crohn's disease in whom pelvic sepsis-related infertility is the direct result of the disease. It is not clear why Scottish women with prior colitis surgery should have had such problems, but the numbers are small.

The menarche usually occurs at a normal age in girls with well-controlled inflammatory bowel disease, but is delayed by a mean of 13 months in those with problematic Crohn's disease and growth retardation.[8] Occasionally, delayed onset of periods is the presenting feature that prompts the investigations leading to a Crohn's diagnosis. Premenstrual worsening of symptoms is very commonly reported (by over 90 per cent of patients) and a cyclical pattern to bowel habit is commoner than in normal controls;[9] the reason for this is unclear. Similarly unclear is the explanation for the slightly premature menopause: about 4 years early in Crohn's disease, and 2 years sooner than in the general population in ulcerative colitis.

PREGNANCY

Fetal outcome

Inflammatory bowel disease typically runs a relatively benign course in pregnancy, and with good fetal outcomes. The north-east Scotland study supported an absence of increase in disease relapse, and indicated that women who, at conception, had active disease were just as likely to have a normal full-term pregnancy as those initially in remission.[7]

However, spontaneous abortion occurred in five pregnancies of women who had both undergone previous surgery for Crohn's and had recurrent disease, which was active in three. This is not statistically significant and probably represents fetal loss within the normal range.[5] Nonetheless, provisional, case-controlled, prospective Italian data also show a non-significant numerical disadvantage to the fetus of an affected mother.[10] There were more preterm deliveries (6.5 versus 1.6 per cent), a lower mean birth weight (2.97 versus 3.34 kg), and more babies with severe congenital abnormalities (3.3 versus 0.8 per cent). Complacency may be unwise.

Maternal outcome

A review of 29 pregnancies in 18 Crohn's patients and 25 in 19 ulcerative colitis patients[11] yielded a gestational incidence of relapse of 14 per cent in Crohn's, and a somewhat surprising 36 per cent in ulcerative colitis. The larger study already referred to[10] was more encouraging with only a 20 per cent relapse rate and a remission rate of 25 per cent in those with active disease at conception. In addition, inflammatory bowel disease may (rarely) present for the first time during pregnancy.

I have found it common for the post-puerperal period to represent a peak time for relapse in both Crohn's disease and ulcerative colitis and, in anticipation of this, routinely book a follow-up appointment for my patients 2–4 weeks after the expected date of delivery. Data from other centres suggest that this may be unnecessarily pessimistic, as post-partum relapses are as infrequent as only 17 per cent and 12 per cent, respectively.[11] Moreover, a significantly improved clinical course was recorded in the 3 years after pregnancy compared with that in the 3 prior years ($P < 0.05$ for both conditions) and compared to age-matched controls. Also, parous Birmingham women have less need for Crohn's disease surgery than their nulliparous neighbours.[12]

IBD drugs in pregnancy

Fortunately, the drugs most often used in inflammatory bowel disease are relatively innocuous in pregnancy. Mesalazine does not cross the placenta to any great extent, and there is much support for its safety at all stages in gestation, including prospective study through pregnancy and into the post-puerperal phase.[13,14] There is only a slight anxiety about larger doses, given a single letter reporting a baby with renal insufficiency born to a mother on mesalazine 4 g/day through the second trimester.[15] All the newer 5-ASA drugs can, in my view, safely be used throughout pregnancy, with the usual proviso that the regulatory authorities (e.g. British Committee on Safety of Medicines) will continue to advise caution. Equally the risk/benefit equation will be shifted away from drug use for situations (such as prophylaxis of Crohn's disease relapse) where the indications are less clear-cut; the prospective parent should clearly be involved in this decision process. Sulphasalazine has the longest track record for safe use in pregnancy, but poses an additional risk of neonatal haemolysis and methaemoglobinaemia because of the sulphonamide component. It is my practice to switch expectant mothers from sulphasalazine to one of the newer agents (or to stop therapy) prior to term to avoid this slight risk.

Steroid use in pregnancy is especially emotive. Hydrocortisone obviously crosses the placenta freely, but prednisolone considerably less so. With daily systemic doses of less than 10 mg prednisolone (or 50 mg hydrocortisone), the risk of adrenal suppression in the infant is negligible because the placenta has such a capacity for steroid metabolism, but adrenal problems can affect the fetus and the neonate if larger doses are required for the mother's health (or if dexamethasone or betamethasone is employed, which do, of course, affect the baby). It is logical to find alternatives to steroids whenever possible, defined liquid diet being an especially attractive option in Crohn's disease,[16] but, as with other potential threats to maternal life and health, the infant is best served by full attention to its mother's needs. Paediatric advice and a reducing steroid regimen for the neonate with actual or potential adrenal suppression should be sought. There have been suggestions that cleft palate and hare lip are more common in the offspring of animals on steroids, but human evidence for this is lacking.

Metronidazole has an established place in obstetric practice for reasons other than Crohn's disease, although there should be a small amount of concern about the more prolonged courses that may be used; there does not appear to be any evidence of peripheral neuropathy in the previously exposed infant. Concerns about congenital abnormalities in animals, and perhaps man, do not seem to deter obstetricians.[17] Ciprofloxacin should not be used because of the potential for neonatal arthropathy.

None of the immunosuppressives should be used in pregnancy unless essential for maternal health. However, there are reassuring data on the use of azathioprine. To Alstead's work summarizing 16 successful pregnancies in 14 women on the drug[18] can now be added data (in abstract form) from Francella *et al.*[4] in respect of no fewer than 155 patients (male and female) with inflammatory bowel disease who had had 6-mercaptopurine (6MP) and had also conceived (on a total of 347 occasions). This constituted about one-third of all their patients on the drug, who in turn represented 17 per cent of all their inflammatory bowel disease patients. There were four groups:

- those who became pregnant having already stopped 6MP (95 pregnancies);
- those who discontinued the drug after pregnancy was established (64 pregnancies);
- those who continued the drug throughout pregnancy (8 pregnancies); and
- a control group who commenced the drug only after completing one or more pregnancies (180 pregnancies).

There were no significant differences between any of the groups in terms of premature delivery, spontaneous abortion, congenital anomaly, neonatal infection or childhood neoplasia. There was, however, a trend towards higher rates for spontaneous abortion (19.2 versus 16.7 per cent), congenital anomaly (4.2 versus 2.8 per cent) and infection (4.2 versus 1.1 per cent) in pregnancies of patients exposed to the drug. Whether the treated parent was the father or the mother seemed to have no influence on outcome, although the one childhood malignancy in the series (a Wilms' tumour) was in the son of a man on 6MP. The numbers of each complication were low and complete confidence is not appropriate, especially given the very small number of women who continued the drug throughout pregnancy, but it is encouraging that all the figures reported are very similar to those for the general healthy population.

Transplant recipients on ciclosporin appear to achieve normal outcomes to their pregnancies, and a single patient with ulcerative colitis received about 3 months of treatment during pregnancy without apparent ill-effect to mother or infant.[19] Methotrexate should never be used in pregnancy because of its capacity to cause chromosomal damage, as a teratogen, and because it is an abortifacient![20,21] What effect the new antibody therapies might have is unknown. Immunosuppression and pregnancy thus remain very uneasy bedfellows. If it is possible to withdraw immunosuppression successfully prior to conception, then this should be done. If attempts at withdrawal lead to rapid and uncontrolled relapse, then it is reasonable for the patient and his or her partner to make an informed choice to remain on the drug, recognizing that there is a risk, but for their particular case that the chance of a successful pregnancy is greater with the patient in remission on the drug than potentially or actually in relapse off it.

Surgery for inflammatory bowel disease may be needed during pregnancy. The desire to avoid potentially toxic drugs paradoxically increases the likelihood that surgery will be considered. There are, unsurprisingly, no controlled data on the safety and success of such surgery in comparison to comparable surgery performed outwith pregnancy, but expectations can be similar. Any abdominal procedure poses risk to fetal viability with very gloomy predictions from the literature of the 1970s and before, but more recent data suggest that this need not be true.[22] The decision to operate for inflammatory bowel disease will only be taken as a lesser of evils and it is most unlikely that a major pelvic procedure such as pouch creation would be considered.

MODE OF DELIVERY

The delivery of the infant will usually be a matter for the woman and her obstetric advisers. Caesarean section is, however, strongly advised in the patient who has active perianal Crohn's, or who has needed previous surgery for anorectal fistula. Questionnaire data suggested that vaginal delivery (especially with episiotomy) poses a substantial risk of provoking perianal Crohn's disease even in those previously unaffected, with a 17.9 per cent frequency of new occurrences of disease occurring within 2 months of pregnancy (n = 179), but these were unvalidated data and probably overestimate the association.[23] Better data now exist.

An 11-year epidemiological, population-based study has examined pregnancies in women with inflammatory bowel disease, and assessed the relationship between perianal disease and mode of delivery, medical records being reviewed in over 90 per cent and questionnaires being completed by a subset of 52 women with Crohn's.[24] The total and elective Caesarean rates were higher for Crohn's disease (20.9 per cent and 9.0 per cent) and for ulcerative colitis (20.8 per cent and 9.3 per cent) than in the general population, for which the rates were 15 per cent and 5.4 per cent ($P < 0.01$ for each). In the subset of 52 women there were 64 deliveries, 54 of which were vaginal. Fifteen of these deliveries had been preceded by perianal disease, which was active in four at the time of delivery; all four reported worsening of their perianal symptoms post-partum. The 11 with inactive perianal disease had no relapse, and of the 39 others only one developed perianal disease in at least 1 year of post-partum follow-up.

Few would argue that elective Caesarean section should be carefully considered in the woman with an ileoanal pouch (see Chapter 4), but good obstetric outcome and subsequent pouch function after vaginal delivery are recorded by at least one prominent centre.[25] There seems to be no other good reason for women with inflammatory bowel disease to undergo Caesarean section more often than the general obstetric population unless they have active perianal disease at the time of birth.

BREAST-FEEDING

All drugs are sources of anxiety for the nursing mother, and with good reason, because most find their way into breast milk, and thus to the infant. Most drugs achieve an equal or lower concentration than that in serum, but a few are concentrated in milk.[26] Amongst those most likely to be used in inflammatory bowel disease there need be no greater anxiety than whilst the mother is pregnant. Even high doses of systemic prednisolone given to the mother pose little risk, as less than 0.1 per cent of the weight-adjusted therapeutic dose reaches the infant.[26] There do not seem to be specific data for the 5-ASA drugs but non-steroidals are safe. Methotrexate should probably remain contraindicated, but there are transplant data that appear to sanction the use of azathioprine and ciclosporin, as the infant blood levels run at less than 5 per cent of those in the mother and clinical problems are not encountered.[26]

Breast-feeding is highly desirable but if it is not possible for the mother to be satisfactorily maintained on a regimen that is obviously safe for the infant, then bottle-feeding is indicated. Nonetheless, the mother with inflammatory bowel disease will wish to know that breast-feeding helps to protect her baby from Crohn's disease.[27]

Paediatric inflammatory bowel disease practice

This volume is plainly inadequate to guide the paediatrician with a specialist interest in inflammatory bowel disease, but since the adult gastroenterologist will occasionally be asked to advise on the management of inflammatory bowel disease affecting children, and since a comprehensive service in paediatric gastroenterology is rarely available, a brief section is included. Referral to a tertiary centre is always wise if any doubt exists. Much of paediatric inflammatory bowel disease practice is, however, remarkably similar to that in adults. The main point of management difference is in respect of growth and growth retardation – an issue in many children with Crohn's disease but more rarely a problem in ulcerative colitis.

The combined incidence of inflammatory bowel disease in those under 16 was around 5 per 100 000 in the mid-1980s in Sweden, with a rough equivalence of ulcerative colitis and Crohn's disease, given the number with unconfirmed Crohn's disease and the 23 per cent with indeterminate colitis at the time of reporting.[28] The British survey recently completed yielded an annual inflammatory bowel disease incidence of 4.7 per 100 000 in those under 16, using data only from paediatricians, and it is recognized that this, consequently, is an underestimate.[29] There is a trend to earlier recognition and diagnosis of inflammatory bowel disease, which probably coincides with a true change in incidence. Numerous centres have confirmed that the continuing increase in incidence of Crohn's disease is most obvious in the paediatric age range, and perhaps most of all in children of immigrants to Western countries from the Indian subcontinent[29] (see also Chapters 1 and 2). It is unlikely, however, that the aetiology of inflammatory bowel disease is different in children.

CLINICAL FEATURES

The clinical features of childhood disease are similar to those of adults with the obvious difference that the very small child is unable to provide the history that is often so important in making a prompt diagnosis. This is evidently an area in which it is difficult to publish, since several of the key references from the past few years remain available only in abstract form. In a series of 31 patients aged 10 or younger[30] there was no striking difference from what might be expected in an adult cohort in terms of distribution of disease, the proportion of ulcerative colitis and Crohn's, or the clinical severity: most were managed as outpatients. In the under-5s, Crohn's disease is more likely to present late with growth retardation alone, whilst features of ulcerative colitis remain more typical.[31] In the latter series, eight under-5s with Crohn's disease had predominantly colonic involvement, with perianal disease in four, and with terminal ileal disease in only one; three had extra-intestinal manifestations. Of 11 patients with ulcerative colitis, nine had pan-colitis and five needed surgery at a mean of 12 months from presentation. In another series, more than 80 per cent of new ulcerative colitics had 'resolution' of their symptoms by 6 months[32] and for any given subsequent year more than half remained symptom free. At 1 year, the risk of colectomy was 1 per cent amongst those with mild disease compared with 8 per cent in moderate/severe disease; at 5 years, the cumulative risks of colectomy were 9 per cent and 26 per cent, respectively.[32] The Leiden group[33] found more anorexia, more general malaise and, predictably, more growth disturbance

in the under-16s. Most of the differences they identify are less striking than the similarities, and the greater delay before diagnosis probably accounts for those that do exist. Puberty may be somewhat delayed, perhaps by over a year in children with Crohn's disease.[8]

There is a general perception that Crohn's disease proves to be the final diagnosis more often than anticipated at first investigation; even when colectomy has been performed for (presumed) ulcerative colitis, the final diagnosis was Crohn's in no less than 53 per cent of a Canadian series.[34] This difficulty is most pronounced for emergency colectomy, in which it reflects adult practice (see Chapters 2 and 4).

The differential diagnosis is a little different in paediatric practice. Adult gastroenterologists are, for example, unlikely to see cows' milk protein (or other allergic) colitis, and will incorrectly assume that this sometimes florid haemorrhagic condition is ulcerative colitis, only to be surprised when a better informed paediatric colleague achieves complete resolution simply by switching the infant to an amended milk formula. An insistence on histological support is recommended, and reference to a paediatric gastroenterologist is wise whenever diagnostic doubt exists.

Disease distribution in children with ulcerative colitis is comparable to that in adults, but there may be a greater tendency for proximal extension of initial ulcerative proctitis. In a five-centre study of 38 children followed over a mean of 4.3 years, the clinical status remained good and/or improved in most (approximately 70 per cent) and only two needed immunosuppression. However, 11 of the total group (29 per cent) exhibited proximal extension, rising to 54 per cent of the 13 followed for more than 5 years.[35]

Children with Crohn's disease are more likely than adults to have extensive and proximal small bowel disease. This is borne out by endoscopic assessment of the upper gastrointestinal tract; abnormalities are typically found in more than two-thirds of children with inflammatory bowel disease if both gastroscopy and colonoscopy are performed, regardless of the localization of symptoms and signs. In one such study, the upper gastrointestinal signs were instrumental in making the diagnosis of Crohn's disease in no less than 41 per cent of patients;[36] this study showed involvement of the upper gastrointestinal tract in 71 per cent, the terminal ileum in 53 per cent and the colon in 86 per cent. There should, however, be care in avoidance of an over-interpretation of ileal lymphoid nodular hyperplasia, which is common in normal children and more so still in those with immunodeficiency (see Chapter 2). The severity of disease probably encompasses the same spectrum as in adult practice.

Growth retardation

Growth retardation is a substantial problem in children with Crohn's disease. More than a third of juvenile patients with inflammatory bowel disease can be expected to fall below the fifth centile for height at some time;[37] two-thirds of those with Crohn's will have a growth velocity more than 2 standard deviations below normal.[38] Final adult height is notably deficient in at least 7 per cent, and falls at least 1 standard deviation below normal in 22–29 per cent.[38,39] Amongst an American cohort of 48 young adults diagnosed with inflammatory bowel disease before completion of puberty (at a mean of 11.8 years), final adult height was compared with that predicted from three different methods.[40] Depending on the method, permanent growth failure had affected 19–35 per cent, and 31 per cent had deficits on two or more diagnostic criteria, a figure rising to 37 per cent if Crohn's disease was considered alone. Nineteen per cent of this group had height below population norms, constituting 'clinically meaningful deficits of ultimate adult height'.

It is therefore important to seek growth retardation, and to do so at a time when useful action might still be taken. Sadly, many units still fail to record the simplest of anthropometric measures on a routine basis.[41] Unfortunately, even if height falling below the third or fifth centile is identified, if this is used as the main criterion for growth failure, many children with subnormal growth will still be missed. Standard deviation-based Z scores (as familiar from bone densitometry), which give a number rather than a percentage, give a more subtle account of height relative to age for the population. It is better still to place reliance on the height velocity, which is most sensitive to small changes and is of greatest relevance to the individual as opposed to the population.[39] Motil *et al.* have shown abnormal Z scores (< -1.64) in 23 per cent at the time of diagnosis in paediatric inflammatory bowel disease and impaired height velocity (< 4 cm/year) in 24 per cent.[37] Concomitant reduction in childhood bone mass and bone density is also demonstrable in Crohn's disease.[42]

Whether growth retardation in inflammatory bowel disease is steroid related is much less clear. The Motil and Griffiths studies[37,39] failed to demonstrate a link with past or present steroids. The Hildebrand and Markowitz studies[38,40] attributed a link to current and cumulative duration of steroid usage respectively, but clearly some of the growth deficit is after the onset of the disease but prior to its diagnosis (and treatment). The Issenman study[42] considered that steroid therapy had no effect on growth, which improved with time whether or not steroids were used. There is an increasing consensus that the main reason for growth failure is caloric insufficiency[43] aggravated by high levels of circulating inflammatory cytokines.

MEDICAL THERAPY

Therapy in children with inflammatory bowel disease is devised to minimize steroid usage, with a favouring of primary nutritional therapy in Crohn's disease, and a somewhat lower threshold for surgical intervention. There is support in paediatric work for the use of a specific formula feed supplemented with transforming growth factor beta (TGF-β), which is now commercially available from Nestlé. In an open study of 29 children, there was a normalization of several cytokines, and 79 per cent came into full clinical remission[44] (see also Chapter 3). Azathioprine and 6MP come under consideration relatively frequently, but there is understandable reserve about their actual use.[45] Safety in fact appears good, and if surgery is not strongly indicated, then they should be utilized more or less as in adults. It is probable that (as for steroids) a higher dose per kilogram body weight is required in the pre-pubertal child; a ratio of 1.5 to 1 is suggested.[46] The Royal Free group in London also advocate intravenous azathioprine (3 mg/kg) on the basis of their good experiences with three particularly sick children (one ulcerative colitis, one indeterminate, one Crohn's).[47]

The actions of infliximab in children are probably similar to those in adults, both on chronic active disease and in fistulation,[48,49] but present knowledge is limited by an absence of controlled data. Etanercept does not seem to have been used in paediatric Crohn's, but might be expected to work safely given successful open-label and placebo-controlled use in children with rheumatoid arthritis.[50]

SURGERY IN CHILDHOOD IBD

Many decisions about surgery in children with inflammatory bowel disease will be taken on similar grounds to those in adults, although the patient's voice will be supported or substituted by that of the parent. However, there is a greater urgency for surgical intervention in the child with Crohn's who is not growing. The St Bartholomew's group have demonstrated major improvement in growth velocity if the bulk of the diseased intestine can be removed, quite apart from the more obvious advantages to be expected from appropriate surgical intervention.[51] It is becoming clear that

the advantages of surgery are most compelling when it is undertaken before puberty is well advanced, or, indeed, when puberty is delayed. An increment of height velocity of only 1 cm per year followed Crohn's surgery at pubertal stage 4 or 5, compared to the more useful response of an increment between 5 and 8 cm per year when operation was performed at pubertal stages 1, 2 or 3.[52] Similar results were reported for ulcerative colitis.[53] A degree of controversy remains, however, the Toronto group considering that surgery made little difference (albeit with the caution that they might reasonably have been otherwise expected to do worse).[39] I believe that it is wise to err on the side of intervention when there is doubt about surgery in a child with Crohn's disease and impaired growth.

As surgical strategy may differ, the distinction of ulcerative colitis from Crohn's disease is clearly important and perhaps more difficult in children.[34] Although some of the Montreal data go back to 1961 and can hardly be considered contemporary, that no fewer than 15 of 28 children treated by colectomy for ulcerative colitis subsequently proved to have Crohn's disease should not be neglected.[34] The reasonable comment is made that error is less likely if preoperative colonoscopy has been performed, especially if the terminal ileum has been visualized and biopsied. This is already preferred practice in most paediatric gastrointestinal units.

In other respects, surgical series indicate strong similarities with adult practice (see Chapter 4). Most units now feel confident to consider pouch creation for the older child with ulcerative colitis, although generally preferring an ileorectal anastomosis in the smallest, with the option to convert to a pouch in adolescence or early adulthood.

Complications of inflammatory bowel disease such as toxic megacolon, sclerosing cholangitis, and the various extra-intestinal manifestations (see also Chapter 6) occur in children at similar frequency. A representative survey of 75 children attending a single clinic identified arthralgia (8 per cent), arthritis (3 per cent), and erythema nodosum, pancreatitis, autoimmune hepatitis, central nervous system and renal symptoms, each in single cases.[54]

NEOPLASIA IN CHILDREN WITH IBD

Malignancy complicating inflammatory bowel disease is almost never seen in children, but this probably simply reflects the major influence of disease duration, and that most children have become adult before becoming at significant risk. Nevertheless, it is precisely those who present in childhood who are ultimately most likely to develop malignancy, and this begins to be of clinical relevance in adolescence (see below).

Adolescence

Adolescents pose problems distinct from both adults and children, and are unfortunately rather neglected by most health care systems. Between 15 and 20 per cent of all patients with inflammatory bowel disease present at this age, so there is little excuse for the continued ignoring of this group. In most cases physicians more used to dealing with adults will be called upon to provide care. The adolescent with inflammatory bowel disease, like the child, remains prey to impaired growth and development, but with a greater desire (and need) for personal autonomy. This can easily lead to rejection of parental advice and encouragement (for example with nutrition) and a poor relationship with professional carers. This area has been nicely explored in 28 young Swedish colitics.[55] Transcriptions of verbatim, semi-structured interviews were analysed according to the so-called constant comparative method for grounded theory. The main outcomes identified were perception of reduced living space, and of inadequate strategies to manage their new situation.

Dependent on the reactions of, and degree of support from, significant others, these adolescents expressed more lack of self-confidence than is normal.

In a partially controlled study of growth-retarded peripubertal individuals, 8 of 14 agreed to and were compliant with an overnight nasogastric tube feed. Linear growth and weight increased significantly over the next 12 months in those 8 (by 7 cm and 11.7 kg, respectively), but remained unchanged in the 6 who declined nasogastric therapy.[56] It is not suggested that this was the only reason for the differences in outcome, as those choosing to reject care may well have a different prognosis for other reasons also; however, it highlights some of the problems that must be tackled in adolescent management. In this context, the results of the Scottish follow-up of growth and development are reassuring for doctors, and should permit useful transmission of that information to adolescents when their anxieties about failed growth are at their peak. The study identified 105 individuals admitted for inflammatory bowel disease during 1968–83. All 87 of those that, by the time of the study, were at least 18 years of age and 5 years or more from the time of admission were contacted.[57] All the patients had become sexually mature and all those with ulcerative colitis were of normal height and body mass index. Patients with Crohn's disease were about 8 kg lighter than their normal contemporaries (mean 67 kg in men, 51 kg in women), but only three were 'pathologically' short. The strong implication is that although the pubertal growth spurt tends to be delayed in Crohn's disease, it is usually, ultimately, effective in achieving normal height.

Concern that immunosuppressive therapy might be unduly hazardous in adolescence has not been borne out by experience,[58] efficacy and safety appearing similar to those recorded in adults. The greater difficulties those I find in persuading this age group to have regular blood counts when on azathioprine and in remission do not seem to translate into problematic myelosuppression, but there must be some concern about this. Steroids are better avoided for all the reasons applicable in paediatric and adult practice, and with the additional pressing need to preserve normal appearance as the patient becomes sexually aware.

Most adults with long-standing ulcerative colitis are now enrolled in endoscopic cancer surveillance programmes (see Chapter 8). However, the entry criterion of 8–10 years' extensive colitis is also readily achieved in adolescents and very young adults when their disease began in childhood; the clinical implications of this have not been clear. The need for dysplasia and cancer screening has now been systematically evaluated in 35 such patients (18 ulcerative colitis, 17 Crohn's colitis; of mean age 21 years and of mean colitis duration of 11 years). No fewer than seven had aneuploidy, of whom two had dysplasia, which was high grade in one ulcerative colitis patient.[59] In addition, one of the aneuploid patients (aged 24 with a 14-year history of ulcerative colitis) came to colectomy within a year, and proved to have a Dukes' C adenocarcinoma. It is clear that the justifications for surveillance are as good as in adults and that the over-riding emphasis should be on the presence of extensive disease of long duration, whatever the age at onset or the present age of the patient.

References

1 Narendranathan M, Sandler RS, Suchindran CM, Savitz DA. Male infertility in inflammatory bowel disease. *J Clin Gastroenterol* 1989; **11**: 403–6.

2 Dejaco C, Mittermaier C, Strohmer H, Gasche C, Moser G. Azathioprine treatment and male fertility in inflammatory bowel disease. *Gut* 1999; **45**(Suppl V): A77.

3 O'Morain C, Smethurst P, Dorre CJ, *et al.* Reversible male infertility due to sulphasalazine. Studies in man and rat. *Gut* 1984; **25**: 1078–80.

4 Francella A, Dayan A, Rubin P, Chapman M, Present D. 6-Mercaptopurine is safe therapy for child bearing patients with inflammatory bowel disease: a case controlled study. *Gastroenterology* 1996; **110**: A909.

5 Burakoff R, Opper F. Pregnancy and nursing. *Gastroenterol Clin North Am* 1995; **24**: 689–98.

6 Mayberry JF, Weterman IT. European survey of fertility and pregnancy in women with Crohn's disease: a case control study by European collaborative group. *Gut* 1986; **27**: 821–5.

7 Hudson M, Flett G, Sinclair TS, Brunt PW, Templeton A, Mowat NA. Fertility and pregnancy in inflammatory bowel disease. *Int J Gynaecol Obstet* 1997; **58**: 229–37.

8 Walker-Smith JA, Murch SH. Crohn's disease and abdominal tuberculosis. In *Diseases of the Small Intestine in Childhood*, 4th edn. Oxford: Isis Medical Media, 1999: 299–328.

9 Kane SV, Sable K, Hanauer SB. The menstrual cycle and its effect on inflammatory bowel disease and irritable bowel syndrome: a prevalence study. *Am J Gastroenterol* 1998; **93**: 1867–72.

10 Bortoli A, Tatarella M, Prada A, *et al.* Pregnancy and inflammatory bowel disease: a prospective case-control study. *Gut* 1999; **45**(Suppl V): A281.

11 Castiglione F, Pignata S, Morace F, *et al.* Effect of pregnancy on the clinical course of a cohort of women with inflammatory bowel disease. *Ital J Gastroenterol* 1996; **28**: 199–204.

12 Nwokolo CU, Tan WC, Andrews HA, Allan RN. Surgical resections in parous patients with distal ileal and colonic Crohn's disease. *Gut* 1994; **35**: 220–3.

13 Trallori G, D'Albasio G, Bardazzi G, *et al.* 5-Aminosalicylic acid in pregnancy: clinical report. *Ital J Gastroenterol* 1994; **26**: 75–8.

14 Bell CM, Habal FM. Safety of topical 5-aminosalicylic acid in pregnancy. *Am J Gastroenterol* 1997; **92**: 2201–2.

15 Colombel JF, Brabant G, Gubler MC, *et al.* Renal insufficiency in infants: side-effect of prenatal exposure to mesalazine? *Lancet* 1994; **344**: 620–1.

16 Teahon K, Pearson M, Levi AJ, Bjarnason I. Elemental diet in the management of Crohn's disease during pregnancy. *Gut* 1991; **32**: 1079–81.

17 Rosa RW, Baum C, Shaw M. Pregnancy outcomes after first trimester vaginitis drug therapy. *Obstet Gynecol* 1987; **69**: 751–9.

18 Alstead EM, Ritchie JK, Lennard-Jones JE, Farthing MJ, Clark ML. Safety of azathioprine in pregnancy in inflammatory bowel disease. *Gastroenterology* 1990; **99**: 443–6.

19 Bertschinger P, Himmelmann A, Risti B, Follath F. Cyclosporine treatment of severe ulcerative colitis during pregnancy. *Am J Gastroenterol* 1995; **90**: 330.

20 Zachariae H. Methotrexate side-effects. *Br J Dermatol* 1990; **122**(Suppl 36): 127–33.

21 Creinin MD. Methotrexate and misoprostol for abortion at 57–63 days gestation. *Contraception* 1994; **50**: 511–15.

22 Boulton R, Hamilton M, Lewis A, Walker P, Pounder R. Fulminant ulcerative colitis in pregnancy. *Am J Gastroenterol* 1994; **89**: 931–3.

23 Brandt LJ, Estabrook SG, Reinus JF. Results of a survey to evaluate whether vaginal delivery and episiotomy lead to perineal involvement in women with Crohn's disease. *Am J Gastroenterol* 1995; **90**: 1918–22.

24 Ilnyckyji A, Blanchard JF, Rawsthorne P, Bernstein CN. Perianal Crohn's disease and pregnancy: role of the mode of delivery. *Am J Gastroenterol* 1999; **94**: 3274–8.

25 Juhasz ES, Fozard B, Dozois RR, Ilstrup DM, Nelson H. Ileal pouch–anal anastomosis function following childbirth. An extended evaluation. *Dis Colon Rectum* 1995; **38**: 159–65.

26 Ito S. Drug therapy for breast-feeding women. *N Engl J Med* 2000; **343**: 118–26.

27 Koletzko S, Sherman P, Corey M, Griffiths A, Smith C. Role of infant feeding practices in development of Crohn's disease in childhood. *Br Med J* 1989; **298**: 1617–18.

28 Hildebrand H, Fredrikzon B, Holmquist L, Kristiansson B, Lindquist B. Chronic inflammatory bowel disease in children and adolescents in Sweden. *J Pediatr Gastroenterol Nutr* 1991; **13**: 293–7.

29 Sawczenko A, Sandhu BK. Results of the first prospective survey of the incidence, presentation and management of inflammatory bowel disease in the United Kingdom and Republic of Ireland. *Arch Dis Child* 2000; **82**(Suppl 1): A2.

30 Chang CH, Heyman MB, Snyder JD. Inflammatory bowel disease in children less than 10 years old: is severe disease common? *Gastroenterology* 1996; **110**: A795.

31 Integlia M, Weiselberg B, Polk B, Grand R, Mobassaleh M. Features of inflammatory bowel disease in children less than 5 years old. *Gastroenterology* 1996; **110**: A807.

32 Hyams JS, Davis P, Grancher K, Lerer T, Justinich CJ, Markowitz J. Clinical outcome of ulcerative colitis in children. *J Pediatr* 1996; **129**: 81–8.

33 Wagtmans MJ, Van Hogezand RA, Mearin ML, Verspaget HW, Lamers CBHW. The clinical course of Crohn's disease differs between children and adults. *Gastroenterology* 1996; **110**: A1041.

34 D'Agata ID, Deslandres C. Outcome of pediatric patients after subtotal colectomy for presumed ulcerative colitis. *Gastroenterology* 1996; **110**: A797.

35 Hyams J, Davis P, Lerer T, *et al.* Clinical outcome of ulcerative proctitis in children. *J Pediatr Gastroenterol Nutr* 1997; **25**: 149–52.

36 Cameron DJ. Upper and lower gastrointestinal endoscopy in children and adolescents with Crohn's disease: a prospective study. *J Gastroenterol Hepatol* 1991; **6**: 355–8.

37 Motil KJ, Grand RJ, Davis-Kraft L, Ferlic LL, Smith EO. Growth failure in children with inflammatory bowel disease: a prospective study. *Gastroenterology* 1993; **105**: 681–91.

38 Hildebrand H, Karlberg J, Kristiansson B. Longitudinal growth in children and adolescents with inflammatory bowel disease. *J Pediatr Gastroenterol Nutr* 1994; **18**: 165–73.

39 Griffiths A, Nguyen P, Smith C, MacMillan, Sherman PM. Growth and clinical course of children with Crohn's disease. *Gut* 1993; **34**: 939–43.

40 Markowitz J, Grancher K, Rosa J, Aiges H, Daum F. Growth failure in pediatric inflammatory bowel disease. *J Pediatr Gastroenterol Nutr* 1993; **16**: 373–80.

41 Ghosh S, Drummond HE, Ferguson A. Neglect of growth and development in the clinical monitoring of children and teenagers with inflammatory

bowel disease: review of case records. *Br Med J* 1998; **317**: 120–1.

42 Issenman RM, Atkinson SA, Radoja C, Fraher L. Longitudinal assessment of growth, mineral metabolism, and bone mass in pediatric Crohn's disease. *J Pediatr Gastroenterol Nutr* 1993; **17**: 401–6.

43 Polk DB, Hattner JA, Kerner JA Jr. Improved growth and disease activity after intermittent administration of a defined formula diet in children with Crohn's disease. *J Parenter Enteral Nutr* 1992; **16**: 499–504.

44 Fell JM, Paintin M, Arnaud-Battandier F, *et al.* Mucosal healing and a fall in mucosal pro-inflammatory cytokine mRNA induced by a specific oral polymeric diet in paediatric Crohn's disease. *Aliment Pharmacol Ther* 2000; **14**: 281–9.

45 Markowitz J, Grancher K, Mandel F, Daum F. Immunosuppressive therapy in pediatric inflammatory bowel disease: results of a survey of the North American Society for Pediatric Gastroenterology and Nutrition. *Am J Gastroenterol* 1993; **88**: 44–8.

46 Cuffari C, Seidman EG, Latour S, Theoret Y. Quantitation of 6-thioguanine in peripheral blood leukocyte DNA in Crohn's disease patients on maintenance 6-mercaptopurine therapy. *Can J Physiol Pharmacol* 1996; **74**: 580–5.

47 Casson DH, Davies SE, Thomson MA, Lewis A, Walker-Smith JA, Murch SH. Low-dose intravenous azathioprine may be effective in the management of acute fulminant colitis complicating inflammatory bowel disease. *Aliment Pharmacol Ther* 1999; **13**: 891–5.

48 Vasiliauskas EA, Schaffer S, Dezenberg CV, *et al.* Collaborative experience of open-label infliximab in refractory pediatric Crohn's disease. *Gastroenterology* 2000; **118**: A178.

49 Braegger CP, Baldassano R, Escher JC, *et al.* A multicenter study of infliximab in the treatment of

children with active Crohn's disease. *Gut* 1999; 45(Suppl V): A262.

50 Lovell DJ, Giannini EH, Reiff A, *et al.* Etanercept in children with polyarticular juvenile rheumatoid arthritis. *N Engl J Med* 2000; **342**: 763–9.

51 Shand WS. Surgical therapy of chronic inflammatory bowel disease in childhood. *Baillières Clin Gastroenterol* 1994; **8**: 149–80.

52 Savage MO, Beattie RM, Camacho-Hubner C, Walker-Smith JA, Sanderson IR. Growth in Crohn's disease. *Acta Paediatr Suppl* 1999; **88**: 89–92.

53 Nicholls S, Vieira MC, Majrowski WH, Shand WS, Savage MO, Walker-Smith JA. Linear growth after colectomy for ulcerative colitis in childhood. *J Pediatr Gastroenterol Nutr* 1995; **21**: 82–6.

54 Stawarski A, Iwanczak F, Iwanczak B, Krzesiek E. Extraintestinal manifestations and complications in children with ulcerative colitis and Crohn's disease. *Gut* 1999; 45(Suppl V): A201.

55 Brydolf M, Segesten K. Living with ulcerative colitis: experiences of adolescents and young adults. *J Adv Nurs* 1996; **23**: 39–47.

56 Aiges H, Markowitz J, Rosa J, Daum F. Home nocturnal supplemental nasogastric feedings in growth-retarded adolescents with Crohn's disease. *Gastroenterology* 1989; **97**: 905–10.

57 Ferguson A, Sedgwick DM. Juvenile onset inflammatory bowel disease: height and body mass index in adult life. *Br Med J* 1994; **308**: 1259–63.

58 Markowitz J, Rosa J, Grancher K, Aiges H, Daum F. Long-term 6-mercaptopurine treatment in adolescents with Crohn's disease. *Gastroenterology* 1990; **99**: 1347–51.

59 Markowitz J, McKinley M, Kahn E, *et al.* Endoscopic screening for dysplasia and mucosal aneuploidy in adolescents and young adults with childhood onset colitis. *Am J Gastroenterol* 1997; **92**: 2001–6.

Extra-intestinal manifestations

The extra-intestinal manifestations of inflammatory bowel disease fall into two broad groups. The conditions that follow an acute course generally also run in parallel with the associated inflammatory bowel disease. The more chronic and potentially progressive extra-intestinal manifestations tend to behave more independently, relatively uninfluenced by the activity of the gastrointestinal disorder. More than a quarter of all inflammatory bowel disease patients can be expected to suffer an extra-intestinal manifestation on a lifetime basis, and the patient with one is more likely to have others.[1] Although it is convenient to consider individual problems according to the particular organ site involved, many of the extra-intestinal manifestations occur in the same patient group.

All of the extra-intestinal manifestations occur preferentially in patients with disease of the colon, and rarely complicate Crohn's disease confined to the small bowel. There are a number of hypotheses for this observation, but no confirmed data. The presence of a faecal stream and disruption of intestinal permeability are implicated (see Chapter 1 and below). The presence of the unoperated ileocaecal region also is associated with a higher incidence of arthropathy than is seen in Crohn's patients after resection.[2] By contrast, those with perforating Crohn's are the most likely to develop extra-intestinal manifestations.[3]

Joints in inflammatory bowel disease

Patients with inflammatory bowel disease are at increased risk of a number of specific joint conditions and remain subject to (for example) degenerative arthritides and rheumatoid arthritis at frequencies typical of the general population. Ankylosing spondylitis (AS) and other spondarthritides are over-represented and there is also the important condition of inflammatory bowel disease-related arthropathy.[4]

Ankylosing spondylitis affecting patients with inflammatory bowel disease runs a relatively independent course typical of spondylitis in patients without gastrointestinal problems[5] (but see below). Modest morning stiffness and low back pain may progress to a stooped posture and an increasingly immobile spine, which can eventually impair ventilation. The sacroiliac joint margins become blurred radiologically, with associated patchy sclerosis, and are later lost; the vertebrae pass through a parallel course from being 'squared', to exhibiting entheses, syndesmophytes and finally the bamboo spine. Patients with ulcerative colitis carry a 30-fold increased risk of spondylitis, but it remains an uncommon association, as AS itself has a prevalence of only 150 per 100 000 in Western populations. Interestingly, although almost all patients with spondylitis have the HLA-B*27 genotype, only between 60 and 80 per cent of those with both ulcerative colitis and spondylitis are positive. The implicated sites appear to be in the HLA class III region.[6] Treatment of progressive spondylitis is never easy, the emphasis resting with physiotherapy and non-steroidal anti-inflammatory drugs (NSAIDs). Unfortunately, the latter are less well tolerated in inflammatory bowel disease; it remains to be seen whether selective inhibition of the cyclo-oxygenase type-2 or COX2 receptor will help here.

Inflammatory bowel disease patients much more frequently develop sacroiliitis without generalized spondylitis. A prevalence of 10–18 per cent based on plain films[7,8] rises to no less than 32 per cent if CT scanning is also included, more or less equally in ulcerative colitis and Crohn's.[8] The condition is often non-progressive and therapy is unnecessary if the patient has no symptoms. Other forms of spondarthritis (psoriatic, etc.) are over-represented in inflammatory bowel disease, but require no special measures. All the above tend to behave independently of the intestinal disorder.

Inflammatory bowel disease-related arthropathy was first described in 1929, and a prevalence between 10 per cent[3] and 22 per cent[9] has been quoted. The Oxford group have made it a special study in the last few years and their publications now present a fairly comprehensive dossier.[10,11] It may present as a polyarthropathy, symmetrically affecting multiple small to medium-sized joints, or in a large-joint pauciarticular form; deforming arthritis is rare. Orchard has classified patients into these two categories on a simple count as to whether five or more joints (type 2) or fewer than five (type 1) have been involved;[10] he makes the distinction between arthritis, where swelling is documented, and arthropathy, where there are symptoms without signs. In a prevalence study of nearly 1000 inflammatory bowel disease patients, type 1 arthritis was recorded in 3.6 per cent of those with ulcerative colitis (83 per cent acute, self-limiting) and in 6.0 per cent of those with

Crohn's (79 per cent self-limiting); 83 per cent and 76 per cent, respectively, of the arthritic episodes were associated with relapses of the inflammatory bowel disease. Type 2 arthritis occurred in 2.5 per cent of patients with ulcerative colitis and 4.0 per cent of those with Crohn's. In 87 per cent and 89 per cent, respectively, arthritis was responsible for persistent symptoms, and 71 per cent and 58 per cent of the episodes of arthritis were independent of inflammatory bowel disease activity. The wide range of incidence and prevalence figures in the literature almost certainly reflects the inclusion criteria and ascertainment bias. We looked deliberately on a symptomatic basis and (unsurprisingly) found a higher point prevalence,[12] with 30 per cent of colitics and 31 per cent of those with Crohn's affected. We identified a higher proportion of young patients with axial (back) pain (6 versus 20 per cent), a higher proportion of smokers with arthropathy (59 versus 29 per cent), and a greater likelihood of other extra-intestinal manifestations.

The rheumatologist with an interest in seronegative arthropathy will find inflammatory bowel disease in at least 50 per cent of such patients. De Vos and her colleagues have reported on 123 patients with well-defined spondyloarthropathy.[13] Patients with AS or previously known intestinal disease were excluded. Eighty-three had histological evidence of proctitis. Nearly 50 of the patients then proceeded to colonoscopy. There was virtual independence of activity of gut and joints in those in whom gastrointestinal disease became overt. However, initial macroscopic and histological inflammation of the intestine predicted a higher risk of progression to formal established AS; of the 19 per cent who progressed, all but one had initial colitis. In 7.3 per cent, frank inflammatory bowel disease developed during follow-up. Sulphasalazine was successfully used for the joint symptoms but had no apparent influence on the likelihood of intestinal symptoms developing. A parallel examination using intestinal scintigraphy in patients with seronegative spondarthropathy yielded abnormal scans in 53 per cent, none of whom was previously considered to have any intestinal involvement.[14]

The potential importance of pouchitis as a human model of inflammatory bowel disease has been discussed in general terms (see Chapter 1); it has relevance also to inflammatory bowel disease-related arthropathy. Although most patients with ulcerative colitis and arthropathy improve after colectomy, a small percentage of those having an ileoanal pouch then develop an arthropathy similar to inflammatory bowel disease-related arthropathy, despite having had no joint symptoms prior to colectomy. In a prospective study of 97 patients with an ileoanal pouch for ulcerative colitis, we found joint symptoms in 31 per cent; 24 per cent had a polyarticular arthralgia affecting primarily the knees and small joints of the hands and in 43 per cent it began only after pouch creation.[15] Clinical findings and radiology were almost exclusively normal. Most patients had mild symptoms and there was no association with positive family history, other extra-intestinal manifestations or with pouchitis, but patients having pouch surgery for polyposis rarely had this problem.

The clinical phenotype of inflammatory bowel disease-related arthropathy (IBDRA) is linked to the patient's genotype via (at least) linkage to the HLA system. In the Oxford data set, patients were compared both with controls and with those with other forms of arthritis.[11] Type 1 IBDRA was positively associated with DRB1*0103 (a DR1 subtype) and with B*27, whereas type 2 IBDRA was linked with B*44. Post-enteric reactive arthritis and ankylosing spondylitis had linkage with B*27 and DRB1*0101, indicating some concordance between these and the type 1, but not the type 2 IBDRA. Interpretation of investigations performed prior to the Oxford classification suggest that type 1 and 2 patients might have different patterns of disordered mucosal immune response also.[16] The observations in pouch patients and the parallel with reactive arthritis suggest a role of abnormal permeability in the pathogenesis of inflammatory bowel disease-related arthropathy.[5] There is now intriguing supportive evidence with the identification of upper gastrointestinal streptococcal antigens (and probably those of other micro-organisms) in the synovial fluid of Crohn's patients with arthritis;[17,18] and in the HLA-B27 transgenic rat arthritis can be prevented by metronidazole.[19]

Osteoporosis in inflammatory bowel disease

The WHO definitions of loss of bone mineral density are based on the T score which refers to number of standard deviations from normal peak bone mass for that sex (rather than the age-corrected Z score); osteopenia exists if the T score is below -1, and osteoporosis if below -2.5. Each integer T score change increases fracture risk by 1.5–3.0 times depending on the bone concerned.

Bone density is undoubtedly reduced in patients with inflammatory bowel disease. This probably reflects mainly the combination of chronic disease activity and cumulative steroid exposure, but there is evidence that the magnitude of bone loss is in part genetically determined through cytokine polymorphisms.[20] Serum calcium is usually normal, but hyperparathyroidism and excess osteoclastic activity are common. It is likely that increased bone turnover (demonstrable by collagen crosslink assay) is the main spontaneous defect, with additional failure of bone formation in steroid-treated patients.[21] TNF-α is implicated as it both activates osteoblasts and matures osteoclasts.[22] There have also been suggestions that concomitant vitamin K deficiency is important, given the vitamin K-dependent activation of osteocalcin to maintain bone mineral density. Preliminary paediatric data suggest that Crohn's patients with osteoporosis have higher uncarboxylated osteocalcin (67.6 per cent of total osteocalcin versus 20–27 per cent in healthy controls) and that this is related to vitamin K deficiency.[23]

Most patients in most studies have negative T scores, more obviously so in Crohn's disease than in ulcerative colitis.[24,25] Osteopenia exists in around 50 per cent and frank osteoporosis exists in at least 10 per cent,[24,25] both are commoner in smokers, and there is evidence that bone loss is more notable in males.[26,27] There is direct linkage between evidence of bone breakdown and inflammatory bowel disease activity.[25] There is a weak but significant association between lower bone density and cumulative exposure to steroids ($r = 0.16$–0.24, depending on bone site),[24] but chronic disease activity and exposure to steroids are clearly not independent variables. The Scottish study of 30 newly diagnosed inflammatory bowel disease patients who had not previously received steroids revealed normal bone mineral density in those presenting with ulcerative colitis, but significant defects were apparent in all of 15 patients with Crohn's disease (mean T scores of below –1).[28] Significantly, in 23 patients reinvestigated after 12 months, there was no marked individual change or significant overall change in score, regardless of whether or not patients had received steroids during this time. Nonetheless, there is an opinion that the time of maximal bone loss is with the very first exposure to steroid.[29] The special issue of failed growth in children is addressed in Chapter 5.

It is possible to reverse osteopenia associated with coeliac disease by dietary intervention,[30] from which should be taken the concept that intervention has the potential to do more than merely to prevent further deterioration. This has not been demonstrated clearly in Crohn's disease, but there are scanty data in support of oestrogens and vitamin D, to which can now be added a useful positive result from a trial of the bisphosphonate alendronate. Half of a group of 32 patients with Crohn's-related osteopenia (T score less than –1) who were in remission and did not

have short bowel syndrome, received alendronate 10 mg daily in a 12-month placebo-controlled trial.[31] The drug was well tolerated and bone mineral density in the lumbar spine and hip increased (by 4.6 per cent and 3.3 per cent), compared respectively to a decrease of 0.9 per cent and an increase of 0.7 per cent in the controls. The changes in the lumbar spine were significant ($P < 0.08$) and markers of bone turnover were substantially diminished ($P < 0.001$). The balancing of the study was not quite equal, and would have been expected to favour the placebo group. This is probably a useful advance; whether the cheaper option of cyclical etidronate would be as good is unknown. Stopping smoking and an impact exercise programme may have some value but compliance was highly disappointing, even in patients recruited to an exercise trial.[32]

There is no convincing evidence that budesonide reduces future bone loss despite the expectation that it should and it is disappointing to discover that even inhaled budesonide is responsible for osteopenia in asthmatics.[33] It is clear, however, that the issue of steroid use and bone loss cannot be ignored by gastroenterologists, as it now appears to be the commonest reason for legal action being taken against us.

Renal and urinary tract problems associated with inflammatory bowel disease

Urinary tract stones, particularly calcium oxalate stones, are over-represented in patients with inflammatory bowel disease. Amongst Crohn's patients needing surgery, the frequency of stones is around 5 per cent,[34] but the patients most at risk are those with extensive small bowel Crohn's yet with a retained colon, in whom the proportion affected by stone formation may exceed 25 per cent.[35] Intestinal luminal oxalate is normally calcium-bound and poorly available. In fat malabsorption calcium becomes preferentially bound to free fatty acids, and oxalate accordingly becomes sodium-bound. Sodium oxalate is soluble and is absorbed in the colon. This increased absorption predisposes to hyperoxaluria, and thus to an increased risk of renal stones.[36] This is particularly a problem in patients with short bowel syndrome (see Chapter 7); avoidance of foodstuffs rich in oxalate such as spinach, parsley, rhubarb, strawberries, beetroot, cocoa and tea should be advised.

Calcium-rich stones might also be a theoretical consequence of the hypercalcaemia that is now identified as a rare complication of Crohn's disease, thought analogous to the hypercalcaemia of sarcoidosis, and which results from the overproduction of 1,25-dihydroxyvitamin D.[37]

Urate stones are less common, and usually reflect continual dehydration associated with high volume intestinal losses. Again, they are seen most often in those with short bowel syndrome, but here the association is with a proximal stoma and high fluid and electrolyte losses.[38] Prevention, from adequate hydration and good urine flow, forms part of standard good management. Nephrologists will often need reminding that advice to drink more is counterproductive (see Chapter 7).

Hydronephrosis and retroperitoneal fibrosis are seen in Crohn's disease. Simple hydronephrosis is evidently not a rare complication, affecting perhaps 2 per cent of all Crohn's patients[39] and 3 per cent of those coming to surgery.[34] It more often affects the right side, and is related to contiguous inflammatory disease.[34] It seems to be benign, and rarely requires action, but intra-ureteric stenting and surgical reconstruction are effective if intervention is necessary.

The continuing question of nephropathy as an important potential complication of aminosalicylate (5-ASA) therapy has been discussed in Chapter 3; most data are reasonably reassuring. It should also be remembered that inflammatory bowel disease itself predisposes to intrinsic renal disease affecting both glomeruli and tubules, independently of therapy.

Morphological changes in the glomeruli of patients with inflammatory bowel disease have long been recognized.[40,41] The prevalence is uncertain but low; reporting authors generally seem to believe that the associations are of a causal nature, and unrelated to pharmacological intervention. Minor elevations of serum creatinine are also often demonstrable in inflammatory bowel disease, but are not progressive and should probably not be considered sufficient to be of major clinical concern.

Pathological enzymuria (corrected for renal excretory function) used as a marker for tubular function proved almost exclusively linked with active disease in ulcerative colitis and not with current or past exposure to 5-ASA.[42] In Crohn's disease there were no obvious relationships. Elevation of urinary β-N-acetyl-D-glucosaminidase (found in 20–25 per cent of cases) suggested that subtle tubular damage is a common feature of inflammatory bowel disease but one that appears independent of both therapy and other extra-intestinal manifestations. The cause is not clear, but it does not appear to have adverse prognostic significance. Two major studies of all-cause mortality failed to demonstrate excess deaths from renal failure (see Chapter 2).

Amyloidosis of the reactive AA type is seen in some patients with long-standing Crohn's disease, but there is probably no increased incidence in ulcerative colitis. The kidney is the commonest site for clinically significant amyloid deposition, affecting up to 1 per cent of patients with Crohn's disease on a lifetime basis.[43] It is probable that it is more frequent when control of Crohn's-related inflammation has not been good, and it is suggested that anti-inflammatory therapy might be justified on this basis even in the asymptomatic patient who continues to exhibit a high level of acute phase reactants.[44] Once renal amyloidosis is established, it is most often responsible for nephrotic syndrome, although the magnitude of this is very variable. It runs a course independent of the Crohn's disease once it has arisen, and occasionally leads to a need for renal replacement therapy.

Skin problems in inflammatory bowel disease

ERYTHEMA NODOSUM

Erythema nodosum presents as painful, raised, red lesions, typically on the shins, in the relatively young patient with active inflammatory bowel disease (Plate 11). It is the commonest dermatological manifestation of inflammatory bowel disease and is more often seen in Crohn's disease than in ulcerative colitis, affecting around 15 per cent of Crohn's patients[45] compared with only about 2 per cent of those with ulcerative colitis.[46] It is the result of a subcutaneous septal panniculitis and is associated with a neutrophil infiltrate that evolves through a more chronic inflammatory process before complete resolution. Biopsy, though of reasonably characteristic nature, is very rarely appropriate given the clear clinical pointers to the diagnosis in inflammatory bowel disease patients. It usually appears during active inflammatory bowel disease (only 10 per cent having inactive colitis[46]), and runs a broadly parallel course that does not normally require specific therapy. Oral potassium iodide has been suggested for resistant cases.[47] Although erythema nodosum may recur with further exacerbations of the intestinal disease, it very rarely recurs after proctocolectomy.

PYODERMA GANGRENOSUM AND ASSOCIATED CONDITIONS

Pyoderma gangrenosum is a form of neutrophilic dermatosis. It affects about 2 per cent of inflammatory bowel disease patients,[46,48] is more

common in long-standing disease, and is usually associated with active colitis in patients with Crohn's disease. A little over half of all patients with pyoderma have underlying inflammatory bowel disease, but it is also seen in a variety of other inflammatory conditions and in isolation.[49] The pathogenesis is not clear, but the strong association of pyoderma lesions with sites of surgical and other trauma (Koebnerization), especially the peristomal area,[50] suggests that pathergy is an important factor (Plate 12).

When it is the presenting feature of inflammatory bowel disease, pyoderma may be misinterpreted because not at first considered in the differential diagnosis. The lesions are single and on a lower limb in just over half of all cases.[49] They characteristically develop into deep ulcers with a necrotic base, undermined purple edges, and a purulent sterile discharge, but there are many exceptions.

The commonest variant of pyoderma presents with numerous small, superficial lesions similar to simple spots, and is then known as pustular pyoderma. A very unusual bullous form, which tends not to ulcerate, is associated with Sweet's syndrome (see below). Pyodermatitis-pyostomatitis vegetans produces a pustular eruption in the oral mucosa and vegetating plaques affecting the groin and axillary folds[51] (stomatitis here refers to the mouth!). A further subtype, in which active ulcerative colitis is accompanied by the disseminated pustular eruption of pustular vacuities and superficial bullous pyoderma, has been described[52] and lends support to the view that all these variants belong on a continuum.[53]

The differential diagnosis for all types of pyoderma is usually infection, although pemphigus may be considered if there are bullae. Biopsy is better avoided because of the potential to aggravate the final magnitude of scarring, but if biopsy of the edges is performed, around three-quarters will have a lymphocytic or leucocytoclastic vasculitis.[49]

Pyoderma gangrenosum may respond to therapy for inflammatory bowel disease, but may require this at an intensity out of proportion to that needed for the bowel. There is good anecdotal support, also, for the use of intralesional steroids, and the application of potent steroid preparations beneath an impermeable dressing seems particularly helpful. Dapsone and minocycline have also been suggested. When the condition is especially troublesome, prolonged high-dose steroids, ciclosporin or other forms of immunosuppression may be indicated. Controlled data do not exist and, whilst I share the caution of another reviewer who counsels against colectomy for extra-intestinal manifestations alone,[54] the occasional mortality associated with the condition should preclude complacence.[49] Regardless of the therapy used, long-term scarring, which has a characteristic cribriform pattern, may remain.

The rare condition of Sweet's syndrome, or acute pyrexial neutrophilic dermatosis, is also described in both ulcerative colitis and Crohn's colitis (usually when active).[55,56] It presents with tender, purple/red nodular or plaque-like lesions of the skin, usually on the upper limbs, face or neck. It takes its name from the association with pyrexia and a high neutrophil count, and may come combined with bullous pyoderma.[53] It is more common in women (> 75 per cent) and is also associated with malignant disorders (especially haematological ones). It is probable that short courses of prednisolone by mouth suffice in most cases, but metronidazole and a variety of other agents have also been suggested.

The explosive onset of fluctuant papulo-nodules on the face, usually in young women, is characteristic of pyoderma faciale. This disorder is neither a true pyoderma nor a variant of acne, but rather a severe form of rosacea, that again is over-represented in inflammatory bowel disease.[57] Isotretinoin and topical steroids appear to be effective therapy.

PSORIASIS

Psoriasis is over-represented in inflammatory bowel disease, partly because of the association with HLA-B27, and is reported in up to 11 per cent of those with ulcerative colitis[58] and 9.6 per cent of those with Crohn's disease,[59] whilst population controls have a frequency around 2 per cent.[59] Its clinical course, the need for therapy and the success rates from therapy are not obviously different in those with inflammatory bowel disease.

A psoriasis-like syndrome incorporating erythema, pustules and fever, with biopsy showing a neutrophil and lymphohistiocytic infiltrate in the dermis, is also reported as a complication of therapy with sulphasalazine.[60]

Ophthalmic complications in inflammatory bowel disease

In common with many of the other extra-intestinal manifestations, involvement of the eye is more often seen in patients with colitis, and on the whole is associated with active intestinal disease.[61,62] It appears to be commoner in Crohn's colitis than in ulcerative colitis, and a disturbing paediatric report suggests that the frequency of asymptomatic anterior uveitis may be as high as 6.2 per cent in Crohn's disease.[63] Iritis and uveitis present clinically, as when unassociated with inflammatory bowel disease, with impaired visual acuity and a painful red eye. The diagnosis can be confirmed by slit-lamp examination if it is not otherwise obvious clinically; topical steroids are usually sufficient therapy (with a mydriatic), but there is a risk of permanent damage if prompt treatment is not initiated. Pain will usually respond to simple analgesics or to non-steroidal anti-inflammatories.[64]

Episcleritis is probably the commonest ophthalmic association of inflammatory bowel disease. It is usually responsible for redness and discomfort with a conjunctivitis-like syndrome, but there are occasionally disturbances of vision and, more rarely still, superficial ulcers may develop. Treatment is not normally required, other than that for the concurrent exacerbation of the intestinal inflammation, but for the more severe cases topical steroids almost always suffice.[64]

In a useful review of 19 Crohn's patients seen in a single eye unit, seven had uveitis, eight had episcleritis, and four had anterior scleritis.[61] Large peripheral corneal infiltrates developed in two patients with scleritis. Activity of the Crohn's disease was associated with episcleritis but not with uveitis or scleritis. In comparison with 93 Crohn's patients without ocular inflammation, ophthalmic complications were more common in those with colitis or ileocolitis (24 per cent), than in those with small bowel involvement alone (3 per cent; $P = 0.013$). Those with arthritis were also more likely to suffer from eye disease (30 versus 7 per cent; $P = 0.003$).

ENT

The otorhinolaryngologist rarely sees patients with inflammatory bowel disease, although the oral manifestations described in Chapter 2 may come to expert attention via this route. There are also various case reports of overlap syndromes with temporal or giant cell arteritis, or (for example) odd presentations of nasal pyoderma gangrenosum, which may simply represent coincidence. Of more likely true association is the apparent link between sensorineural deafness and both ulcerative colitis[65] and Crohn's disease.[66] An autoimmune mechanism is postulated and our own unpublished data suggest that subclinical forms are not rare (up to 10 per cent of those under 50 having abnormal audiograms). It is important to identify this at the earliest symptomatic stage if prompt steroid therapy is to be instituted and permanent deafness avoided.

Neurological

There is increasing understanding of the linkage between intestinal inflammation and the effects on

motility (see Chapter 2), and there is a steady trickle of neuromuscular phenomena associated with inflammatory bowel disease in individual case reports, but, apart from those that reflect the thrombotic tendencies of inflammatory bowel disease patients (see Chapter 7), it is uncertain that the problems described are other than chance associations. There are suggestions from a better documented series that a form of pupillary autonomic neuropathy and exaggerated sinus arrhythmia (without cardiac neuropathy) is over-represented amongst patients with ulcerative colitis and Crohn's disease.[67,68] Such phenomena may reflect an autoimmune process affecting the small vessels supplying both central and peripheral nerves.[69] Reliable data are not yet available but there has been for some time a suggestion that multiple sclerosis is over-represented in inflammatory bowel disease;[70] our own as yet unpublished survey of 1000 patients suggests that this is a true association. Overall, more than 3 per cent of patients in our survey had important neurological diagnoses, a similar total to that of an Israeli study which associated peripheral neuropathy with ulcerative colitis and myelopathy with Crohn's disease at levels that are probably statistically significant.[71]

Cardiopulmonary

Clinical manifestations of pulmonary disease are not common in inflammatory bowel disease, but the evidence now suggests that chronic respiratory disease in those below middle age is, despite initial impressions, more likely to be a consequence of the gastrointestinal disease than a second diagnosis such as sarcoid[72] or Wegener's.[73] No reliable epidemiological data exist, but ulcerative colitis seems more often complicated by respiratory problems than Crohn's disease.[74] Gas transfer (TLCO) is reduced in up to 57 per cent of selected patients with both ulcerative colitis and Crohn's,[75] perhaps especially during active phases of disease,[76] and lymphocyte subsets in induced sputum are abnormal in 65 per cent of non-smoking inflammatory bowel disease patients.[77] The principal pathologies are obstructive bronchiolitis and granulomatous bronchiolitis in Crohn's disease, and a form of otherwise idiopathic bronchiectasis or bronchiolectasis in ulcerative colitis.[74,78,79] Diagnostic information comes mainly from pulmonary function tests and CT scanning.[74] Fortunately, rapid progression is not the rule and many patients will prove to be steroid responsive.[74]

Cardiac disease is most uncommon in association with inflammatory bowel disease, but there is a link to pericarditis, which may be the presenting feature,[80] and to myocarditis, which may be fatal.[81] A Swiss study identified no fewer than 68 patients with at least one episode of pericarditis or myocarditis; no strong link to inflammatory bowel disease activity was identifiable and there was usually a good response to steroid therapy.[81] A proportion of inflammatory bowel disease-associated pericarditis is related to sensitivity to 5-ASA drugs and these should always be withdrawn even when they have been used apparently safely for many years.

Hepatobiliary disease in inflammatory bowel disease

CHOLELITHIASIS

Gallstones are commoner in patients with ileal Crohn's disease and particularly so when there has been terminal ileal resection. The prevalence in Birmingham was 28 per cent in relatively unselected patients with Crohn's disease screened by ultrasonography,[82] if those who had already had a cholecystectomy were included, and reaches 45 per cent in those with established short bowel syndrome.[83] A population-controlled study suggests, at first sight, that these figures may overemphasize the attributable risk, as 9.7 per cent

of the normal population also had stones.[84] After age and sex matching, however, the odds ratio (OR) for cholelithiasis proved significant for both ulcerative colitis (OR: 2.5; CI: 1.2–5.2) and Crohn's disease (OR: 3.6; CI: 1.2–10.4), with, as expected, the highest rate in those with ileal involvement (OR: 4.5). The duration of the intestinal disorder also correlates with the risk of stone formation. The Birmingham group were unable to demonstrate a direct link with ileal involvement,[82] but, curiously, found an association with the number of laparotomies rather than with the cumulative magnitude of intestinal resection, and suggested that biliary stasis and/or dysmotility are therefore more important than the bile salt malabsorption and reduced bile salt pool that have previously been implicated. In general, patients with previous intestinal resection for Crohn's disease have low biliary cholesterol saturation, and a higher than normal ratio of ursodeoxycholic to deoxycholic acid.[85] Cholesterol stones are not therefore to be expected in Crohn's disease, and gallstones in inflammatory bowel disease are indeed usually predominantly of pigment type. Predominantly cholesterol stones are, however, described in patients with ileoanal anastomoses.[86] Crohn's-induced stones may also result from a competition for binding between excess (malabsorbed) colonic bile salts and bilirubin, promoting an enterohepatic circulation of bilirubin, a higher concentration of bilirubin in gallbladder bile and a predisposition to pigment stones.[87] The management of cholelithiasis in patients with inflammatory bowel disease is that of cholelithiasis in general, but it may prove difficult or impossible safely to perform laparoscopic cholecystectomy in the patient who has already had extensive surgical intervention for Crohn's disease.

INTRINSIC LIVER DISEASE

Parenchymal liver disease occurs to some extent in primary sclerosing cholangitis (see below) but is also over-represented in other respects, with upwards of 10 per cent of patients with inflammatory bowel disease having abnormal liver function tests at some time.[88] In most cases, these reflect active intestinal disease and have no other significance. Patients with inflammatory bowel disease appear similarly susceptible to viral hepatitis and the effects of alcohol abuse, but those with ulcerative colitis in particular are more prone to certain hepatic disorders. Liver disease tends to affect those with more severe inflammatory bowel disease, so the 50 per cent with abnormal liver histology at prospective liver biopsy in a series of patients having colectomy for ulcerative colitis might be thought to be unrepresentative,[89] were it not for a 50 per cent rate of abnormal histology in biopsies from 74 colitics with normal liver function.[90] There were, however, higher proportions of specific diagnoses in Mattila's study,[89] with steatosis affecting 28 per cent, sclerosing cholangitis 41 per cent, hepatitis 21 per cent, and only 10 per cent with the ill-defined abnormalities more typical of the Swedish study.[90]

Steatosis is accordingly a common intrinsic condition of the liver in inflammatory bowel disease, and is found in Crohn's as well as in ulcerative colitis. It probably reflects chronic inflammation and possibly a degree of malnutrition, and does not appear to be progressive. Hepatic fibrosis and cirrhosis may be seen as complications of long-term parenteral nutrition, and will, as such, occasionally be seen in patients with Crohn's disease who have had massive resections, but they also occur in unresected inflammatory bowel disease. The incidence of cirrhosis attributable to the intestinal disorder is not known, given confounding factors such as transfusion-related hepatitis, sclerosing cholangitis and alcohol abuse, but is probably in the region of 1 per cent on a lifetime basis. Appropriate management and prognosis are most probably those of cirrhosis in general.

Chronic active hepatitis affects patients with ulcerative colitis more than those with Crohn's disease – at a frequency in the region of 2 per cent.

There has been some confusion in the literature over the distinction between chronic active hepatitis and pericholangitis, not least since the two may occur together. It is increasingly recognized that the latter is predominantly a feature of primary sclerosing cholangitis, and is of little consequence in its own right. From a large series of patients with severe autoimmune chronic hepatitis, Perdigoto *et al.* identified no less than 16 per cent with associated ulcerative colitis, half of whom also had sclerosing cholangitis.[91] The colitics appeared to have more severe disease and worse prognosis than those with isolated liver disease, but this adverse influence was lost when the patients with sclerosing cholangitis were excluded. Such patients usually respond to steroids and azathioprine similarly to those without intestinal disease.

The only hepatic lesion that appears commoner in Crohn's disease than in ulcerative colitis is granulomatous hepatitis. The prevalence is not certain, there having been no biopsy study of unselected patients comparable to the Swedish studies in ulcerative colitis. Clinically significant disease affects about 1 per cent of those with Crohn's, with a cholestatic enzyme profile, sometimes associated with hepatic discomfort and pyrexia.[92]

PRIMARY SCLEROSING CHOLANGITIS

Primary sclerosing cholangitis (PSC) is a chronic cholestatic condition variable both in its severity and in its tendency to progress. At least 70 per cent of patients with PSC also have ulcerative colitis, the diagnosis of PSC occasionally preceding the diagnosis of colitis.[93,94] In a Swedish study of 76 patients with PSC, 65 were previously known to have inflammatory bowel disease. Nine of the remaining 11 agreed to be investigated by colonoscopy. This revealed ulcerative colitis in six, Crohn's disease in one, and non-specific changes in two.[93] Concomitantly PSC can be expected in about 2.5 per cent of colitics. It is also described in

Crohn's disease. The colitis is usually extensive, and often relatively inactive.

Potential aetiological associations

The strong association between PSC and the HLA haplotype A1B8-DR3DQ2 has been refined to the subtype haplotype DRB1*1301, DQA1*0103, DQB1*0603,[95] genetic probing indicating that the determinant for this lies close to the DRB locus.[96]

An association has also been established between PSC and the presence of antineutrophil cytoplasmic antibodies. This exceeds the expected degree of association for their prevalence in ulcerative colitis alone in some series (see Chapter 1) and has been reported at frequencies from 26 per cent to 85 per cent.[97] It is probable that (as in the colon) the antibody has no clinical, pathogenic or prognostic significance.[98] Detectable pANCA has also been described, however, in 25 per cent of healthy relatives of those with PSC.[99] Other autoantibodies are also demonstrable and the presence of anticardiolipin may have adverse prognostic significance.[100]

The association of non-smoking with ulcerative colitis (see Chapter 1) holds good for patients with PSC, whether or not they also have ulcerative colitis, although it should be conceded that few patients with PSC and without colitis have been studied.[101,102] There may be an association of PSC with sarcoidosis – present in 0.7 per cent of PSC cases in one meeting abstract.[103]

Clinical features

PSC should be considered in all colitic patients who develop abnormal liver biochemistry. In the absence of firmly established useful therapy it is not justifiable to seek it routinely in patients with normal liver function. Early PSC is almost always asymptomatic. With progression the patient describes periodic cholestasis (pruritus, dark urine, pale stools), with or without evidence of cholangitis and right upper quadrant abdominal pain.

There are no characteristic physical signs before the advent of portal hypertension, liver failure and decompensated cirrhosis. Osteopenia is common in PSC,[104] but not necessarily more so than in other patients with inflammatory bowel disease. Diagnosis of PSC requires moderately invasive procedures and it is therefore appropriate to check first for other causes of liver dysfunction that are identifiable by serology or biochemical tests.

Imaging

PSC can be inferred from biliary abnormalities identified on ultrasonographic scanning,[105] but the reliability is insufficient to yield confident positive or negative outcomes. Magnetic resonance imaging of the biliary tree is at an exciting phase of its evolution, and may reduce the need for diagnostic endoscopic retrograde cholangiopancreatography (ERCP), but its resolution is probably still insufficient to confirm or refute the diagnosis.[106] The radiological diagnosis of PSC requires evidence of biliary changes at at least two sites, with evidence of mucosal damage and a combination of stenosis and dilatation of the biliary tree (Figure 6.1). It is conventional to confine the diagnosis to individuals in whom there has been no history of cholelithiasis, as the changes of sclerosing cholangitis secondary to chronic duct stone retention cannot be distinguished from those of PSC. The sclerosing cholangitis peculiar to HIV infection and AIDS[107] deserves brief comment as this variant almost certainly has an infective aetiology. The radiological features of AIDS-related sclerosing cholangitis are virtually identical to those of PSC apart from the AIDS-related condition being associated at times with intraluminal polypoidal lesions, which are not seen in PSC. Although the radiographic similarity might suggest comparable aetiopathogenesis in PSC, it may simply reflect the fact that the biliary tree (indeed, like the liver) has only a limited repertoire of responses to chronic inflammation of whatever cause.

Figure 6.1 ERCP in primary sclerosing cholangitis. The distended gallbladder is characteristic and helps to confirm that the scrawny stenotic intrahepatic ducts are diseased and that the appearances are not simply those of an under-filled system. In this case the slight irregularities of the common bile duct should anyway lead to the correct diagnosis.

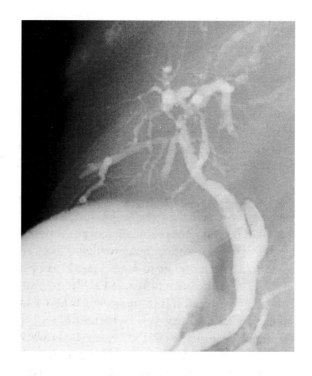

Pathology

When only small biliary radicals are involved, ERCP will be normal, and liver biopsy is accordingly necessary to make the diagnosis of PSC in nearly 10 per cent of cases.[94] Nonetheless, a majority of initially normal ERCPs become characteristically abnormal with time. Some authorities would always seek histological support for a radiographic diagnosis, but this is not necessarily a productive course. Large duct disease may be associated with virtually normal histology, or produces changes simply confirming distal cholestasis without providing further evidence as to its cause. When present, the specific histological findings are, however, characteristic. The so-called onion-skin or lamellar periportal fibrosis is unmistakable, and is associated with a variable degree of chronic inflammatory response, progressing to hepatic fibrosis and cirrhosis in its later stages. Although the rate of progression is variable, Markov modelling from sequential biopsy data predicts progression from stage II disease in 42 per cent at 1 year and over 90 per cent by 5 years compared with 14 per cent and 52 per cent at the same intervals in those with initially stage III disease; more than occasional (15 per cent) patients can be expected to improve.[108]

Therapy

Treatment of PSC was not hitherto possible other than by liver transplantation for end-stage liver failure. Two alternative strategies are now under active exploration. If a single dominant stricture is identified at ERCP, it is technically possible to dilate it with trans-endoscopic balloons (with or without infusion of steroids), and with the possibility of subsequent stenting.[109] Endoscopic therapy may also be appropriate for patients with a small number of major strictures if a single long stent can be expected to span them all. The use of the expandable metal stent has been taken up with enthusiasm, as the smaller calibre of the unexpanded stent allows negotiation of tighter strictures, and its larger final lumen leads to improved flow properties and less troublesome follow-up. Following numerous case reports, a retrospective study of 71 patients with dominant strictures (from 1009 PSC patients seen over 10 years) documented 34 patients undergoing dilatation, and 37 with dilatation and stenting (roughly equally percutaneous and endoscopic). More procedure-related complications and acute cholangitis were seen in the stent group with no apparent advantage.[110] There are still no controlled data. This is of more than average concern, as PSC usually follows a remitting and relapsing course, and will tend to provoke intervention at times of maximal expression, when spontaneous improvement is concurrently also at its most likely.

A number of pharmacological agents have been employed in PSC but with very limited success. The Dutch multicentre study of ursodeoxycholic acid[111] yielded reductions in enzyme levels, with no change in bilirubin or synthetic markers of liver function over 2 years. The similar Mayo Clinic study (14 mg/kg) demonstrated an improvement in albumin and bilirubin levels as well as enzymes, but the intervention had no impact on histological progression or on rates of transplantation or death over 2 years.[112] Given these very modest results, a larger dose (25–30 mg/kg) was evaluated in a pilot study of 30 patients.[113] Only 22 completed the intended 12 months. Liver enzymes markedly improved, but the bilirubin was again unchanged and the albumin rose only from 41 to 43 g/L; the overall prognostic risk score did nevertheless fall. Whilst there may be some who will still wish to treat their patients, this is clearly not strongly indicated and it is doubtful that additional data will be sufficient to alter this disappointing conclusion.

Published use of the immunosuppressant tacrolimus (FK-506) is uncontrolled and only in very small numbers but may deserve mention because its use has been associated with a fall in serum bilirubin and thus possibly with prognostic gain.[114]

Prognosis

Some patients have little trouble from their PSC, whilst others follow a rapidly deteriorating course culminating in cirrhosis, hepatic failure and death if successful liver transplantation is not possible. Several prognostic models have accordingly been devised based on standard clinical criteria, with or without inclusion of liver biopsy data.[94,115–117] Each is fallible,[115] but there is some measure of agreement that female gender, increasing age, decreasing albumin, and increasing bilirubin level are poor prognostic markers. It does not seem to matter whether there is small or large duct involvement, or both.[94] Although said to be inferior to the more complex Mayo score,[116] a simple implementation of the Childs–Pugh score has been found entirely satisfactory by others.[117] High cholesterol and anaemia may also be of adverse prognostic value, but the data come from a predominantly symptomatic population (70 per cent) and may not be generalizable.[118]

Activity of associated colitis has little, if any, bearing on the progress of PSC, and even colectomy affects the biliary status very little. Patients with established parenchymal liver disease run a greater operative risk if they come to later colectomy, however, with three of eight such patients perishing in one series.[119] Overall transplant-free survival has improved since early studies and is now typically in excess of 75 per cent at 10 years,[120] which probably reflects earlier diagnosis and better case ascertainment rather than any influence of therapeutic strategies.

Unfortunately, ulcerative colitis tends to run an aggressive course after transplantation for PSC. Thirty patients surviving for at least 12 months post-transplant have been reviewed.[121] Amongst 18 who had a prior diagnosis of ulcerative colitis, the colitis became troublesome in four with previously quiescent disease, substantially deteriorated in four with preoperatively active disease, and two required colectomy (despite the transplant-related immunosuppression in each case). Three new cases of ulcerative colitis emerged in transplant follow-up from amongst 12 patients with no preoperative diagnosis,[121] but there was no evidence of neoplasia in this series.

Neoplasia in primary sclerosing cholangitis

Patients with PSC are at substantially increased risk of cholangiocarcinoma, and also at an increased risk of colorectal malignancy over and above the increased risk determined by their extent and duration of colitis. This is discussed in more detail in Chapter 8.

References

1 Veloso FT, Carvalho J, Magro F. Immune-related systemic manifestations of inflammatory bowel disease. A prospective study of 792 patients. *J Clin Gastroenterol* 1996; **23**: 29–34.

2 Orchard TR, Jewell DP. The importance of ileocaecal integrity in the arthritic complications of Crohn's disease. *Inflamm Bowel Dis* 1999; **5**: 92–7.

3 Maeda K, Okada M, Yao T, *et al*. Intestinal and extra-intestinal complications of Crohn's disease: predictors and cumulative probability of complications. *J Gastroenterol* 1994; **29**: 577–82.

4 De Vos M, De Keyser F, Mielants H, Cuvelier C, Veys E. Review article: bone and joint diseases in inflammatory bowel disease. *Aliment Pharmacol Ther* 1998; **12**: 397–404.

5 Keat A. Spondyloarthropathies. *Br Med J* 1995; **310**: 1321–4.

6 Brown MA, Pile KD, Kennedy LG, *et al*. A genome-wide screen for susceptibility loci in ankylosing spondylitis. *Arthritis Rheum* 1998; **41**: 588–95.

7 Gravellese EM, Kantrowitz FG. Arthritic manifestations of inflammatory bowel disease. *Am J Gastroenterol* 1988; **83**: 703–9.

8 McEniff N, Eustace S, McCarthy C, O'Malley M, O'Morain CA, Hamilton S. Asymptomatic sacroiliitis in inflammatory bowel disease. Assessment by computed tomography. *Clin Imaging* 1995; **19**: 258–62.

9 Münch H, Purrmann J, Reis HE, *et al*. Clinical features of inflammatory joint and spine manifestations in Crohn's disease. *Hepatogastroenterology* 1986; **33**: 123–7.

10 Orchard TR, Wordsworth BP, Jewell DP. Peripheral arthropathies in inflammatory bowel disease: their articular distribution and natural history. *Gut* 1998; **42**: 387–91.

11 Orchard TR, Thiyagaraja S, Welsh KI, Wordsworth BP, Hill Gaston JS, Jewell DP. Clinical phenotype is related to HLA genotype in the peripheral arthropathies of inflammatory bowel disease. *Gastroenterology* 2000; **118**: 274–8.

12 Yahia B, Dave U, Keat A, Forbes A. Arthropathy in inflammatory bowel disease, an underestimated problem? *Gastroenterology* 1996; **110**: A1048.

13 De Vos M, Mielants H, Cuvelier C, Elewaut A, Veys E. Long-term evolution of gut inflammation in patients with spondyloarthropathy. *Gastroenterology* 1996; **110**: 1696–703.

14 Alonso JC, Lopez-Longo FJ, Lampreave JL, *et al*. Different abdominal scintigraphy pattern in patients with ulcerative colitis, Crohn's disease and seronegative spondylarthropathies. *Br J Rheumatol* 1995; **34**: 946–50.

15 Thomas PD, Keat AC, Forbes A, Ciclitira PJ, Nicholls RJ. Extraintestinal manifestations of ulcerative colitis following restorative proctocolectomy. *Eur J Gastroenterol Hepatol* 1999; **11**: 1001–5.

16 Cuvelier C, Mielants H, De Vos M, Veys E, Roels H. Immunoglobulin containing cells in terminal ileum and colorectum of patients with arthritis related gut inflammation. *Gut* 1988; **29**: 916–25.

17 Baker SJ, Jacob E, Bowden GH. Crohn disease arthropathy: antigens in synovial fluid share epitopes with strains of two species of viridans streptococci. *Scand J Gastroenterol* 2000; **35**: 287–92.

18 Lichtman SN. Translocation of bacteria from gut lumen to mesenteric lymph nodes – and beyond? *J Pediatr Gastroenterol Nutr* 1991; **13**: 433–4.

19 Rath HC, Ikeda JS, Linde HJ, Scholmerich J, Wilson KH, Sartor RB. Varying cecal bacterial loads influences colitis and gastritis in HLA-B27 transgenic rats. *Gastroenterology* 1999; **116**: 310–19.

20 Nemetz A, Toth M, Zagoni T, *et al*. Interleukin-1 gene polymorphisms stimulate steroid induced

bone loss in inflammatory bowel diseases. *Gut* 1999; **45**(Suppl V): A15.

21 Schulte C, Dignass AU, Mann K, Goebell H. Bone loss in patients with inflammatory bowel disease is less than expected: a follow-up study. *Scand J Gastroenterol* 1999; **34**: 696–702.

22 Azuma Y, Kaji K, Katogi R, Takeshita S, Kudo A. Tumor necrosis factor-alpha induces differentiation of and bone resorption by osteoclasts. *J Biol Chem* 2000; **275**: 4858–64.

23 Chawla A, Iofel E. Vitamin K status and bone mineral density in children with Crohn's disease. *Gastroenterology* 2000; **118**: A63.

24 Silvennoinen JA, Karttunen TJ, Niemelä SE, Manelius JJ, Lehtola JK. A controlled study of bone mineral density in patients with inflammatory bowel disease. *Gut* 1995; **37**: 71–6.

25 Bischoff SC, Herrmann A, Goke M, Manns MP, von zur Muhlen A, Brabant G. Altered bone metabolism in inflammatory bowel disease. *Am J Gastroenterol* 1997; **92**: 1157–63.

26 Ardizzone S, Bollani S, Bettica P, Bevilacqua M, Molteni P, Bianchi Porro G. Altered bone metabolism in inflammatory bowel disease: there is a difference between Crohn's disease and ulcerative colitis. *J Intern Med* 2000; **247**: 63–70.

27 Robinson RJ, al-Azzawi F, Iqbal SJ, *et al.* Osteoporosis and determinants of bone density in patients with Crohn's disease. *Dig Dis Sci* 1998; **43**: 2500–6.

28 Ghosh S, Cowen S, Hannan WJ, Ferguson A. Low bone mineral density in Crohn's disease but not in ulcerative colitis at diagnosis. *Gastroenterology* 1994; **107**: 1031–9.

29 Valentine JF, Sninsky CA. Prevention and treatment of osteoporosis in patients with inflammatory bowel disease. *Am J Gastroenterol* 1999; **94**: 878–83.

30 Valdimarsson T, Löfman O, Toss G, Ström M. Reversal of osteopenia with diet in adult coeliac disease. *Gut* 1996; **38**: 322–7.

31 Haderslev KV, Tjellesen L, Sorensen HA, Staun M. Alendronate increases lumbar spine bone mineral density in patients with Crohn's disease. *Gastroenterology* 2000; **119**: 639–46.

32 Robinson RJ, Krzywicki T, Almond L, *et al.* Effect of a low-impact exercise program on bone mineral density in Crohn's disease: a randomized controlled trial. *Gastroenterology* 1998; **115**: 36–41.

33 Boulet LP, Milot J, Gagnon L, Poubelle PE, Brown J. Long-term influence of inhaled corticosteroids on bone metabolism and density. Are biological markers predictors of bone loss? *Am J Resp Crit Care Med* 1999; **159**: 838–44.

34 Sato S, Sasaki I, Naito H, *et al.* Management of urinary complications in Crohn's disease. *Surg Today* 1999; **29**: 713–17.

35 Andersson H, Bosaeus I, Fasth S, Hellberg R, Hultén L. Cholelithiasis and urolithiasis in Crohn's disease. *Scand J Gastroenterol* 1987; **22**: 253–6.

36 Chadwick VS, Modka K, Dowling RH. Mechanism for hyperoxaluria in patients with ileal dysfunction. *N Engl J Med* 1973; **289**: 172–6.

37 Bosch X. Hypercalcemia due to endogenous overproduction of 1,25-dihydroxyvitamin D in Crohn's disease. *Gastroenterology* 1998; **114**: 1061–5.

38 Grossman MS, Nugent FW. Urolithiasis as a complication of chronic diarrheal disease. *Am J Dig Dis* 1967; **12**: 491–3.

39 Present D, Rabinowitz JG, Banks PA, Janowitz HD. Obstructive hydronephrosis – a frequent but seldom recognized complication of granulomatous disease of the bowel. *N Engl J Med* 1969; **280**: 523–8.

40 Glassman M, Kaplan M, Spivak W. Immune-complex glomerulonephritis in Crohn's disease. *J Pediatr Gastroenterol Nutr* 1986; **5**: 966–9.

41 Wilcox GM, Aretz HT, Roy MA, Roche JK. Glomerulonephritis associated with inflammatory bowel disease. *Gastroenterology* 1990; **98**: 786–91.

42 Kreisel W, Wolf LM, Grotz W, Grieshaber M. Renal tubular damage: an extra-intestinal manifestation of chronic inflammatory bowel disease. *Eur J Gastroenterol Hepatol* 1996; **8**: 461–8.

43 Greenstein AJ, Sachar DB, Panday AK, *et al.* Amyloidosis and inflammatory bowel disease. A 50-year experience with 25 patients. *Medicine* 1992; **71**: 261–70.

44 Lovat LB, Madhoo S, Pepys MB, Hawkins PN. Long-term survival in systemic amyloid A amyloidosis complicating Crohn's disease. *Gastroenterology* 1997; **112**: 1362–5.

45 Jorizzo JL. Blood vessel-based inflammatory disorders. In Moschella SL, Hurley HJ, eds. *Dermatology*, 3rd edn. Philadelphia: Saunders, 1992: 584–6.

46 Mir-Madjlessi SH, Taylor JS, Farmer RG. Clinical course and evolution of erythema nodosum and

pyoderma gangrenosum in chronic ulcerative colitis: a study of 42 patients. *Am J Gastroenterol* 1985; **80**: 615–20.

47 Marshall JK, Irvine EJ. Successful therapy of refractory erythema nodosum associated with Crohn's disease using potassium iodide. *Can J Gastroenterol* 1997; **11**: 501–2.

48 Schoetz DJ Jr, Coller JA, Veidenheimer MG. Pyoderma gangrenosum and Crohn's disease. Eight cases and a review of the literature. *Dis Colon Rectum* 1983; **26**: 155–9.

49 von den Driesch P. Pyoderma gangrenosum: a report of 44 cases with follow-up. *Br J Dermatol* 1997; **137**: 1000–5.

50 Tjandra JJ, Hughes LE. Parastomal pyoderma gangrenosum in inflammatory bowel disease. *Dis Colon Rectum* 1994; **37**: 938–42.

51 Soriano ML, Martinez N, Grilli R, Farina MC, Martin L, Requena L. Pyodermatitis-pyostomatitis vegetans: report of a case and review of the literature. *Oral Surg Oral Med Oral Pathol Oral Radiol Endosc* 1999; **87**: 322–6.

52 Lazarov A, Amichai B, Halevy S. Pustular vasculitis and superficial bullous pyoderma gangrenosum in a patient with ulcerative colitis. *Cutis* 1995; **56**: 297–300.

53 Salmon P, Rademaker M, Edwards L. A continuum of neutrophilic disease occurring in a patient with ulcerative colitis. *Australas J Dermatol* 1998; **39**: 116–18.

54 Lamers CB. Treatment of extraintestinal complications of ulcerative colitis. *Eur J Gastroenterol Hepatol* 1997; **9**: 850–3.

55 Fett DL, Gibson LE, Su WPD. Sweet's syndrome: systemic signs and symptoms and associated disorders. *Mayo Clin Proc* 1995; **70**: 234–40.

56 Travis S, Innes N, Davies MG, Daneshmend T, Hughes S. Sweet's syndrome: an unusual cutaneous feature of Crohn's disease or ulcerative colitis. The South West Gastroenterology Group. *Eur J Gastroenterol Hepatol* 1997; **9**: 715–20.

57 Rosen T, Unkefer RP. Treatment of pyoderma faciale with isotretinoin in a patient with ulcerative colitis. *Cutis* 1999; **64**: 107–9.

58 Yates VM, Watkinson G, Kelman A. Further evidence for an association between psoriasis, Crohn's disease, and ulcerative colitis. *Br J Dermatol* 1982: **106**: 323–5.

59 Lee FI, Bellary SV, Francis C. Increased occurrence of psoriasis in patients with Crohn's disease

and their relatives. *Am J Gastroenterol* 1990; **85**: 962–3.

60 Kawaguchi M, Mitsuhashi Y, Kondo S. Acute generalized exanthematous pustulosis induced by salazosulfapyridine in a patient with ulcerative colitis. *J Dermatol* 1999; **26**: 359–62.

61 Salmon JF, Wright JP, Murray AD. Ocular inflammation in Crohn's disease. *Ophthalmology* 1991; **98**: 480–4.

62 Billson FA, De Dombal FT, Watkinson G, Goligher JG. Ocular complications of ulcerative colitis. *Gut* 1967; **8**: 102–6.

63 Hofley P, Roarty J, McGinnity G, *et al.* Asymptomatic uveitis in children with chronic inflammatory bowel disease. *J Pediatr Gastroenterol Nutr* 1993; **17**: 397–400.

64 Soukiasian SH, Foster CS, Raizman MB. Treatment strategies for scleritis and uveitis associated with inflammatory bowel disease. *Am J Ophthalmol* 1994; **118**: 601–11.

65 Kumar BN, Walsh RM, Wilson PS, Carlin WV. Sensorineural hearing loss and ulcerative colitis. *J Laryngol Otol* 1997; **111**: 277–8.

66 Bachmeyer C, Leclerc-Landgraf N, Laurette F, *et al.* Acute autoimmune sensorineural hearing loss associated with Crohn's disease. *Am J Gastroenterol* 1998; **93**: 2565–7.

67 Straub RH, Andus T, Lock G, *et al.* Kardiovaskulare und pupillare autonome und somatosensible Neuropathie bei chronischen Erkrankungen mit Autoimmunphanomenen. *Med Klin* 1997; **92**: 647–53.

68 Straub RH, Antoniou E, Zeuner M, Gross V, Scholmerich J, Andus T. Association of autonomic nervous hyperreflexia and systemic inflammation in patients with Crohn's disease and ulcerative colitis. *J Neuroimmunol* 1997; **80**: 149–57.

69 Elsehety A, Bertorini TE. Neurologic and neuropsychiatric complications of Crohn's disease. *South Med J* 1997; **90**: 606–10.

70 Purrmann J, Arendt G, Cleveland S, *et al.* Association of Crohn's disease and multiple sclerosis. Is there a common background? *J Clin Gastroenterol* 1992; **14**: 43–6.

71 Lossos A, River Y, Eliakim A, Steiner I. Neurologic aspects of inflammatory bowel disease. *Neurology* 1995; **45**(3 Pt 1): 416–21.

72 Fellermann K, Stahl M, Dahlhoff K, Amthor M, Ludwig D, Stange EF. Crohn's disease and

sarcoidosis: systemic granulomatosis? *Eur J Gastroenterol Hepatol* 1997; **9**: 1121–4.

73 Stebbing J, Askin F, Fishman E, Stone J. Pulmonary manifestations of ulcerative colitis mimicking Wegener's granulomatosis. *J Rheumatol* 1999; **26**: 1617–21.

74 Mahadeva R, Walsh G, Flower CD, Shneerson JM. Clinical and radiological characteristics of lung disease in inflammatory bowel disease. *Eur Respir J* 2000; **15**: 41–8.

75 Kuzela L, Vavrecka A, Prikazska M, *et al.* Pulmonary complications in patients with inflammatory bowel disease. *Hepatogastroenterology* 1999; **46**: 1714–19.

76 Tzanakis N, Bouros D, Samiou M, *et al.* Lung function in patients with inflammatory bowel disease. *Respir Med* 1998; **92**: 516–22.

77 Fireman Z, Osipov A, Kivity S, *et al.* The use of induced sputum in the assessment of pulmonary involvement in Crohn's disease. *Am J Gastroenterol* 2000; **95**: 730–4.

78 Vandenplas O, Casel S, Delos M, Trigaux JP, Melange M, Marchand E. Granulomatous bronchiolitis associated with Crohn's disease. *Am J Respir Crit Care Med* 1998; **158**: 1676–9.

79 Spira A, Grossman R, Balter M. Large airway disease associated with inflammatory bowel disease. *Chest* 1998; **113**: 1723–6.

80 Sarroŭj BJ, Zampino DJ, Cilursu AM. Pericarditis as the initial manifestation of inflammatory bowel disease. *Chest* 1994; **106**: 1911–12.

81 Kupferschmidt H, Langenegger T, Krahenbuhl S. Perikarditis bei chronisch entzundlicher Darmerkrankung: Grundkrankheit oder Nebenwirkung der Therapie? Ein 'clinical problem solving'. *Schweiz Med Wochenschr* 1996; **126**: 2184–90.

82 Hutchinson R, Tyrrell PN, Kumar D, Dunn JA, Li JK, Allan RN. Pathogenesis of gall stones in Crohn's disease: an alternative explanation. *Gut* 1994; **35**: 94–7.

83 Nightingale JM. The short-bowel syndrome. *Eur J Gastroenterol Hepatol* 1995; **7**: 514–20.

84 Lorusso D, Leo S, Mossa A, Misciagna G, Guerra V. Cholelithiasis in inflammatory bowel disease. A case-control study. *Dis Colon Rectum* 1990; **33**: 791–4.

85 Lapidus A, Einarsson K. Effects of ileal resection on biliary lipids and bile acid composition in patients with Crohn's disease. *Gut* 1991; **32**: 1488–91.

86 Mibu R, Makino I, Chijiiwa K. Gallstones and their composition in patients with ileoanal anastomosis. *J Gastroenterol* 1995; **30**: 413–15.

87 Brink MA, Slors JFM, Keulemans YC, *et al.* Enterohepatic cycling of bilirubin: a putative mechanism for pigment gallstone formation in ileal Crohn's disease. *Gastroenterology* 1999; **116**: 1420–7.

88 Broomé U, Glaumann H, Hellers G, Nilsson B, Sörstad J, Hultcrantz R. Liver disease in ulcerative colitis: an epidemiological and follow up study in the county of Stockholm. *Gut* 1994; **35**: 84–9.

89 Mattila J, Aitola P, Matikainen M. Liver lesions found at colectomy in ulcerative colitis: correlation between histological findings and biochemical parameters. *J Clin Pathol* 1994; **47**: 1019–21.

90 Broomé U, Glaumann H, Hultcrantz R. Liver histology and follow up of 68 patients with ulcerative colitis and normal liver function tests. *Gut* 1990; **31**: 468–72.

91 Perdigoto R, Carpenter HA, Czaja AJ. Frequency and significance of chronic ulcerative colitis in severe corticosteroid-treated autoimmune hepatitis. *J Hepatol* 1992; **14**: 325–31.

92 Maurer LH, Hughes RW Jr, Folley JH, Mosenthal WT. Granulomatous hepatitis associated with regional enteritis. *Gastroenterology* 1967; **53**: 301–5.

93 Broomé U, Löfberg R, Lundqvist K, Veress B. Subclinical time span of inflammatory bowel disease in patients with primary sclerosing cholangitis. *Dis Colon Rectum* 1995; **38**: 1301–5.

94 Angulo P, Maor-Kendler Y, Donlinger JJ, Lindor KD. Small-duct primary sclerosing cholangitis: prevalence and natural history. *Gastroenterology* 2000; **118**: A 902.

95 Olerup O, Olsson R, Hultcrantz R, Broomé U. HLA-DR and HLA-DQ are not markers for rapid disease progression in primary sclerosing cholangitis. *Gastroenterology* 1995; **108**: 870–8.

96 Underhill JA, Donaldson PT, Doherty DG, Manabe K, Williams R. HLA DPB polymorphism in primary sclerosing cholangitis and primary biliary cirrhosis. *Hepatology* 1995; **21**: 959–62.

97 Bansi DS, Bauducci M, Bergqvist A, *et al.* Detection of antineutrophil cytoplasmic antibodies in primary sclerosing cholangitis: a comparison of the alkaline phosphatase and immunofluorescent techniques. *Eur J Gastroenterol Hepatol* 1997; **9**: 575–80.

98 Lo SK, Fleming KA, Chapman RW. A 2-year follow-up study of anti-neutrophil antibody in

primary sclerosing cholangitis: relationship to clinical activity, liver biochemistry and ursodeoxycholic acid treatment. *J Hepatol* 1994; **21**: 974–8.

99 Seibold F, Slametschka D, Gregor M, Weber P. Neutrophil autoantibodies: a genetic marker in primary sclerosing cholangitis and ulcerative colitis. *Gastroenterology* 1994; **104**: 532–6.

100 Angulo P, Peter JB, Gershwin ME, *et al.* Serum autoantibodies in patients with primary sclerosing cholangitis. *J Hepatol* 2000; **32**: 182–7.

101 Loftus EV Jr, Sandborn WJ, Tremaine WJ, *et al.* Primary sclerosing cholangitis is associated with non-smoking: a case-control study. *Gastroenterology* 1996; **110**: 1496–502.

102 Van Erpecum KJ, Smits SJHM, Van de Meeberg PC, *et al.* Risk of primary sclerosing cholangitis is associated with nonsmoking behaviour. *Gastroenterology* 1996; **110**: 1503–6.

103 Joseph JK, Porayko MK, Steers JL, *et al.* The association of primary sclerosing cholangitis and sarcoidosis. *Gastroenterology* 1996; **110**: A1224.

104 Angulo P, Therneau TM, Jorgensen A, *et al.* Bone disease in patients with primary sclerosing cholangitis: prevalence, severity and prediction of progression. *J Hepatol* 1998; **29**: 729–35.

105 Majoie CB, Smits NJ, Phoa SS, Reeders JW, Jansen PL. Primary sclerosing cholangitis: sonographic findings. *Abdom Imaging* 1995; **20**: 109–12.

106 Ponchon T. Diagnostic endoscopic retrograde cholangiopancreatography. *Endoscopy* 2000; **32**: 200–8.

107 Forbes A, Blanshard C, Gazzard B. Natural history of AIDS related sclerosing cholangitis: a study of 20 cases. *Gut* 1993; **34**: 116–21.

108 Angulo P, Larson DR, Therneau TM, LaRusso NF, Batts KP, Lindor KD. Time course of histological progression in primary sclerosing cholangitis. *Am J Gastroenterol* 1999; **94**: 3310–13.

109 Gaing AA, Geders JM, Cohen SA, Siegel JH. Endoscopic management of primary sclerosing cholangitis: review and report of an open series. *Am J Gastroenterol* 1993; **88**: 2000–8.

110 Kaya M, Peterson BT, Angulo P, Lindor KD. Balloon dilation compared to stenting of dominant strictures in primary sclerosing cholangitis. *Gastroenterology* 2000; **118**: A902.

111 Van Hoogstraten HJF, Wolfhagen FJH, Van de Meeberg PC, *et al.* Ursodeoxycholic acid therapy for primary sclerosing cholangitis: results of a 2-year randomized controlled trial to evaluate single versus multiple daily doses. *J Hepatol* 1998; **29**: 417–23.

112 Lindor KD, for Mayo Clinic Primary Sclerosing Cholangitis Study Group. Ursodiol for primary sclerosing cholangitis. *N Engl J Med* 1997; **336**: 691–5.

113 Harnois DM, Angulo P, Jorgensen RA, *et al.* High-dose ursodeoxycholic acid as a therapy for patients with primary sclerosing cholangitis. *Gastroenterology* 2000; **118**: A902–3.

114 Van Thiel DH, Carroll P, Abu-Elmagd K, *et al.* Tacrolimus (FK 506), a treatment for primary sclerosing cholangitis: results of an open-label preliminary trial. *Am J Gastroenterol* 1995; **90**: 455–9.

115 Broomé U, Eriksson LS. Assessment for liver transplantation in patients with primary sclerosing cholangitis. *J Hepatol* 1994; **20**: 654–9.

116 Kim WR, Poterucha JJ, Wiesner RH, *et al.* The relative role of the Child–Pugh classification and the Mayo natural history model in the assessment of survival in patients with primary sclerosing cholangitis. *Hepatology* 1999; **29**: 1643–8.

117 Shetty K, Rybicki L, Carey WD. The Child–Pugh classification as a prognostic indicator for survival in primary sclerosing cholangitis. *Hepatology* 1997; **25**: 1049–53.

118 Okolicsanyi L, Fabris L, Viaggi S, *et al.* Primary sclerosing cholangitis: clinical presentation, natural history and prognostic variables: an Italian multicentre study. *Eur J Gastroenterol Hepatol* 1996; **8**: 685–91.

119 Post AB, Bozdech JM, Lavery I, Barnes DS. Colectomy in patients with inflammatory bowel disease and primary sclerosing cholangitis. *Dis Colon Rectum* 1994; **37**: 175–8.

120 Loftus EV, Sandborn WJ, Tremaine WJ, *et al.* Risk of colorectal neoplasia in patients with primary sclerosing cholangitis. *Gastroenterology* 1996; **110**: 432–40.

121 Papatheodoris GV, Hamilton M, Mistry PK, *et al.* Ulcerative colitis has an aggressive course after orthotopic liver transplantation for primary sclerosing cholangitis. *Gut* 98; **43**: 639–44.

Complications of inflammatory bowel disease

Intra-abdominal sepsis and abscess formation in Crohn's disease

The perianal and perineal abscesses, fissures and superficial fistulae of Crohn's disease can usually be treated adequately by local measures. More complex perineal disease and the multiple fistulous openings of the 'watering can perineum' pose more difficulty and will often only respond to defunctioning by a more proximal stoma. Chronic intra-abdominal and pelvic abscesses may represent still greater problems.

Drainage of septic foci is as necessary in Crohn's disease as in other situations, but whether drainage alone can be sufficient therapy is controversial. Several major centres consider that drainage should be considered only as an immediate measure to overcome septicaemia and restore cardiovascular stability and general well-being, before proceeding to later more definitive surgery to resect the implicated segment of bowel. There is a related debate as to the place of open surgery as opposed to non-surgical methodologies to achieve drainage. The argument in favour of drainage alone is supported by the general desire to minimize surgery and quantity of bowel resection, and by the fact that many of these patients appear to do extremely well in the short term, and are then keen to avoid further intervention when they seem to have recovered.

The relatively limited numerical scale of the problem is clear from the literature, but the difficulty of management should not be underestimated. The Birmingham group published a surgical series on sepsis in Crohn's disease[1] referring to 124 resections in 111 patients, 13 of whom had abscesses preoperatively (unsuspected in 8). These were mostly localized and all affected 13 patients 'requiring urgent surgery'. A further 17 abscesses (6 multiple) occurred postoperatively, 5 in patients with preoperative lesions. In New York, Ribeiro et al.[2] recorded 129 abscesses (21 per cent) in 610 patients with small bowel Crohn's disease which were intraperitoneal in 109 cases and retroperitoneal in the remainder; all were considered to have required operative intervention. Fifteen required further surgery for abscess and 26 developed postoperative enterocutaneous fistulae; there were three deaths from sepsis.

The particular case of psoas abscess has attracted attention because of its potential to mislead clinically (presenting, for example, with pain in the knee or hip rather than with an obviously abdominal problem), and also because it may be the presenting feature of Crohn's disease (11 of 46 cases in one series).[3] Although Crohn's disease is probably the single commonest predisposing factor for psoas abscess, it still accounts for less than half of those that occur, the 14 of 43 in one series being typical.[4]

At St Mark's, having excluded perineal abscesses and those occurring within 3 months of surgery (because it was otherwise difficult to make the distinction from postoperative wound infection), we identified 35 patients with Crohn's-related abscesses from a prospective database of 531 Crohn's patients admitted a total of 1156 times in a 4-year period.[5] The age and sex distributions (14 male, median age 35 years) were typical of our patient group and the affected patients had had Crohn's disease for a median of 12 years. The abscesses were abdominal in 61 per cent, retroperitoneal in 22 per cent, and pelvic in 17 per cent, and were associated with abdominal masses in 64 per cent of cases and with enterocutaneous fistula in 26 per cent (see below). Three-quarters of the patients had chronically active Crohn's disease and 18 per cent had subacute obstruction at the time of presentation with abscess. Nearly half had been on steroids for more than 6 months and most had had previous surgery (in 36 per cent of cases for previous abscess or fistula). A communication between the bowel and the abscess was demonstrable in 61 per cent, in 35 per cent originating from a previous anastomosis. Similar observations have been made in Montreal.[6] Microbiological investigation is not particularly helpful in these patients as mixed growths are usual. In almost all cases, aerobic intestinal organisms will be demonstrated, with anaerobes as well in about a third.

There is no ideal method to investigate and localize abscesses in Crohn's disease, nor are there controlled trials to guide the clinician. There is an obvious case for ultrasonographic scanning given its availability and non-invasiveness,[7] but this may yield poor views in the patient with intestinal distension and when there has been a recent abdominal incision. Protagonists for the CT scan[8] will probably soon concede that the ability of MR scanning to detect inflammation relatively specifically (on spin-echo sequences) is preferable (see also Chapter 2), when adequate information is unavailable from ultrasound. It is unclear whether endoscopic ultrasound will be useful to the general radiologist but Tio provides encouraging data from one specialist centre, which compare well with all other forms of imaging and with surgical assessment.[9]

PERCUTANEOUS AND SURGICAL DRAINAGE OF CROHN'S-RELATED ABSCESSES

Percutaneous drainage of a Crohn's-related abscess was first described by Bluth in 1985,[10] and by Millward in 1986,[11] with success in three of these four patients. Doemeny reviewed its use in nine cases and reported technical and short-term success in eight, with long-term resolution in five, only three patients needing elective surgery at some stage.[12] Percutaneous drainage was also technically possible in the London and Montreal series (see above) when attempted, and led to resolution of the acute problem in around half the treated patients, the others coming to later surgery.[5,6]

The results for percutaneous drainage were, of course, in selected patients, and conclusions should be guarded, but it is instructive to examine the results in the contemporaneous patients at St Mark's treated initially by open surgery. Of 23 such patients, 10 had a drainage procedure, and 13 a more definitive resection (with stoma creation in four). There were nine postoperative recurrences, recurrent fistulae in two, new enterocutaneous fistulae in two, and new presentation of short bowel syndrome in six, two of whom remain on long-term home parenteral nutrition. There were no deaths, but at 3 months only two-thirds were well and free from sepsis and fistula.[5] Surgical data from other centres, with a substantial rate of new enterocutaneous fistula[2] and relapse in 19 of 26 surgically drained patients compared with only 4 of 18 resected,[3] taken together with the St Mark's data, begin to suggest that surgical drainage should be avoided. Given that none of the data sets is controlled, and that in each case a considered clinical decision was taken to follow one option or another, it is pertinent to examine other possible prognostic factors and alternative therapeutic strategies.

Pre-intervention steroids have not appeared to influence outcome. Even when an abdominal mass was identified and high-dose steroids were used in therapy (albeit in the absence of overt sepsis), Felder was able to reassure us that of 24 patients so treated, none required urgent surgery or developed life-threatening sepsis even though 13 of the 24 masses were finally shown to include an abscess component.[13] No other generalizable factors have emerged.

Drainage by radiologically guided percutaneous methods is technically possible in the great majority of Crohn's-related abscesses, and although a clinically useful result is usual, nearly 50 per cent of patients will need surgical intervention nevertheless. Similar success, but a higher complication rate, is associated with surgical drainage procedures. Controlled trial of the two forms of drainage is probably feasible, but will not be easy given the relative rarity of the condition and the great difficulty in ensuring matching between groups (these are not especially homogeneous groups of patients) and may never be done. A pragmatist might reasonably take the view that within the limitations indicated, percutaneous drainage is no more or less successful than open surgical drainage. As percutaneous drainage is less invasive and possibly has a lower complication rate than open drainage, it should be the first choice if the surgical option would (at that time) be drainage alone. A percutaneous approach would seem especially appropriate for the patient who is unfit for surgery, or who is still recovering from previous intervention. Percutaneous drainage is less likely to be helpful in patients with obviously multilocular abscesses and those in whom fistulation has already occurred. In each case, there should be a plan for more definitive surgery once the acute septic event has resolved, with the intention of minimizing the chance of recurrence. When there is a reasonable prospect of definitive surgery at the first intervention, then immediate excisional surgery offers the best chance of long-term remission and may be a sensible course to follow. Reconstructive surgery with primary closure in the presence of current sepsis is less likely to be wise, however, and defunctioning stoma creation will often be necessary, reducing the apparent benefit of combining drainage with resection.

Perianal fistula (fistula *in ano*)

The perianal fistula is the commonest of the fistulae seen in Crohn's disease, with a lifetime incidence perhaps as high as 35 per cent, and these are also seen in ulcerative colitis (see Chapter 2). Their relationship to the sphincter muscle complex may be elucidated by the exploring finger, but even in the early days of endoanal ultrasound this proved itself equal to the expert clinician[14] and is almost certainly superior.[15] A clear classification is critical when surgical intervention is considered, and inclusion of pelvic MR scanning with or without endoluminal coils will often help in difficult cases.[16]

A surgical retrospective at St Mark's included 59 patients with perianal Crohn's disease who had been treated by laying the fistula open (*n* = 27; 81 per cent success), or by insertion of a loose seton (*n* = 27; 85 per cent success).[17] Only five more complex cases had diversionary stomas as part of an operative sequence. Physicians are rarely familiar with the modest seton which is simply a suture of non-absorbable material drawn through the fistula track and tied outside on the perineum, thus providing continued drainage for as long as is necessary. Other enlightened centres also promote the use of setons in these patients.[18] A cutting seton – which is gradually tightened to provide, in effect, a gradual laying open – is rarely needed.

However, the first therapeutic step will usually be the use of antibiotics. There are no reliable data to support this, the literature relying on uncontrolled observations from the 1970s and 1980s. Nor are there trustworthy data to support the use of 5-ASA drugs or steroids. Azathioprine/6-mercaptopurine has a more secure track record in this context, achieving closure in 6 of 18 perirectal fistulae over about 3 months,[19] and aggressive use of ciclosporin or the combination of azathioprine with tacrolimus may have a role in the intractable case.[20,21]

There has been a great deal of excitement about the use of infliximab in fistulating Crohn's disease, and in fact the data to which this applies are almost exclusively in the context of anorectal fistulae. In a well-controlled multicentre study, 85 patients with chronic perianal fistulae received antibody or placebo at weeks 0, 2 and 6. There were side effects in a majority, albeit mainly of a minor nature. Over 60 per cent of the treated patients achieved a sustained reduction, by 50 per cent or more, of the number of draining fistulae compared with only 26 per cent of controls ($P < 0.002$); however, in only 46 per cent did all fistulae close (versus 13 per cent; $P < 0.001$) and in most of these the fistulae subsequently recurred.[22] Most surgeons are singularly unimpressed with closure of a fistula for only a few months and would regard this as a fistula that has 'closed over' rather than resolved. I share this important reservation in respect of the infliximab data and add two further concerns. Many of the patients included might well have been satisfactorily (or dare one say better) managed by surgical laying open, with or without seton insertion. There is also increasing concern about septic complications, to the extent that those using infliximab in this context are now very reluctant to commence infusions without preliminary MRI scanning to exclude pelvic sepsis; the reassuring absence of serious local sepsis in the trial patients may prove to be a reflection of selection or of small numbers.

Enterocutaneous and enterovesical fistulae

ENTEROCUTANEOUS FISTULA

The management of an enterocutaneous fistula is heavily influenced by the underlying aetiology and its anatomical nature, which together mainly determine the likelihood of resolution without surgical intervention. A simple single fistula with no obstruction which follows colectomy for ulcerative colitis, for example, stands a much better chance of closing with good medical care than multiple complex fistulae occurring spontaneously in Crohn's disease. Closure is impeded by continuing sepsis, malnutrition and, particularly, by distal obstruction or bowel discontinuity.

Enterocutaneous fistulae always have their origins in adherent, abscess-related disorders and sepsis. There is always an associated penetrating bowel disorder, and the commonest single association is with recent surgery. Fistulae may be conveniently classified according to their anatomy, taking into account both the site of the intestine involved and the nature of the openings on the skin. Simple, single openings clearly have less significance than the more complex fistula where the two ends of bowel have become disrupted or where communication with the skin is via a continuing abscess cavity (Figure 7.1).

We do not know the true incidence of postoperative fistulae in inflammatory bowel disease as they are considered by many surgeons to be indicative of a technical failing and are therefore not widely reported. The data available come from referral centres, which are unlikely to be representative, as is borne out by the results of one such series[23] in which 6.3 per cent of enterocutaneous fistulae were in patients with Crohn's disease, and 4.2 per cent in ulcerative colitis, a condition not normally associated with this complication. I am sure that the 11.8 per cent frequency in my own

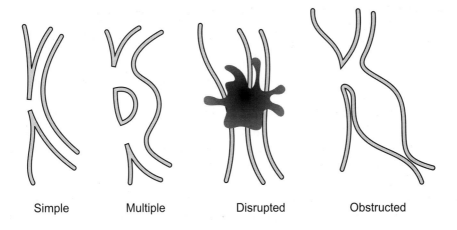

Simple　　　Multiple　　　Disrupted　　　Obstructed

Figure 7.1 A classification of enterocutaneous fistulae. In the disrupted (or complex) fistula the two ends of intestine are no longer in direct contact or communicate only via an abscess cavity.

Crohn's disease practice is heavily biased. Perhaps the best figure yet is the 3.4 per cent prevalence of enterocutaneous fistulae amongst 502 consecutive Crohn's disease patients seen in a single Italian centre.[24] Enterocutaneous fistulae are associated with significant mortality (around 4 per cent), but this is rarely a direct result of the fistula itself, more a reflection of the patient's overall poor state. In Crohn's disease, fistulae can be expected in up to 15 per cent of patients at some stage in their disease.[25] At least 80 per cent of these episodes occur shortly after surgery and up to 25 per cent of laparotomies may be complicated in this way. The fistula is usually at the site of the surgical incision.[26] It is valuable to distinguish the relatively straightforward fistula occurring after satisfactorily comprehensive surgery (Plate 13) from those occurring in patients with extensive Crohn's and involving actively diseased bowel (Plate 14). The former stands a reasonable chance of closing with medical therapy, whereas the latter will very rarely heal without surgical intervention. Failure to make this distinction has led to conflicting statements in the literature claiming spontaneous closure in anything from 0 to 60 per cent of cases. There is

also the frequent occurrence of a fistula closing over but without true resolution, which can lead to over-estimations of therapeutic success if follow-up is inadequate.[27]

The imaging of enterocutaneous fistulae is far from ideal, but ultrasound scanning, barium studies, CT and MR scanning all have a place, the last of these gradually coming to predominate.[15] Endoscopic evaluation is not normally very contributory. The 'fistulogram', in which water-soluble contrast is instilled into the cutaneous opening, is, however, helpful in most cases (see Chapter 2), and a variant of this using hydrogen peroxide has the advantage of avoiding radiation. However, the originators' enthusiasm for the superiority of the latter type is not entirely supported by their data, as not all patients had investigation by all the methods described.[24]

The immediate management of the patient with an acute enterocutaneous fistula begins with resuscitation, which may require fluid replacement and the drainage of abscesses (see above). Care of the skin around the fistulous opening should be an early priority, especially when the fistula is from the jejunum and the effluent rich in enzymes and acid. The patient will then usually also need nutritional support. Total parenteral nutrition may be necessary, but when the fistula is low ileal or colonic, enteral feeding will often allow sufficient bowel rest without the hazards of the parenteral approach or the loss of the protective/trophic effects that luminal nutrients have on the small bowel mucosa. The high-output fistula may lead to grave problems in assessment of fluid and sodium balance, but the principles outlined for management of short bowel syndrome can then usefully be applied (see below). Patients with less than 1 metre of reasonably normal intestine above the fistula will generally require parenteral support. If the fistula patient is not nil by mouth, the 'antisecretory' regimen proposed for short bowel syndrome patients will usually be indicated (see below).

In a survey of similar patients treated either with parenteral nutrition or with enteral tube-based regimens, there was no difference in mortality, or an obvious difference in fistula outcome.[28] There were, however, almost 50 per cent more septic episodes in the patients treated with parenteral nutrition compared with those with the enterally based regimens. Enteral regimens are most likely to be successful when given slowly (and in most cases continuously) by nasogastric or gastrostomy tube. The volume should be kept low and additional sodium will often need to be added. High-energy feeds (those with more than 1 kcal/mL) are less appropriate as they may provoke an osmotic diarrhoea and increase the fistula output.

The place of parenteral nutrition in enterocutaneous fistula may be summarized as being mandatory in patients in whom true intestinal failure is present, and in whom it is impossible to achieve positive nutritional balance with enteral regimens. It is usually indicated in those with a high fistula site and/or output (> 2000 mL daily). Parenteral nutrition will probably be indicated if spontaneous closure of the fistula is a reasonable

expectation since then the time needed to that closure can be expected to be shorter. It may be indicated if the patient is malnourished since the duration of malnutrition may then be shortened, but it is unlikely to be appropriate in the patient with a fistula low in the bowel, when the output is low and the fistula well tolerated. Standard regimens with modification to allow for the greater requirements for fluid (up to 6 L daily), sodium (up to 400 mmol/day) and magnesium can be used. Even when parenteral nutrition is being employed, the patient should continue oral 'antisecretory' therapy.

Immunosuppressive agents such as azathioprine may be valuable in selected patients with enterocutaneous fistulae complicating active Crohn's disease.[19] The place of ciclosporin[20] is less clear, as the small number of patients apparently helpfully treated is insufficient to provide confidence that the potential for impaired healing has truly been overcome. There are no controlled data.

Infliximab shows considerable promise in the management of fistulating Crohn's disease,[22] but there are few readily interpretable data in respect of enterocutaneous fistulae at present. The single major controlled trial[22] included only a very small number of affected patients and it is difficult to be sure how representative they were of the more complex patients seen in surgical practice. The concerns about worsening sepsis if comprehensive drainage has not been established prior to infliximab for perianal fistulae have been described, and there is not that often an equivalent to the seton or another effective mode of drainage for most abdominal sites.[29] Anecdotal reports already suggest that there can be a problem if infliximab is used; at St Mark's there has been one near-fatality from overwhelming abdominal wall sepsis.

Somatostatin and its more stable analogue, octreotide, reduce intestinal and pancreatic secretion and the speed of intestinal transit. As they also increase water and electrolyte absorption, it is understandable that therapeutic trials have been conducted in patients with high fistulae. Both agents will reduce fistula output reliably and reproducibly by about 500 mL per day[30] and the addition of octreotide may be considered for this reason. However, in three placebo-controlled studies of patients with postoperative fistulae, there was no improvement in the percentage of fistulae which healed without surgery, even though the speed at which this healing took place was faster (by about 10 days).[31] There were also fewer infective complications in the patients treated with octreotide.

A somewhat more controversial approach is taken by one group who report the beneficial use of reinfusion of intestinal secretions lost from the fistula site to reduce hepatic dysfunction, perhaps via a reduction in endotoxaemia.[32] This is not a technique with which most units have felt comfortable, and it is probably significant that there have been no more recent publications on its use.

Surgery is often required in patients with enterocutaneous fistulae. It is particularly strongly indicated if the fistula is unrelated to recent surgery, if the bladder is involved, and when the fistula is high in the bowel or of particularly high output. The results of surgery can be expected to be good when there is localized disease and when it is possible to excise the involved bowel and the fistula track completely. Drainage procedures are probably not sufficient alone, although they may form a part of initial resuscitation.

ENTEROVESICAL FISTULA

The literature suggests a frequency of Crohn's-related enterovesical fistula of between 2 and 5 per cent, but again there is referral centre bias and the overall lifetime risk is probably much less. Not all enterovesical fistulae are obviously symptomatic and up to a third will be found at surgery or in investigation of other aspects of complicated Crohn's disease.[33] Most are ileal or from the

sigmoid colon and they tend to coexist with fistulous complexes involving multiple intestinal loops and communication to the skin or vagina. The combination of cystoscopy[33] and MR scanning[34] is probably most efficacious in investigation. Azathioprine has a place in the non-surgical management but most patients will require surgical intervention. Unfortunately, there is a high rate of operative complications and recurrent fistula (12 per cent in the Birmingham series,[33] 4 per cent in the larger similar study from the Cleveland Clinic[35]). This seems mainly to be predicated upon perioperative sepsis.

FISTULA SUMMARY

The best results from fistula surgery are achieved when it is unhurried and follows meticulous preoperative attention to fluid and sodium balance, adequate nutrition and good skin care. At St Mark's it is strongly advised that no patient with a fistula should have elective surgery within 6 weeks of a previous laparotomy.[36] It must be emphasized that the management of the patient with an enterocutaneous or enterovesical fistula is a team effort. No one discipline, however skilled, can hope to manage these patients to their best advantage. The skills of the physician, surgeon and ward nurse need the supplementary skills of the stoma care therapist, the nutrition nurse and often members of the psychological support team, given the chronic and emotionally damaging nature of these unpleasant conditions.

Short bowel syndrome

Intestinal failure or short bowel syndrome (SBS) results from a deficiency in the ability of the intestine to handle nutrients and its own secretions. Excessive water and electrolyte losses and malnutrition result. SBS usually follows major resection, typically leaving less than 200 cm of small bowel, but also when the relatively intact intestine is unable to function because of severe inflammation (or disorders of motility). In many Crohn's patients with SBS, both causes coexist.

Short bowel syndrome is unusual, with a prevalence of less than one case per 100 000 population in the UK and North America, and with an incidence around one-tenth of that. Crohn's disease accounts for around half of all benign causes of long-term intestinal failure. Short-term intestinal failure is, of course, seen in many postoperative inflammatory bowel disease patients with prolonged 'ileus', and in a few patients after the apparently straightforward creation of an end-ileostomy for ulcerative colitis. It is also a relatively frequent cause for medical referral in the patient after one-stage pouch surgery (see Chapter 4), who seems at above-average risk of this complication, presumably from the combination of a lengthy procedure (with more than average handling of the small intestine) with a modest loss of effective small bowel length from the creation of the pouch.

The management of SBS is influenced by the expected duration of the problem. In the short term, parenteral nutrition will be required for any patient unable to achieve nutritional adequacy with enteral feeding, but many such patients will later achieve sufficient intestinal function to become partially or totally independent of parenteral nutrition. The ileum is more adaptable than the jejunum, and the continued presence of the colon also helps in attainment of fluid/electrolyte balance and to some extent in nutrition. The process of intestinal adaptation begins soon after injury, and continues for at least 6 months and probably up to 2 years.[37]

Short bowel syndrome is best managed when anticipated. The length of the remaining small bowel should be measured at the time of surgery, and both its anatomical identity and integrity recorded. The variable length of the normal small intestine and the frequent history of previous resections in patients with Crohn's disease make measurements of the resected segment much less helpful. When there is no record of the length of remaining bowel, an approximate measurement can be made on barium follow-through.

Patients with a high jejunostomy can be expected to lose upwards of 3 L of fluid each day with a sodium loss of at least 90 mmol/L. This follows from the physiological, secretory response of the upper gastrointestinal tract and jejunum, as only when the luminal sodium concentration reaches 90 mmol/L or more does net absorption commence. Since almost all spontaneously consumed drinks have a very low sodium content, salt and water deficiency becomes almost inevitable. Unfortunately, the consequent onset of thirst will exacerbate the problem. As the patient drinks more, yet more intestinal secretion is provoked, amplifying the already high stomal losses. Daily parenteral fluid and electrolyte supplements are likely to be required in all those with less than 100 cm of small bowel above a stoma.[38] If all or part of the colon remains in continuity with the small intestine, then there is more opportunity for restitutive distal reabsorption of sodium and water, and regular intravenous fluids are less likely to be necessary.

Absorption of nutrients also correlates inversely with jejunal length. In Nightingale's study,[39] every patient with less than 85 cm of small bowel terminating in a stoma required parenteral nutrients as well as intravenous fluids. Those with a healthy length of small bowel in excess of 100 cm can often be maintained in reasonable nutrition with oral food and supplements. If a short small bowel remains in continuity with a functional large intestine, the colon may be harmed by non-reabsorbed bile salts and food components, but it is also able to utilize short-chain fatty acids derived from unabsorbed carbohydrate as a source of energy.[40] There is accordingly advantage in ensuring a higher proportion of total oral energy from carbohydrate in these patients. For the same total energy provision, the SBS patient with a colon will absorb more when the diet contains more carbohydrate and less fat, in contrast to the SBS patient who lacks a colon, in whom the distribution of fat and carbohydrate calories in the diet makes no difference to retention of energy.[41] Although there may also be a theoretical advantage in avoiding fats in SBS patients to reduce steatorrhoea, this is rarely a clinical issue and most patients should be encouraged to eat as they wish.[42,43]

Retention of all or most of the colon may be considered roughly equivalent to an additional 50 cm of small bowel in respect of the absorption of nutrients (as well as the more dramatic advantage in respect of easier fluid and electrolyte management alluded to above).[39] All of 71 patients studied with greater than 50 cm of small bowel and retained colons were supported with enteral supplements alone at 5-year follow-up. It is probable that part of this benefit is vested in the functional ileocaecal valve, and unfortunate that this is the part of the bowel most often resected in Crohn's disease. The greater potential of the terminal ileum for adaptation, the preservation of the 'ileal brake' and normal absorption of bile salts and vitamin B_{12} are also usually denied the postoperative patient with Crohn's.

SYMPTOMS AND SIGNS

Weight loss despite good appetite and food consumption, especially in the presence of profuse diarrhoea (or high stomal losses), will be obvious pointers to intestinal failure, but the early symptoms of sodium deficiency are often missed, as patients find them difficult to describe and may not volunteer them. In addition to features suggestive of postural hypotension, thirst and relative oliguria, patients may experience curious echo-like sensations. Examination will include weight and height, enabling computation of the body mass index, but taking into account the presence of dehydration or oedema, the latter in particular being a source of potential confusion. A search for

signs of specific nutrient deficiencies is appropriate but will usually be unproductive, as intestinal failure presents with obvious macronutrient deficiency before the more subtle features from lack of micronutrients become apparent. Salt and water deficiency is more reliably indicated by postural hypotension than assessment of skin turgor or venous filling. Tetany provoked by the sphygmomanometer cuff provides confirmation of calcium or (much more often) magnesium deficiency.

Arguably the most important (and one of the most underutilized) investigations in SBS is the urine sodium concentration. This need not be a timed collection, as random samples will usually give the necessary information. If the sodium content is less than 20 mmol/L, salt deficiency is likely. Only in the presence of established renal failure does the urine sodium content become unreliable. Other laboratory data are almost superfluous. It is difficult to monitor fluid and sodium balance in short bowel syndrome, especially if there are stomal or fistula leakages, but daily weighing (on the same scales), lying and standing blood pressure, and daily urine sodiums are reproducible, practical and sufficiently informative in most cases.

THERAPY

Nutrients

The aim of SBS management is to provide a good quality of life, with effective but minimally invasive medical interventions which prevent thirst and dehydration and permit maintenance of an acceptable body weight. It is often difficult for Crohn's disease patients to achieve pre-morbid body weight, but it should always be possible to attain a weight that is acceptable to patient and physician, and it is practical to aim for a body mass index of around 20 kg/m^2. Additional quantifiable objectives include an average stomal output of no more than 2 L/day, or the absence of disabling diarrhoea in the patient without a stoma. The daily urine output should ideally exceed 1 L, although in practice as little as 700 mL is acceptable as long as the patient is healthy in other respects and has a urine sodium of at least 20 mmol/L. The serum magnesium should be in the normal range. Normal levels of other nutritional markers are usually achieved surprisingly easily.

Many SBS patients will come to attention whilst still in serious trouble from their inflammatory bowel disease, with uncontrolled stoma or enterocutaneous fistula output and problematic skin care (see above). The immediate involvement of the stoma therapist is an essential part of good intestinal failure management, and may be the team's first opportunity to gain the patient's trust and confidence. This is especially true when referral follows a long sequence of unsuccessful or partially successful operative interventions. The peri-stoma/fistula skin needs careful handling, with preventative methods to protect it from necrosis or infection. Correction of zinc deficiency may be particularly helpful in this context whether or not the characteristic rash is seen. Even in the absence of SBS, deficiencies of such micronutrients as zinc, selenium and vitamins A, C, D and E are common in Crohn's disease.[44]

Most patients with a short bowel will take food orally despite their substantially incomplete absorption. Only if eating causes severe symptoms, or if in the management of a high fistula there has been a decision to continue a deliberate nil-by-mouth policy to maximize chances of closure, should it not be positively encouraged. Patients should be advised to concentrate on normal foods high in energy and protein,[45] and most will need to avoid large fluid volumes. Aside from the advantage from colonic fermentation of carbohydrate (see above), they need not avoid fatty food, since the high-energy content is valuable, tolerance is rarely a problem, and excess losses of divalent cations do not occur as was once thought.[43] Elemental feeds should not be used as their high

osmolarity will increase the stomal output. Certain foods such as tomatoes or onions will also have this effect in some individuals. Patients with a high jejunostomy should add salt to their food within the limits of palatability to minimize sodium secretion into the gut and thereby to minimize stomal losses of both sodium and water. This may be the only nutritional measure required in patients in whom the stomal losses average less than 1200 mL/day.

Patients who are unable to maintain their normal weight on a high-calorie diet with frequent meals and between-meal snacks may achieve this goal by use of one of the specially prepared liquid or semi-solid food supplements, perhaps given overnight via a nasogastric or gastrostomy tube, as the slower but more continuous administration maximally utilizes the absorptive potential of the remaining bowel. There has been concern about the use of percutaneous gastrostomy tube insertion in Crohn's disease given the high frequency of upper gastrointestinal disease and a perceived risk of gastrocutaneous fistula. Our experience at St Mark's Hospital has, however, been uniformly positive, and although numbers and duration of follow-up are modest, we are increasingly optimistic that gastrostomy feeding can be utilized safely when it seems indicated in inflammatory bowel disease.[46]

When absorption falls below about one-third of all energy taken enterally, it becomes impossible to achieve positive nutritional balance, or to maintain a satisfactory weight.[38] Parenteral supplements then become necessary. For practical purposes, any patient with a stomal output of greater than 2500 mL/day is likely to be dependent on fluids, electrolytes and nutrients, all given by the parenteral route.[47] The nutrient regimens to be considered reflect the frequent need for large volumes and generous amounts of magnesium and sodium rather than specific nutritional issues. Parenteral nutrition is almost inevitably a long-term concern in these patients and should always be administered via a dedicated tunnelled catheter inserted into a central vein, or via one of the implantable devices. It is usual to commence with a continuous 24-hour infusion regimen, but quickly increasing the rate to permit a steadily lengthening nutrition-free period each day. This cyclical regimen has many advantages, enables mobility and is surprisingly important in psychological rehabilitation.[48]

The concept of non-total parenteral nutrition is important and not always fully appreciated even by those engaged in the regular care of patients such as these. Most patients with intestinal failure from Crohn's disease are able to eat, and most are able to absorb a useful proportion of the nutrients that are taken orally, even if this is inadequate to sustain life without intravenous support. These patients accordingly do not require *total* parenteral nutrition, as they can and do absorb some of their daily requirements from the gut. Enteral feeding is encouraged also to help maintain normal gastrointestinal flora, to increase gastrointestinal adaptation, and to prevent gall bladder sludge accumulation. Once malnutrition is corrected, unless there is a compelling daily need for fluids and electrolytes, it will often prove possible to reduce the parenteral feeding to three or four nights a week.

Fluid and electrolyte balance

Fluid balance in SBS patients is frequently poorly managed. This results from basic misapprehensions and inappropriate extrapolation from other conditions in which thirst and dehydration coexist. The remedy in the patient with intestinal failure is almost always to restrict fluid intake, and to prescribe a glucose–electrolyte solution to drink whenever thirsty, or on a regular basis to prevent thirst in the more severely affected individual.[49] The more crucial element of the strategy is the restriction of sodium-poor fluids, but the prescription of a rehydration solution is often easier to explain and compliance easier to ensure.

Experimental work indicates that the solution should contain at least 90 mmol of sodium/L, but it must also be palatable, easy to prepare and (preferably) cheap, to promote its long-term use by the patient. Studies at St Mark's Hospital have suggested that the use of the World Health Organization formula (without potassium chloride) is a good compromise on theoretical and experimental grounds.[50]

The St Mark's oral rehydration solution consists of: glucose powder, 20 g (110 mmol); sodium chloride, 3.5 g (60 mmol); sodium bicarbonate, 2.5 g (30 mmol), measured using standard scoops, and made up to 1 L in tap water. The inclusion of sodium bicarbonate is to increase palatability (and perhaps absorption)[50] rather than for an effect on pH, and may be replaced by sodium citrate (2.9 g = 30 mmol) if the patient prefers. Most find it easiest to drink if chilled, but palatability can also be improved by flavouring with fruit drink concentrates or pure lemon juice. Restriction of all other fluids to 500–750 mL each day, but with emphasis on drinking at least as much of the electrolyte solution, is recommended.

Intravenous fluids will often be required in the initial resuscitation of short bowel patients. These should be given mainly as sodium chloride 0.9 per cent (150 mmol/L of sodium) as sodium deficiency is as much a problem as lack of water. For practical purposes, the patient with overt clinical dehydration, postural hypotension, or biochemical evidence of pre-renal uraemia can be considered to need intravenous fluids. If these features are absent, an oral regimen should at least be attempted. Sodium should be replaced to provide around 90 mmol for each litre of measured urine and gastrointestinal losses from the previous 24 hours. Potassium will often not be needed if the patient continues to receive enteral nutrition, but magnesium is frequently necessary. If it proves impossible to wean from parental fluids, training in the self-administration of intravenous supplements becomes necessary, unless adequate control can be reliably achieved with the addition of less than 1 L daily. In this case the simpler and safer option of self-administration of subcutaneous saline can be employed.

Magnesium deficiency is common in SBS patients with a terminal jejunostomy, and will be confused with hypocalcaemia (which it renders untreatable until the low magnesium is corrected). Once recognized, its deficiency can rapidly be remedied by the administration of intravenous magnesium, 10–12 mmol, repeated as necessary until the serum magnesium has returned to within the normal range. Oral magnesium supplements at a dose of 12–24 mmol daily will usually be tolerated without worsening diarrhoea or increasing stomal output. If the patient requires more magnesium, then the dose can be increased until side effects become intolerable or the therapeutic dose is reached. Heavy magnesium oxide capsules (160 mg) are found easier and no less effective than magnesium glycerophosphate; nevertheless, tolerance is variable, and therapeutic trials are worthwhile if the first salt tried is not acceptable. In some patients tolerance is so poor that compliance is negligible; intravenous magnesium becomes necessary, and in some cases is the main justification for long-term parenteral access. Up to 8 mmol can, however, be administered daily via a subcutaneous fluid regimen.

Opioids provide some control over the absence of the ileal brake, rapid gastric emptying and consequent rapid intestinal transit.[51] They act on receptors in the gastrointestinal tract, reduce loss of water and electrolytes[52,53] and may contribute to increased nutrient absorption.[54] Loperamide is preferred as it acts only on the opioid receptors in the gut, and not centrally. Codeine phosphate is frequently used either alone or in combination with loperamide as it is preferred by some patients. Diphenoxylate is prescribed occasionally as, although double-blind trial has shown it to be less effective,[55] some patients find it helpful. Encephalinase inhibitors such as racecadotril have been found effective in acute diarrhoea and deserve attention in the SBS context.[56]

Very large doses of opioids may be required. A prescription for 64 mg loperamide *and* 480 mg codeine phosphate each day is neither unusual nor inappropriate in SBS patients without a colon. The resultant reduction in stool or stomal losses can make a crucial difference to quality of life (as, for example, by permitting an undisturbed night's sleep), without risk of physical or psychological dependence. The drugs should be taken 30–60 minutes before meals for maximal effect.

Proton pump inhibitors reduce gastric acid secretion, but there is also a parallel reduction in the volume of gastric secretion, rendering these agents of considerable value in SBS. Reduced jejunostomy output and increased absorption of nutrients can be achieved.[57] Although neither effect is itself dramatic (typically a jejunostomy output will be reduced by no more than 15 per cent or 500 mL/day), it can be sufficient to have meaningful impact on quality of life. For reasons that are not entirely clear, doses much larger than in standard therapeutic regimens are frequently needed to obtain maximal benefit.

Somatostatin and its analogues reduce gastric, biliary and pancreatic secretions[58] and slow gastrojejunal transit time.[59] Although there is also evidence that they have an adverse effect on the uptake of nutrients, possibly on wound healing, and may interfere with the physiological process of adaptation to resection,[60] it is natural that their effects on stomal and fistula output have been studied (see above). Sodium and water losses are not significantly affected in patients who are net absorbers (or in positive gastrointestinal balance), but a reproducible reduction in stomal output can be achieved in net secretors, averaging around 500 mL/day. There does not seem to be any difference in efficacy between somatostatin and the more convenient octreotide. Twice or thrice daily subcutaneous injections of octreotide 50–100 μg have usually been used, with little evidence for greater effect from daily doses in excess of 300 μg. Major side effects are not recorded, although the high risk of gallstone formation is important, given the already increased frequency of gallstones in SBS patients. There is no evidence as yet that lanreotide, introduced as a longer-acting version of octreotide and permitting fortnightly injection, has a role in SBS, but it is similarly effective in control of symptoms and preferred by patients with carcinoid syndrome.[61]

A series of other agents thought of potential use in SBS have been tried and found to be of very limited effect. The bulking agents such as ispaghula decrease the fluidity of gut effluent, but increase the loss of water and electrolytes and aggravate their depletion.[52] Cholestyramine is of value in patients with a retained colon with either bile salt-related diarrhoea without steatorrhoea, or with hyperoxaluria. Its negative influence on absorption of fat-soluble vitamins and its lack of palatability militate further against its use.

Professionals more peripherally involved in the care of SBS patients are often ill-informed and intimidated by the problems posed, leading to suboptimal care. The most damaging effects arise when the dehydrated patient is incorrectly advised to drink more fluid. Each patient should be educated about the condition and its management, and should have written details which can be shown to new health care personnel. The anger and general distress of patients and relatives should not be underestimated; formal psychological support and counselling may be appropriate in some cases.

New treatment modalities for short bowel syndrome

No degree of meticulous attention to the management strategies outlined above will be sufficient to reverse established short bowel syndrome once the 6–24-month period of intestinal adaptation is complete. Various surgical procedures have been devised to lengthen the abbreviated small bowel in paediatric practice but these have not become established in adults, not least because of the concerns that any operative intervention has the potential to worsen an already parlous situation. Combinations of human growth hormone and glutamine have been claimed to permit weaning from intravenous nutrition,[62] but it is probable that most of the gain in those patients was from implementation of best practice in a tertiary centre, given that a similar strategy applied in a controlled fashion in two other centres had no effect.[63,64] We are holding out some hope for a therapeutic impact from glucagon-like peptide 2, which has important trophic effects *in vitro*[65] and may be useful in SBS.[66]

Intestinal transplantation is now being performed in around 100 patients per year world wide.[67] Approximately half of these are in the under-16s group, in whom inflammatory bowel disease is not frequently represented, but about 16 per cent of all adult transplant recipients have Crohn's disease. The results are improving and almost all patients successfully treated become independent of intravenous nutrition. However, the graft survival is currently only just over 50 per cent at 2 years and patient survival around 60 per cent, with most (55 per cent) deaths being directly from sepsis, and a frequency of lymphoproliferative disease of around 10 per cent. There is also the interesting spectre of recurrent Crohn's disease in the transplanted bowel to be considered. Only 6 months after surgery a patient immunosuppressed with tacrolimus, methylprednisolone, bone marrow infusions, and OKT3 antibody, represented with abdominal pain that proved to be the result of unequivocal recurrent Crohn's disease in the donor intestine.[68]

Anaemia in inflammatory bowel disease

It may seem odd to include a separate section on anaemia as a complication of inflammatory bowel disease, this being a common presenting feature of the new patient, which usually responds rapidly to the control of inflammation and curtailed intestinal blood loss. Short- to medium-term supplementation with the appropriate haematinics will provide the necessary support, with indefinite vitamin B_{12} for those with no terminal ileum. However, there are patients in whom chronic low-grade blood loss, or the anaemia of chronic disease, is not easily overcome. This will sometimes be sufficient to justify colectomy in the chronic colitic, but poses even greater problems in the patient with extensive Crohn's who has anaemia partly because of an existing degree of intestinal failure. It is obviously important to define the nature of the anaemia. Vitamin B_{12} deficiency is easily diagnosed and overcome, but will normally have been anticipated and pre-empted in patients with terminal ileal resection. Folate and iron deficiency often coexist in patients with extensive small bowel Crohn's, and an apparently normocytic anaemia should not be attributed to chronic disease until their status has been established (the patient with folate and iron deficiency will normally have an elevated red cell distribution width even if there is not overt anaemia). Adequate folate restitution, also, is usually straightforward with oral or intravenous restitution as appropriate.

Iron replacement is more often problematic. Many inflammatory bowel disease patients find iron salts intolerable, and many have specific gastrointestinal side effects that limit use. It is worth trying a variety of formulations including liquid oral iron (Sytron© in the UK), which some patients seem to tolerate better and which may lead to useful absorption even in those with a short bowel. Transfusion is of limited application, tends to be of short-lived value, and has its own hazards. Similar strictures apply to the use of total-dose iron therapy by infusion, and to prolonged courses of intramuscular injections. Although intravenous iron is effective in around 75 per cent of otherwise intractable iron-deficient patients, it is not without risk. In a small unpublished audit at St Mark's,

25 per cent of Crohn's patients treated with intravenous iron developed a clinically significant anaphylactoid reaction. As, in the view of the supervising physician, half of these required adrenaline therapy, alternatives are clearly needed!

Ferric hydroxide sucrose (or iron saccharate) is a novel iron formulation said to be free of risk of anaphylaxis. It has been widely and effectively used in the chronic anaemia of renal failure[69] and is finding a place in inflammatory bowel disease therapy.[70] Unfortunately, it is recommended that doses of no more than 200 mg are given at a single infusion. There does not seem to be a strong evidence base for this and 500 mg at a time may be safe and permit typical full replacement in as few as two infusions.[69]

Study of anaemic patients with Crohn's disease demonstrates a defect in erythropoietin production which is inadequate for the magnitude of anaemia, regardless of iron status or the current degree of disease activity.[71] In other medical contexts, both intractable iron deficiency and the anaemia of chronic disease have been significantly helped by exogenous erythropoietin. There may be a place for this expensive parenteral therapy in difficult inflammatory bowel disease cases also.[72,73] In Schreiber's study, 15 patients with ulcerative colitis and 19 with Crohn's disease were randomized to oral iron with or without sub-cutaneous erythropoietin (150 units/kg twice weekly).[72] Over 12 weeks there was a mean 1.7 g/dL gain in haemoglobin in those receiving both drugs compared to a loss of 0.85 g/dL in those on iron alone. Significance was achieved for both Crohn's disease and ulcerative colitis. Disappointingly, there was less value from the addition of erythropoietin to intravenous iron,[74] most of the gains in a controlled trial coming from the iron, albeit with advantage from erythropoietin to the poor responders.

Iron deficiency in the absence of anaemia, however, is probably best left untreated given evidence from the management of rheumatoid arthritis. Administration of iron in this context leads to an increase in inflammation and an overall adverse effect on morbidity presumably via an iron-catalysed pro-oxidant effect.[75] It is also suggested that oral iron may (rarely) directly provoke presentation with colitis.[76]

Thrombosis and thromboembolic phenomena in inflammatory bowel disease

Thrombosis and thromboembolic phenomena are important causes of morbidity and mortality in active inflammatory bowel disease.[77] Although strict comparative data have been lacking, there has been an impression that deep vein thrombosis in the legs and pelvis, pulmonary embolism, mesenteric and intracranial thromboses are all commoner than in other groups of patients with benign disease. An Austrian group have now provided key missing data in a retrospective cohort study of over 350 patients with inflammatory bowel disease.[78] Almost six times as many patients had had thromboembolic events (6.8 per cent) as had age- and sex-matched controls (1.2 per cent; $P < 0.0001$; odds ratio: 6.0; CI: 2–17). Most events were in the over-40s at times of increased risk (postoperative or active disease); deep vein thrombosis and pulmonary emboli were the usual manifestations. Radiological verification was sought for all volunteered episodes but there is a possibility that recall bias may have exaggerated the differences from controls.

Mesenteric microvascular thrombosis, postulated as a pathogenic factor for inflammatory bowel disease, and possible abnormalities in heparan status (see Chapters 1 and 3) may be contributory factors, as may the thrombocytosis typical of the patient with active disease. Spontaneous platelet aggregation, and high levels of thromboxane B2, platelet factor 4,

fibrinopeptide A and β-thromboglobulin are demonstrable in Crohn's disease.[77,79] There are substantially reduced, and therefore prothrombotic, levels of antithrombin III in some but not all patients with active inflammatory bowel disease.[80,81] Acquired deficiency of proteins C and S may also occur. There is evidence for abnormality also of the tissue plasminogen system.[79] In one study, patients with Crohn's disease were found to have pathological levels of plasma factor VII:C, lipoprotein(a) and fibrinogen.[82] In ulcerative colitis, levels of lipoprotein(a) and fibrinogen were normal, but factor VII:C again exceeded the normal range. The probable increased risk of arterial thrombosis in inflammatory bowel disease may be linked to an increased prevalence of IgG anticardiolipin antibodies in inflammatory bowel disease: 15.6 per cent in Crohn's disease and 18.1 per cent in ulcerative colitis compared with 3 per cent of matched controls.[83] Mutation of factor V Leiden has not generally been found to be implicated,[84,85] but might be important in some populations.[86]

The issue of thrombosis in inflammatory bowel disease is beginning to take on medicolegal significance and it will be difficult to refute future claims arising from thrombotic events if prophylactic measures were not taken, since it will be argued that such an event was sufficiently predictable that these measures should have been taken, or that the reason for not so doing should have been recorded. All patients admitted for inflammatory bowel disease should be on a prophylactic regimen (quite apart from any potential therapeutic benefit from heparin in ulcerative colitis; see Chapter 3); those with septic or other complications of their disease appear to be at especial risk.[3] If thrombosis occurs, however, there does not appear to be any particular need for inflammatory bowel disease patients to be managed differently from those with thrombosis complicating other medical conditions. Apart from during the immediate postoperative period, standard anticoagulation with heparin and then a coumarin such as warfarin is safe and will not normally lead to excessive gastrointestinal bleeding (indeed, the opposite is suggested for heparin in ulcerative colitis; see Chapter 3). Patients with SBS are sometimes difficult to anticoagulate satisfactorily, but cautious use of warfarin with haematological monitoring at a fixed interval from exposure to nutrient solutions (particularly lipid) will usually suffice. Difficulty in achieving anticoagulation with heparin in inflammatory bowel disease probably reflects concurrent antithrombin III deficiency; it is possible that leeches may be able to help here as their anticoagulant, hirudin, unlike heparin, is independent of antithrombin III![87]

References

1 Keighley MRB, Eastwood D, Ambrose NS, *et al.* Incidence and microbiology of abdominal and pelvic abscess in Crohn's disease. *Gastroenterology* 1982; **83**: 1271–5.

2 Ribeiro MB, Greenstein AJ, Yamazaki Y, Aufses AH Jr. Intra-abdominal abscess in regional enteritis. *Ann Surg* 1991; **213**: 32–6.

3 Ricci MA, Meyer KK. Psoas abscess complicating Crohn's disease. *Am J Gastroenterol* 1985; **80**: 970–7.

4 Leu SY, Leonard MB, Beart RW Jr, Dozois RR. Psoas abscess: changing patterns of diagnosis and etiology. *Dis Colon Rectum* 1986; **29**: 694–8.

5 Jawhari A, Kamm MA, Ong C, Forbes A, Bartram CI, Hawley PR. Intra-abdominal and pelvic abscesses in Crohn's disease: results of non-invasive and surgical management. *Br J Surg* 1998; **85**: 367–71.

6 Sahai A, Belair M, Gianfelice D, Cote S, Gratton J, Lahaie R. Percutaneous drainage of intra-abdominal abscesses in Crohn's disease: short and long-term outcome. *Am J Gastroenterol* 1997; **92**: 275–8.

7 Maconi G, Parente F, Bollani S, *et al.* High resolution bowel ultrasound for the detection of intestinal complications in Crohn's disease. *Gut* 1999; **45**(Suppl V); A201.

8 Gore RM, Cohen MI, Vogelzang RL, Neiman HL, Tsang TK. Value of computed tomography in the detection of complications of Crohn's disease. *Dig Dis Sci* 1985; **30**: 701–9.

9 Tio TL, Mulder CJJ, Wijers OB, *et al.* Endosonography of peri-anal and pericolorectal fistula and/or abscess in Crohn's disease: a study of 36 patients. *Gastrointest Endosc* 1990; **36**: 331–6.

10 Bluth EI, Ferrari BT, Sullivan MA. Abscess drainage with the aid of pelvic real-time ultrasonography. *Dis Colon Rectum* 1985; **28**: 262–3.

11 Millward SF, Ramesewak W, Fitzsimons P, Frost R, Tam P, Toi A. Percutaneous drainage of iliopsoas abscess in Crohn's disease. *Gastrointest Radiol* 1986; **11**: 289–90.

12 Doemeny JM, Burke DR, Meranze SG. Percutaneous drainage of abscesses in patients with Crohn's disease. *Gastrointest Radiol* 1988; **13**: 237–41.

13 Felder JB, Adler DJ, Korelitz BI. The safety of corticosteroid therapy in Crohn's disease with an abdominal mass. *Am J Gastroenterol* 1991; **86**: 1450–5.

14 Choen S, Burnett S, Bartram CI, Nicholls RJ. Comparison between anal endosonography and digital examination in the evaluation of anal fistulae. *Br J Surg* 1991; **78**: 445–7.

15 Orsoni P, Barthet M, Portier F, Panuel M, Desjeux A, Grimaud JC. Prospective comparison of endosonography, magnetic resonance imaging and surgical findings in anorectal fistula and abscess complicating Crohn's disease. *Br J Surg* 1999; **86**: 360–4.

16 deSouza NM, Gilderdale DJ, Coutts GA, Puni R, Steiner RE. MRI of fistula-in-ano: a comparison of endoanal coil with external phased array coil techniques. *J Comput Assist Tomogr* 1998; **22**: 357–63.

17 Scott HJ, Northover JM. Evaluation of surgery for perianal Crohn's fistulas. *Dis Colon Rectum* 1996; **39**: 1039–43.

18 McCourtney JS, Finlay IG. Setons in the surgical management of fistula in ano. *Br J Surg* 1995; **82**: 448–52.

19 Korelitz BI, Present DH. Favorable effect of 6-mercaptopurine on fistulae of Crohn's disease. *Dig Dis Sci* 1985; **30**: 58–64.

20 Present DH, Lichtiger S. Efficacy of cyclosporine in treatment of fistula of Crohn's disease. *Dig Dis Sci* 1994; **39**: 374–80.

21 Lowry PW, Weaver AL, Tremaine WJ, Sandborn WJ. Combination therapy with oral tacrolimus (FK506) and azathioprine or 6-mercaptopurine for treatment-refractory Crohn's disease perianal fistulae. *Inflamm Bowel Dis* 1999; **5**: 239–45.

22 Present DH, Rutgeerts P, Targan S, *et al.* Infliximab for the treatment of fistulas in patients with Crohn's disease. *N Engl J Med* 1999; **340**: 1398–405.

23 Lévy E, Frileux P, Cugnenc PH, Honiger J, Ollivier JM, Parc R. High output external fistulae of the small bowel: management with continuous enteral nutrition. *Br J Surg* 1989; **76**: 676–9.

24 Maconi G, Parente F, Bianchi-Porro G. Hydrogen peroxide enhanced ultrasound-fistulography in the assessment of enterocutaneous fistulas complicating Crohn's disease. *Gut* 1999; **45**: 874–8.

25 Rinsema W, Gouma DJ, Von Meyenfeldt MF, Van der Linden CJ, Soeters PB. Primary conservative management of external small-bowel fistulas. *Acta Chir Scand* 1990; **156**: 457–62.

26 Kelly JK, Preshaw RM. Origin of fistulas in Crohn's disease. *J Clin Gastroenterol* 1989; **11**: 193–6.

27 Driscoll RH Jr, Rosenberg IH. Total parenteral nutrition in inflammatory bowel disease. *Med Clin North Am* 1978; **62**: 185–201.

28 Von Meyenfeldt MF, Meijerink WJHJ, Rouflart MMJ, *et al.* Perioperative nutritional support: a randomised clinical trial. *Clin Nutr* 1992; **11**: 180–6.

29 Joseph M, Hewett PJ, Hill H. The use of setons in the management of complex enterocutaneous fistulae of the abdominal wall. *Aust N Z J Surg* 1994; **64**: 628–9.

30 Nubiola P, Sancho J, Seguira M, *et al.* Blind evaluation of the effect of octreotide, a somatostatin analogue, on small bowel fistula output. *Lancet* 1987; **2**: 672–4.

31 Scott NA, Finnegan S, Irving MH. Octreotide and gastrointestinal fistulae. *Digestion* 1990; **45**: 66–71.

32 Rinsema W, Gouma DJ, Von Meyenfeldt MF. Reinfusion of secretions from high-output proximal stomas or fistulas. *Surg Gynecol Obstet* 1988; **167**: 372–6.

33 Yamamoto T, Keighley MRB. Enterovesical fistulas complicating Crohn's disease: clinicopathological features and management. *Int J Colorectal Dis* 2000; **15**: 211–15.

34 Boudghene F, Aboun H, Grange JD, Wallays C, Bodin F, Bigot JM. L'imagerie par resonance magnetique dans l'exploration des fistules abdominales et ano-perineales de la maladie de Crohn. *Gastroenterol Clin Biol* 1993; **17**: 168–74.

35 McNamara MJ, Fazio VW, Lavery IC, Weakley FL, Farmer RG. Surgical treatment of enterovesical fistulas in Crohn's disease. *Dis Colon Rectum* 1990; **33**: 271–6.

36 McIntyre P, Ritchie J, Hawley P, Bartram C, Lennard-Jones J. Management of enterocutaneous fistulas: a review of 132 cases. *Br J Surg* 1984; **71**: 293–6.

37 Gouttebel MC, Saint Aubert B, Colette C, Astre C, Monnier LH, Joyeux H. Intestinal adaptation in patients with short bowel syndrome. *Dig Dis Sci* 1989; **34**: 709–15.

38 Nightingale JMD, Lennard-Jones JE, Walker ER, Farthing MJG. Jejunal efflux in short bowel syndrome. *Lancet* 1990; **336**: 765–8.

39 Nightingale JMD, Lennard-Jones JE, Gertner DJ, Wood SR, Bartram CI. Colonic preservation reduces need for parental therapy, increases incidence of renal stones, but does not change prevalence of gall stones in patients with a short bowel. *Gut* 1992; **33**: 1493–7.

40 Royall D, Thomas MS, Wolever BM, Jeejeebhoy KN. Evidence for colonic conservation of malabsorbed carbohydrate in short bowel syndrome. *Am J Gastroenterol* 1992; **87**: 751–6.

41 Nordgaard I, Hansen BS, Mortensen NPB. Colon as a digestive organ in patients with short bowel. *Lancet* 1994; **343**: 373–6.

42 Woolf GM, Miller C, Kurian R, Jeejeebhoy KN. Nutritional absorption in short bowel syndrome. *Dig Dis Sci* 1987; **32**: 8–15.

43 Woolf BM, Miller C, Kurian R, Jeejeebhoy KN. Diet for patients with a short bowel: high fat or high carbohydrate? *Gastroenterology* 1983; **84**: 823–8.

44 Geerling BJ, Badart-Smook A, Stockbrugger RW, Brummer RJ. Comprehensive nutritional status in patients with long-standing Crohn disease currently in remission. *Am J Clin Nutr* 1998; **67**: 919–26.

45 McIntyre PB, Fitchew M, Lennard-Jones JE. Patients with a high jejunostomy do not need a special diet. *Gastroenterology* 1986; **91**: 25–33.

46 Anstee QM, Forbes A. The safe use of percutaneous gastrostomy for enteral nutrition in patients

with Crohn's disease. *Eur J Gastroenterol Hepatol* 2000; **12**: 1089–93.

47 Forbes A, Chadwick C. Short bowel syndrome. In Merritt RJ, ed. *ASPEN Nutrition Support Practice Manual*. Silver Spring: American Society for Parenteral and Enteral Nutrition, 1998.

48 Matuchansky C, Messing B, Jeejeebhoy KN, Beau P, Beliah M, Allard J. Cyclical parenteral nutrition. *Lancet* 1992; **340**: 588–92.

49 Griffin GE, Fagan EF, Hodgson HJ, Chadwick VS. Enteral therapy in the management of massive gut resection complicated by chronic fluid and electrolyte depletion. *Dig Dis Sci* 1982; **27**: 902–8.

50 Newton CR, McIntyre PB, Lennard-Jones JE, Gonvers JJ, Preston DM. Effect of different drinks on fluid and electrolyte losses from a jejunostomy. *Proc R Soc Med* 1985; **78**: 27–9.

51 Nightingale JMD, Kamm MA, Van Der Sijp JRM, *et al.* Disturbed gastric emptying in the short bowel syndrome. Evidence for a 'colonic brake'. *Gut* 1993; **34**: 1171–6.

52 Newton CR. Effect of codeine phosphate, Lomotil and Isogel on ileostomy function. *Gut* 1978; **19**: 377–83.

53 Tytgat GN, Huibregtse K, Dagevos J, Van Den Ende A. Effect of loperamide on fecal output and composition in well-established ileostomy and ileorectal anastomosis. *Dig Dis* 1977; **22**: 669–75.

54 McIntyre PB. The short bowel. *Br J Surg* 1985; **72**: S92–3.

55 Pelemans W, Vantrappen G. A double blind crossover comparison of loperamide with diphenoxylate in the symptomatic treatment of chronic diarrhea. *Gastroenterology* 1976; **70**: 1030–4.

56 Vetel JM, Berard H, Fretault N, Lecomte JM. Comparison of racecadotril and loperamide in adults with acute diarrhoea. *Aliment Pharmacol Ther* 1999; **13**(Suppl 6): 21–6.

57 Cortot J, Fleming CR, Malagelada JR. Improved nutrient absorption after cimetidine in short-bowel syndrome with gastric hypersecretion. *Med Intell* 1979; **300**: 79–81.

58 O'Keefe SJD, Peterson ME, Fleming CR. Octreotide as an adjunct to home parenteral nutrition in the management of permanent end-jejunostomy syndrome. *J Parent Enteral Nutr* 1994; **18**: 26–36.

59 Cooper JC, Williams NS, King RFGJ, Barker MCJ. Effects of a long-acting somatostatin

analogue in patients with severe ileostomy diarrhoea. *Br J Surg* 1986; **73**: 128–31.

60 O'Keefe SJD, Haymond MW, Bennet WM, Oswald B, Nelson DK, Shorter RG. Long-acting somatostatin analogue therapy and protein metabolism in patients with jejunostomies: *Gastroenterology* 1994; **107**: 379–88.

61 O'Toole D, Ducreux M, Bommelaer G, *et al.* Treatment of carcinoid syndrome: a prospective crossover evaluation of lanreotide versus octreotide in terms of efficacy, patient acceptability, and tolerance. *Cancer* 2000; **88**: 770–6.

62 Byrne TA, Morrissey TB, Nattakom TV, *et al.* Growth hormone, glutamine and a modified diet enhance nutrient absorption in patients with severe short bowel syndrome. *JPEN J Parenter Enteral Nutr* 1995; **19**: 296–302.

63 Scolapio JS. Effect of growth hormone, glutamine, and diet on body composition in short bowel syndrome: a randomized, controlled study. *JPEN J Parenter Enteral Nutr* 1999; **23**: 309–12.

64 Szkudlarek J, Jeppesen PB, Mortensen PB. Effect of high dose growth hormone with glutamine and no change in diet on intestinal absorption in short bowel patients: a randomised, double blind, crossover, placebo controlled trial. *Gut* 2000; **47**: 199–205.

65 Kitchen PA Fitzgerald AJ, Goodlad RA, *et al.* Glucagon-like peptide-2 increases sucrase-isomaltase but not caudal-related homeobox protein-2 gene expression. *Am J Physiol: Gastrointest Liver Physiol* 2000; **278**: G425–8.

66 Jeppesen PB, Hartmann B, Thulesen J, *et al.* Treatment of short bowel patients with glucagon-like peptide 2, a newly discovered intestinotrophic, anti-secretory, and transit modulating peptide. *Gastroenterology* 2000; **118**: A1009–10.

67 Intestinal Transplant Registry. Current results. 1999. www.lhsc.on.ca/itr/.

68 Sustento-Reodica N, Ruiz P, Rogers A, Viciana AL, Conn HO, Tzakis AG. Recurrent Crohn's disease in transplanted bowel. *Lancet* 1997; **349**: 688–91.

69 Barker A, Denning J, Turney J. A haemoglobin optimisation clinic for peritoneal dialysis patients. *Br J Renal Med* 1999; **4**: 23–4.

70 Reffitt DM, Meenan J, Powell JJ, Thompson RPH. Sustained improvement in the quality of life of patients with anaemia and inflammatory bowel

disease given intravenous iron. *Gut* 1999; 45(Suppl V): A132.

71 Gasche C, Reinisch W, Lochs H, *et al.* Anemia in Crohn's disease. Importance of inadequate erythropoietin production and iron deficiency. *Dig Dis Sci* 1994; **39**: 1930–4.

72 Schreiber S, Howaldt S, Schnoor M, *et al.* Recombinant erythropoietin for the treatment of anemia in inflammatory bowel disease. *N Engl J Med* 1996; **334**: 619–23.

73 Dohil R, Hassall E, Wadsworth LD, Israel DM. Recombinant human erythropoietin for treatment of anemia of chronic disease in children with Crohn's disease. *J Pediatr* 1998; **132**: 155–9.

74 Gasche C, Dejaco C, Waldhoer T, *et al.* Intravenous iron and erythropoietin for anemia associated with Crohn disease. A randomized, controlled trial. *Ann Intern Med* 1997; **126**: 782–7.

75 Winyard PG, Blake DR, Chirico S, Gutteridge JM, Lunec J. Mechanism of exacerbation of rheumatoid synovitis by total-dose iron-dextran infusion: in-vivo demonstration of iron-promoted oxidant stress. *Lancet* 1987; **1**: 69–72.

76 Kawai M, Sumimoto S, Kasajima Y, Hamamoto T. A case of ulcerative colitis induced by oral ferrous sulfate. *Acta Paediatr Jpn* 1992; **34**: 476–8.

77 Webberley MJ, Hart MT, Melikian V. Thromboembolism in inflammatory bowel disease: role of platelets. *Gut* 1993; **34**: 247–51.

78 Novacek G, Miehsler W, Woginer S, *et al.* Thromboembolism in inflammatory bowel disease – preliminary results of a case-control study. *Gut* 1999; **45**(Suppl V): A196.

79 Chamouard P, Grunebaum L, Duclos B, Wiesel L, Cazenave JP. Biological manifestations of a prethrombotic state in developmental Crohn's disease. *Gastroenterol Clin Biol* 1990; **14**: 203–8.

80 Knot EA, Ten Cate JW, Bruin T, Iburg AH, Tytgat GN. Antithrombin III metabolism in two colitis patients with acquired antithrombin III deficiency. *Gastroenterology* 1985; **89**: 421–5.

81 Bohe M, Genell S, Ohlsson K. Protease inhibitors in plasma and faecal extracts from patients with active inflammatory bowel disease. *Scand J Gastroenterol* 1986; **21**: 598–604.

82 Hudson M, Chitolie A, Hutton RA, Smith MSH, Pounder RE, Wakefield AJ. Thrombotic vascular risk factors in inflammatory bowel disease. *Gut* 1996; **38**: 733–7.

83 Koutroubakis IE, Petinaki E, Anagnostopoulou E, *et al.* Anti-cardiolipin and anti-beta2-glycoprotein I antibodies in patients with inflammatory bowel disease. *Dig Dis Sci* 1998; **43**: 2507–12.

84 Zauber NP, Sabbath-Solitare M, Ragoria G, *et al.* Factor V Leiden mutation is not increased in patients with inflammatory bowel disease. *J Clin Gastroenterol* 1998; **27**: 215–16.

85 Jackson LM, O'Gorman PJ, O'Connell J, Cronin CC, Cotter KP, Shanahan F. Thrombosis in inflammatory bowel disease: clinical setting, procoagulant profile and factor V Leiden. *Q J Med* 1997; **90**: 183–8.

86 Over H, Ulgen S, Tuglular T, *et al.* Thrombophilia and inflammatory bowel disease: does factor V mutation have a role? *Eur J Gastroenterol Hepatol* 1998; **10**: 827–9.

87 Turpie AGG. Hirudin and thrombosis prophylaxis. *Lancet* 1996; **347**: 632–3.

Malignancy complicating inflammatory bowel disease

Colorectal carcinoma in ulcerative colitis

There is general agreement that colorectal carcinoma is more common in those with long-standing extensive ulcerative colitis. Historically, risks of 5–10 per cent at 20 years, rising to 12–30 per cent at 30 years, and a 20-fold increased lifetime risk were suggested. As the frequency of sporadic colorectal carcinoma is around 3 per cent in most developed countries, this lifetime risk is both discordant with the two former figures and internally inconsistent, as this would imply that nearly two-thirds of all patients with unresected extensive colitis develop malignancy. Newer data are more secure and somewhat less gloomy.

The death rate in the Swedish population is only three (not 20) times background,[1,2] and in Denmark there appears to be no excess in colorectal carcinoma after 25 years of extensive colitis (probably at least in part because of an aggressive surgical policy).[3] The more recent studies confirm the absence of increased risk if the disease remains confined to the rectum and sigmoid, and continue to place the patient with left-sided disease at intermediate risk.[4] A note of caution is required here, given the possibility of proximal extension of colitis (see Chapter 2).

When colorectal carcinoma complicates ulcerative colitis it shares many features with its sporadic counterpart, but the St Mark's study of 157 tumours in 120 patients[5] illustrates some of the differences. The distribution of tumours was predominantly left-sided (56 per cent rectosigmoid, 12 per cent descending/splenic flexure), but the 32 per cent of lesions which were proximal is a higher figure than for most sporadic series; 67.5 per cent of all patients had a rectosigmoid tumour. The overall 5-year survival in the St Mark's patients of 59.4 per cent was consistent with contemporaneous UK survival data for colorectal carcinoma in general. For each Dukes' stage, too, results seemed comparable (Table 8.1).

Table 8.1 Five-year survival data for patients with colorectal carcinoma complicating ulcerative colitis

Overall	59.4%
Dukes' A	90.6%
Dukes' B	87.8%
Dukes' C	28.3%
Disseminated	Nil

n = 157 tumours in 120 patients.[4]

Colorectal carcinoma in Crohn's disease

In Crohn's disease, one population-based study showed an increased risk of colorectal cancer,[6] whilst seven others indicated no overall increase,[2,7–11] or were inconclusive.[12] Amongst a total of 374 individuals considered by the Copenhagen IBD group,[13] there were two colonic and two rectal cancers, yielding a relative risk for all colorectal carcinomas of 1.04, compared with the Danish population. The more recent Swedish study revealed an even more comforting standardized mortality ratio of 0.3.[2] Referral centre studies in general, however, show consistently increased frequencies of colorectal carcinoma, with relative risks varying between 3.0 and 20.[14–20] In New York, of 18 deaths related to Crohn's disease, neoplasia (including colorectal carcinoma) was responsible in six.[21] Only two units report an absence of increased risk.[22,23] There is obviously uncertainty here, but patients with Crohn's disease attain secure immunity from colorectal carcinoma only by proctocolectomy.

The Crohn's patient at particular risk of colorectal carcinoma has extensive colitis (> 50 per cent involvement) of long duration (> 10 years) and of early onset (in childhood or before 20 years).[19,20,24] Nonetheless, despite a median Crohn's duration of 15–18 years at cancer diagnosis, nearly a third have had Crohn's for less than 10 years. Those with stricturing disease and those with bypassed segments of intestine are also at risk, although it is likely that the 30 per cent risk attributed to the latter group reflects several of the other risk factors also.[16,18,19] Malignant transformation may also affect the Crohn's-related enterocutaneous fistula. Although adenocarcinoma of the fistula track has only recently been described definitively for the first time,[25] the long-term fistula probably constitutes another high-risk context. The pathologists at the Karolinska Hospital believe that the incidence of Crohn's-related colorectal carcinoma is increasing (0.2 cases per year in 1951–89; 1.7 per year since then) and is now more common than as a complication of ulcerative colitis (probably because of surveillance of the latter).[24]

When colorectal carcinoma complicates Crohn's, it follows a course that diverges from that of the general population. The median age at cancer diagnosis is around 50 years, and approximately 40 per cent of patients have right-sided lesions. Presumably because early symptoms are attributed to exacerbations of Crohn's disease (and perhaps because of the excess of right-sided lesions), diagnosis tends to be late, and is often only made at surgery even now. The overall prognosis is poorer than for colorectal carcinoma unassociated with inflammatory bowel disease, with typical 5-year survivals in the region of 20 per cent, and it is probable that Crohn's patients with colorectal carcinoma have a worse prognosis than patients with sporadic neoplasms matched for Dukes' stage.[14,16,18,22,26]

Pathogenesis of increased colorectal carcinoma in inflammatory bowel disease

The increased rate of colorectal carcinoma in inflammatory bowel disease requires explanation, but an adequate understanding of the mechanisms that lead from chronic inflammation to neoplasia, which can account for the timing and distribution of tumours, does not yet exist.

There are changes in glycosylation of the mucosa in ulcerative colitis and Crohn's disease, including increased expression of a range of specific oncofetal antigens. These changes are shared by sporadic adenomas and colorectal carcinomas.[27] In each case the mucosal alterations are widespread and probably of functional consequence. They lead to altered binding (mostly increased) to dietary and microbial lectins.

Peanut lectin binds selectively to the Thomsen Friedereich carbohydrate antigen, which is over-expressed in inflammatory bowel disease (and colorectal carcinoma), and increases cell proliferation. A similar effect can be seen in normal volunteers eating 100 g peanuts per day for 5 days, in whom rectal mucosal proliferation is increased if lectin receptors are present but not in their absence.[28] Interestingly, the opposite effect can be shown with a mushroom-derived Thomsen Friedereich antigen *in vitro*.[29] Rhodes postulates that galactose-binding lectins (whether dietary or microbial in origin) increase the cancer risk.[30] This effectively means all lectins other than mushroom. The accepted protection from cancer through healthy eating is thus explained by the high galactose content of fruit and vegetables (as opposed to cereal fibre, which is low in galactose): galactose in the gut lumen can bind to and inactivate the lectins. Hence a high-galactose diet offers protection against colorectal carcinoma in the general population and also, putatively, in inflammatory bowel disease. There is limited epidemiological support for this hypothesis from its originator.[31]

Dysregulation of the epithelial cell adhesion molecules may also play an important role in the pathogenesis of colitis-related colorectal carcinoma. We have shown substantial changes in the expression of E-cadherin (downregulated or mutated) and P-cadherin (upregulated and especially so in dysplasia) in colitis tissues, which we suspect are of functional consequence.[32]

There was more evidence of epithelial cell proliferation in rectal biopsies from colitics whether the disease was active or in remission with associated atrophy, but not in remission with normal histology.[33] Over-expression of the *ras* p21 oncoprotein was most notable in those with atrophy. This may become of clinical importance in terms of surveillance strategy. Proliferation may also be inhibited usefully by dietary folate supplementation.[34]

Study of the expression of the transforming growth factor (TGF) regulatory peptides in inflammatory bowel disease has also been informative. TGF-α is of considerable importance in the response of the intestinal epithelium to injury, and perhaps also in the pathogenesis of neoplasia. Although its expression was indistinguishable from normal in Crohn's disease and in active ulcerative colitis, the levels were enhanced to up to three times control values in inactive ulcerative colitis.[35] This phenomenon is not easily explained and still requires confirmation by others, but if true may help us to understand the independence of cancer risk from the clinical severity of colitis, since chronic over-expression of TGF-α might be expected to provoke epithelial hyperproliferation and to be (partly) causative in the increased incidence of neoplasia. Some additional support for this view comes from the authors' observation that TGF-α expression was at its highest level in patients with the greatest duration of colitis (i.e. those at most risk of neoplasia).

There is some evidence that the expression of the mismatch repair gene *MLH1* is different in patients with inflammatory bowel disease from that in the normal population.[36] As mutations and differential allelic expression at this site are strongly associated with hereditary non-polyposis colonic cancer, this observation could be of aetiological significance in the increased cancer risk in inflammatory bowel disease. Chromosomal instability associated with telomere shortening is also implicated in ulcerative colitis-associated dysplasia and colorectal carcinoma.[37] These aspects have potential value in screening as well as in improving understanding of pathogenesis value. More work is needed.

The study of apoptosis in inflammatory bowel disease has led to conflicting results. It is unclear whether changes seen in acute inflammation are merely secondary to that inflammation, but it is likely that dysfunctional programmed cell death is of some relevance to cancer risk. Representatively perplexing studies include those showing:

- increased apoptosis in active ulcerative colitis;[38,39]
- increased apoptosis in quiescent ulcerative colitis;[38]
- increased apoptosis in active Crohn's disease;[40]
- normal levels of apoptosis in ulcerative colitis;[40,41] and
- decreased apoptosis in active Crohn's disease and active ulcerative colitis.[42]

Cancer surveillance – introduction and principles

Cancer surveillance in inflammatory bowel disease has unfortunately become somewhat controversial. This is mainly because of its expense and the absence of controlled trial data. Patients and their doctors see clear advantage in regular clinical assessment; this was central to the first series of guidelines on management of inflammatory bowel disease from the British Society of Gastroenterology[43] and will remain in the new edition due shortly. The value of regular hospital contact in the context of cancer avoidance is strongly supported (admittedly not causally) by the Leicester data; two or more hospital attendances each year were associated with an odds ratio (OR) for development of colitis-related colorectal carcinoma of 0.16 (CI: 0.04–0.6; $P = 0.007$) compared with those seen less frequently.[44] Cancer surveillance, however, differs from this traditional follow-up model in several particulars and must be specifically considered.

Cancer surveillance must satisfy a number of criteria if it is to be justifiable. It must be able to identify early cancers, or (better) high-risk lesions that will progress to tumours if left untreated. There must be curative therapy available for these early lesions when detected. The surveillance method must be safe and acceptable to the subjects to whom it is to be offered, who must in turn be available to the surveyors. To avoid the medical, emotional and financial problems that arise from false-positive and false-negative results, there should be perfect sensitivity and specificity, but as this will never be achieved the methodology should ensure that an appropriate balance is drawn, to ensure maximal benefit at least cost in terms of missed cancers, against prolonged and potentially hazardous further investigation in those not at risk. The ideal surveillance programme will not only lead to its subjects avoiding cancer, but will also save money for their health care system. It is most unusual for a standard diagnostic test to satisfy the more stringent requirements of a surveillance procedure.

Patients with inflammatory bowel disease constitute an identifiable and medically accessible population at high risk for colorectal carcinoma, and colonoscopy is a potential surveillance tool. However, it is only moderately satisfactory in this capacity, being unpleasant, time-consuming, expensive, and not without risk. Furthermore, although the experienced colonoscopist will recognize almost all sporadic colorectal carcinomas and their premonitory polyps, an important proportion of early mass lesions will be missed in inflammatory bowel disease, lost amidst the abnormalities of the colitic bowel. The colonoscopist is also unlikely to recognize premalignant changes in flat or moderately irregular mucosa from their macroscopic appearances. Multiple colonic biopsies are therefore integral to the use of colonoscopy as a surveillance tool for inflammatory bowel disease-related cancer.

Surveillance in ulcerative colitis

Surveillance of patients with long-standing ulcerative colitis has been conducted over the past quarter century by many centres, on the *a priori* assumption that it would be obviously beneficial. The results have not been clear-cut, however, and the lack of controlled data from the time of its introduction is now greatly regretted.

Axon's critical analysis of 1994[45] attracted much attention and had a perhaps unduly negative influence on surveillance strategy. By his account, 476 surveillance colonoscopies were required for each useful result, consequently comparing poorly with the likely benefits from random colonoscopy seeking adenomatous polyps and early cancers in an unselected middle-aged population. He accordingly concluded that colonoscopic surveillance in ulcerative colitis was not justified. He had correctly excluded advanced cancers and those found at surgery, but it was perhaps unnecessarily harsh to discount abnormalities found at the first 'screening' procedure since, while to do so is strictly correct in terms of surveillance definition, these patients would not have had any procedure were it not for the initiation of their personal programme. There was a historic justification for excluding colectomy for low-grade dysplasia, to which we will return. It is difficult to be sure how much surveillance was influenced by symptoms, and the 17 patients from the 12 series in whom procedures were linked to symptoms would still have had a (positive) colonoscopy within a maximum of 24 months and might reasonably be counted as successes. There are still no unshakable supportive data, but the theme to be drawn from many centres and various contexts is more positive than Axon allowed.

A 1994 update on the St Mark's surveillance programme reported on 332 patients with macroscopically right-sided ulcerative colitis of more than 10 years' duration.[46] Colonoscopy with multiple biopsies was performed every 2 years, with a rigid sigmoidoscopy and rectal biopsy in the intervening years. The overall colorectal carcinoma rate was 6.0 per cent ($n = 20$), occurring at a median age of 51, in patients with colitis for a median of 21 years; 60 per cent of the tumours were in the rectosigmoid. Only 11 of the tumours were detected by the surveillance programme (eight Dukes' A; one B; two C). Nine of these were therefore 'useful' diagnoses, although the two Dukes' Cs were still alive and disease-free at 3 and 7 years. Surveillance missed six cancers, all of which were advanced at the time of diagnosis (four Dukes' C; two disseminated), with an interval of 10–23 months from the most recent colonoscopy. These six patients were younger (median 38 years), but had the same median duration of disease as the whole group of patients with tumours. Three further cancers occurred in patients who had left the programme for a variety of reasons. Surveillance detected dysplasia in 21 patients, nine of whom had cancer; these cancers were found at the same colonoscopy in four, and only after resection in five. Twelve patients with dysplasia had no cancer at resection. Surveillance therefore usefully detected nine early cancers, and a further 12 very high-risk patients. Benefit to these 21 patients required a total of 1316 colonoscopies, and as one diagnosis was made by planned interval sigmoidoscopy, 66 colonoscopies were required for each useful result, at a cost of around £35 000 ($\approx$US\$50 000) per case detected. There were no major complications.

Comparable Swedish data from 1999 report on 43 patients with extensive, long-standing colitis surveyed between 1973 and 1996.[47] The median time of follow-up was 6 years. Low-grade dysplasia was found at least once in 24 patients, high-grade dysplasia in four and a carcinoma (Dukes' A) in one. Eleven patients underwent colectomy because of dysplasia and one additional patient was found to have a carcinoma (also Dukes' A) at surgery. No surveyed patient died form colorectal carcinoma during this period. The actuarial risk of having dysplasia after 25 years of disease was 16 per cent.

A parallel Swedish paper approached surveillance from an epidemiological standpoint, and is supportive of the endeavour.[48] The study base comprised all patients with ulcerative colitis for the Stockholm and Uppsala areas (for 1955–84 and 1965–83, respectively), representing 4664 prevalent cases in a population of three million. Cases of fatal colorectal carcinoma occurring after 1975 were identified from cancer registry data (almost 100 per cent inclusive), and were included if ulcerative colitis had been present for 5 years or more prior to cancer death. Forty such patients were found, and 102 colitic controls matched for age, sex, disease duration, and disease extent, were selected. It was required that controls were still alive at the time of death of the matching case, and had not undergone panproctocolectomy in the 5 years prior to the case's cancer diagnosis. Cases were then compared with controls for the utilization of surveillance colonoscopy. Colonoscopies performed for diagnosis, index examinations and those for clinical indications were excluded. These assessments were made retrospectively from clinical notes and may not be entirely free from error and/or bias. Although just failing to reach statistical significance, the results are nevertheless impressive. Only two of the 40 cancer patients had ever received a surveillance colonoscopy (5 per cent) compared with 18 of the 102 controls (17.6 per cent) (OR: 0.29; CI: 0.06–1.31). Furthermore, 12 controls compared with only one case had received more than one surveillance procedure (OR: 0.22; CI: 0.03–1.74), indicating a 'dose response'. In Leicester, repeated (more than two) colonoscopies in an informal surveillance programme yielded an OR for fewer cancers of 0.42, which just failed to reach significance, but again without evident hazard (CI: 0.16–1.1; $P = 0.08$).[44]

As far as can be ascertained, provision of surveillance colonoscopy (at tertiary centres) is more beneficial than harmful, but it cannot be considered mandatory. The evidence in its favour is, however, such that no major centre will now feel able to sanction its controlled trial against routine care.

INTERPRETATION OF DYSPLASIA

The identification of dysplasia is an imperfect science, with problems in its definition, and with marked between-observer variation, the latter reaching 66 per cent as recently as 1988.[49] Tighter histological criteria have reduced, but not eliminated, these problems.[50] It is also recognized that some patients develop malignancy apparently without prior dysplasia. Despite double reporting by skilled gastrointestinal pathologists using standardized criteria, in around 25 per cent of colitis-related cancers no dysplasia can be found at a site separate from the malignancy, even though the whole resected colon is available for examination.[46,51] In Connell's study, 18 per cent had no evidence of dysplasia at the site of malignancy, or on any previous surveillance biopsy.[46] It is unknown whether prior dysplasia was truly absent at the tumour site or was simply missed in the pre-invasive phase of neoplasia, but in either case this is a practical failing of current surveillance protocols.

Many samples historically categorized as borderline and mild or low-grade dysplasia are now downgraded. Even now, biopsies scored by non-experts will much more often be reclassified by the colorectal pathologist: dysplastic to non-dysplastic rather than the converse. This has the effect of increasing the clinical significance of the smaller number that retain a diagnosis of low-grade or high-grade dysplasia.

High-grade dysplasia is undoubtedly an informative marker for future malignancy.[51] Approximately half of those affected can be expected on statistical grounds to develop frank malignancy within 5 years if, for some reason, surgery is not performed.[52] The recognition, from several centres, that around a third of those with ulcerative colitis complicated by high-grade dysplasia are found to have otherwise unsuspected cancer in the resected colon is also of considerable importance. The significance of low-grade dysplasia is more often but probably unjustifiably questioned. Several centres have reported on the frequency at which low-grade dysplasia progresses to high-grade dysplasia or cancer.[46,51,52] The risk is always at least 1 in 5, and in one case was over 50 per cent at 5 years,[46] as long as clear histological criteria for dysplasia are employed (see above). It is, accordingly, current practice at St Mark's to advise colectomy for all patients with confirmed low-grade dysplasia. Confirmed in this context does not mean separate sites or separate occasions, but confirmed by two expert pathologists. With the information we have on the likely risk of progression of low-grade dysplasia to malignancy, it merely confuses things if a second colonoscopy is performed and reveals no areas of dysplasia. It is reasonable to defer colectomy only if the patient understands the substantial risk being taken.

If the expert pathologist is uncertain about the presence of dysplasia (most likely if there is a great deal of inflammation), then a verdict of 'indefinite for dysplasia' can be recorded. This should be interpreted as an invitation to repeat colonoscopy with further biopsies, preferably at a time of clinical quiescence.

THE DYSPLASIA-ASSOCIATED LESION OR MASS AND THE BENIGN ADENOMA

The dysplasia-associated lesion or mass (DALM) has caused confusion and consternation. As described in the literature, this has a very high predictive value for concurrent or imminent malignancy and is generally considered to be a strong indication for colectomy whatever the grade of dysplasia. Unfortunately, it can be difficult for the pathologist to decide whether a dysplastic lesion seen histologically is indeed part of a DALM or whether it forms part of a discrete polypoid adenoma.

Schneider and Stolte classified a total of 136 neoplastic lesions demonstrated in 76 patients with confirmed ulcerative colitis on the basis of a series of suggested pathological and morphological criteria.[53] They considered that 41 per cent of patients had adenomas, 55 per cent had dysplastic lesions and 4 per cent had both. Clearly their criteria are open to interpretation, but there were striking differences in the populations presenting with the two different types of lesion. Patients with adenomas were of mean age 66 years whereas those with DALMs were, on average, only 43.4, but had had their colitis for longer (12.6 versus 7.2 years). The site of the lesion and the extent of colitis were, however, unhelpful in making any distinction. Multiple lesions were common in both groups and a mere 27 per cent of patients with a DALM had only a single lesion.

Following on from this, there has been an endoscopic feeling that one should be safe in assuming that a lesion is a 'simple' adenoma if it has a stalk and that, therefore, snare polypectomy rather than colectomy is sufficient therapy. Many gastroenterologists feel reasonably comfortable if the histology reports adenoma of whatever grade of dysplasia if the stalk is free of dysplasia, but concomitantly wary if the base is wide and/or dysplasia extends to the margins of the excision. There is perhaps no place for submucosal resection in the patient with ulcerative colitis.

A recent paper from Boston has tried to help with a study in colitics with dysplastic lesions. The conclusions are somewhat limited by the relatively small numbers considered ($n = 34$), but are reassuring. The outcome, at a mean of nearly 4 years, in 24 cases in which the endoscopist and pathologist together considered that the lesion was an 'adenoma-like DALM' was compared with that in 10 cases where the lesion was thought to be a 'coincidental sporadic adenoma'.[54] The definition of coincidental is taken here to mean arising outside the areas of the bowel known to be involved with colitis. All lesions were treated endoscopically. Just over half the 24 developed new but similar polypoid lesions during follow-up, but only a single patient developed a focus of dysplasia other than in this form; no patient developed a carcinoma. Half the patients with a 'sporadic' adenoma developed new similar lesions (in line with the group's own non-colitic control population). Colectomy does not seem to be warranted in any of these patients for reasons of neoplastic potential, but care is required in assigning the correct appellation of a lesion in a given patient. There is an interesting correlation with the Schneider and Stolte series, as both Boston patient groups were relatively elderly (mean age over 60). I have preferred to think of patients having either a DALM or an adenomatous polyp (sporadic and colitis-associated being grouped together). If there is a stalked polyp that has been confidently and completely excised on endoscopic and histological criteria, then I consider this in much the same light as a sporadic polyp, but I am wary if the base is wide and/or dysplasia extends to the margins of the excision. The new data support this stance. There is perhaps no place for submucosal resection in the patient with ulcerative colitis, and if there is a dysplastic lesion that is associated with a mass, then this is a mandate for early colectomy without repeated investigation.

IMPLEMENTATION OF SURVEILLANCE

Allied to this we must ask what is actually being done. The Leicester group performed a questionnaire study of British gastroenterologists.[55] A commendable 83 per cent response rate was achieved and 94 per cent of responders claimed to operate some form of surveillance for long-standing ulcerative colitis, but only 35 per cent maintained a register of those patients. Typically, patients are recruited at just over 9 years, and a quarter of units are including patients with left-sided disease, who begin surveillance at around 12 years. Disturbingly, only 53 per cent routinely recommend colectomy when high-grade dysplasia is found and only 4 per cent on the basis of low-grade dysplasia. The nature of the study limits interpretation somewhat, since it is not clear how well verified either condition was. In particular, only 45 per cent of biopsies appear to reach even a single specialist pathologist. However, the authors' conclusion that there is disorganization and inconsistency is inescapable and this is almost certainly to the disadvantage of many patients.

HOW CAN SURVEILLANCE BE IMPROVED?

Better implementation of intended strategy

The Leicester data[55] and the development of cancers in patients who have been lost to follow-up[46] indicate that procedural aspects to ensure that patients designated at high risk actually have the follow-up and procedures intended are crucial. This is becoming easier as most units introduce some form of inflammatory bowel disease database, but there is inevitably a manpower component that is not always readily funded, even in these days of clinical governance and accountability. Every colitis-related colorectal cancer death ought to be considered potentially avoidable.

Nonetheless, it is evident that correctly implemented colonoscopic surveillance in isolation is insufficient, and that strategies intended to improve surveillance should be sought and tested.

Better colonoscopy

There is a little potential for better conventional colonoscopy from the continual improvements in endoscopic technology and more effective training. A higher yield of tissue will help the pathologist. Although it is estimated that 30 endoscopic biopsies sample only 0.15 per cent of mucosal surface, it is speculated that this might yield a 90 per cent confidence of detecting dysplasia. The evidence base for this is unclear. In any event, it is currently impractical to consider more than 15–20 biopsies per examination.

Performing colonoscopy at greater frequency might help to improve the positive pick-up rate, and switching to annual colonoscopy is a rational response to the failings of the St Mark's 1994 analysis. This would be unlikely to have identified all five tumours missed between 12 and 24 months and could not have influenced detection of that at 10 months. It also has very major implications in terms of numbers of procedures (and therefore the cost of the programme) (see below). We should accordingly be looking for alternative means to supplement the existing data, aiming to identify patients at an especially high risk who can be most aggressively targeted, and conversely to identify those at relatively low risk in whom efforts may legitimately be less (e.g. colonoscopy every 5 years).

The possible value of tissue characterization from optical coherence tomography at colonoscopy and laser-induced fluorescence in identifying areas of especial risk (or acutely pinpointing dysplasia) were addressed in Chapter 2, and data specific to colitis are eagerly awaited. It does not seem that simple dye-spray techniques are sufficiently discriminatory to help in this context, given my own experience and an extraordinary dearth of reports in the literature favouring a technique that is otherwise widely promoted for detection of small cancers. Alternative imaging modalities that provide an indication of tissue thickening were described in Chapter 2 but it is unlikely that these will be sufficient to depose methods that allow tissue collection for histological examination.

Additional markers of malignancy and premalignancy

Potentially useful additional markers identified from their actual or putative value in sporadic colorectal carcinoma or other solid tumours include the presence of aneuploidy, mutations of oncogenes, of tumour suppresser genes, or of mismatch repair genes.

Aneuploidy

Aneuploidy (disturbance of the cell's normal diploid state) can be demonstrated in colonic biopsies from patients with dysplasia and/or malignancy. Most authors favour a progressive sequence: aneuploidy preceding dysplasia, itself in turn preceding carcinoma,[56] but this is recognized to be a generalization.[57] There is usually a positive correlation with histological grading, and a high proportion of patients with aneuploidy and without dysplasia seem likely to progress relatively quickly (5 of 5 within 2.5 years in Rubin's study[56]), but progression is not inevitable. It is possible that the apparent high degree of protection (good negative predictive value) for patients in whom there is no aneuploidy may be more valuable from a prognostic viewpoint. Prospective assessment was made in the Swedish study referred to above.[47] From 1982, flow-cytometric analysis for the detection of DNA-aneuploidy was included. Aneuploidy preceded dysplasia in seven patients, occurred simultaneously in nine and only after dysplasia in two. The actuarial risk of having aneuploidy after 25 years of disease was 29 per cent. A retrospective subgroup analysis showed that patients who had had three consecutive colonoscopies negative for dysplasia and/or DNA-aneuploidy formed a lower-risk group, and the authors suggest that these patients might have their surveillance interval increased to a colonoscopy every fifth year.

Protein p53

Inactivating mutations of the p53 tumour suppressor gene are very frequent in most solid tumours, but also a relatively late event in the neoplastic process. There has been debate as to the frequency of p53 mutations in colitis-related colorectal carcinoma, and whether changes at this locus occur sufficiently early in the neoplastic process to provide additional or earlier information than is possible from detection of dysplasia.[58] A consensus has, however, emerged that p53 mutations are both early features (sooner than in sporadic carcinomas) and strongly correlated with aneuploidy.[59] In another series there was p53 over-expression in 12.5 per cent of examples of low-grade dysplasia, in 80.0 per cent in high-grade dysplasia and in 90.9 per cent of colitis-related carcinomas (compared with only 54.5 per cent in their sporadic carcinomas); also non-dysplastic mucosa showed p53 over-expression in one colitis cancer.[60] Prospective assessment is still needed to clarify whether a routine search for aberrant p53 expression in surveillance biopsies is warranted.

Markers of tissue proliferation

Markers of proliferative activity in the colonic mucosa have also been examined. The Ki67 anti-gen is a proliferation marker (expressed in all stages of the cell cycle except G0) and is expressed most at times of maximal cell proliferation. Newer antibodies make its immunohistochemical evalua-tion in routine formalin/paraffin sections relatively straightforward. Nuclear antigens associated with cell proliferation have also been identified and can be demonstrated similarly, and in a single paper Kullmann *et al.* examined both Ki67 and prolifer-ating cell nuclear antigen (PCNA) in biopsies from patients with ulcerative colitis with and with-out dysplasia compared with normal controls.[61] Although there were strongly supportive trends and good statistical correlation, there was insuffi-cient discrimination between the labelling indices for either marker used alone to be other than a further guide, these data favouring Ki67 as the better option. There was more PCNA in high-grade than in low-grade dysplastic samples (PCNA index 81 versus 44 per cent) and similarly for Ki67 (55 versus 31 per cent). However, the study took dysplasia to be a gold standard, which it is not. It will be instructive to examine proliferation mark-ers as independent predictors of neoplasia, not least since there are possible routes to their thera-peutic manipulation.[62]

The mucin-associated carbohydrate antigen sialosyl-Tn, which has been linked to sporadic colorectal carcinoma, was expressed more often in patients with carcinoma complicating ulcerative colitis (44 per cent of biopsies) than in controls without carcinoma or dysplasia (11 per cent).[63] The antigen appeared up to 7 years before neo-plasia and its expression was not compromised by active inflammation. In a prospective study of six patients who were repeatedly colonoscoped, and who at some time developed aneuploidy, a preva-lence of sialosyl-Tn positivity of 10 per cent was found – roughly double that of aneuploidy – with only two biopsies from one patient showing dysplasia.[64] In all but one instance the sialosyl-Tn expression preceded aneuploidy. These data suggest a complementary role in identifying the highest-risk patients, but prospective analysis is required; alone it is clearly an inadequate alterna-tive to established methods. Curiously, this anti-gen is also expressed in Crohn's disease uncomplicated by neoplasia and, at 7 per cent in a resection series, too frequently to be useful in predicting risk of neoplasia in this context.[64]

Apoptosis

The expression of programmed cell death in inflammatory bowel disease is posing an investiga-tory challenge (see above). It is, nonetheless, likely that markers of apoptotic activity will prove to be helpful in assessing cancer risk in the future.

To date none of the above options has been adequately tested in the context of its impact on a surveillance programme, and there are no controlled data to judge whether a programme including such additional markers is more effec-tive than one without. Hopefully this will change.

Better targeting of patients for colonoscopy

Family history

Better targeting of colonoscopy, or at least the frequency at which it is performed, is desirable to maximize the cost-effectiveness of surveillance. The importance of long duration and the extent of colitis are built into all existing surveillance strategies, coupled now with evidence that confirmed dysplasia is a sufficiently valid measure of cancer risk to warrant surgical intervention. In sporadic colorectal carcinoma there are very clear links with the prior presence of adenomas and of a positive family history (at their most dramatic in the hereditary polyposis syndromes).[65] Until very recently there have been scant data to indicate whether these factors apply equally in patients with ulcerative colitis, and they have not been included as separate risk factors in determining frequency or intensity of investigation in any of the surveillance programmes that have reported to date.

The Mayo Clinic group has recently studied family history in 174 patients with colorectal carcinoma complicating ulcerative colitis in a questionnaire-based case–control fashion.[66] There were no population data, but selection and recall bias were apparently slight (the latter judged by cross-checking for familial stroke). A family history of colorectal cancer existed in 14.3 per cent of cases compared with only 6.7 per cent in matched colitics without colorectal carcinoma (much as in the general population) (OR: 2.33; CI: 1.06–5.14; P = 0.03). By logistic regression, a family history of sporadic colorectal cancer was an independent risk factor for cancer in ulcerative colitis, and for an increased risk of colorectal carcinoma in relatives of colitics with colorectal carcinoma. Most of the cancers in relatives were, of course, sporadic rather than colitis-related. Similar findings emerged from the Leicester study,[44] in which any family history of colorectal carcinoma (not only in colitic relatives) increased the cancer risk in patients, with an OR of 5.0 (CI: 1.1–22.8; P < 0.04) (an effect which failed to reach significance in first-degree relatives probably because of small numbers). It is therefore rational to

include the family history in determining surveillance strategy, but the magnitude of the effect requires further analysis before changes are implemented.

Other high- and low-risk groups

It is probable that adenomas are associated with an increased risk of malignancy in colitis, but there are no reliable data. As they are associated with a 50 per cent risk of adenoma recurrence within 4 years,[54] it seems reasonable to assume that they are also associated with increased cancer risk. The risk is not sufficient to warrant a change in frequency of colonoscopy if the patient is already due for a procedure every 2 years, but a patient with left-sided colitis and adenomas is currently considered in my practice to have 'earned' surveillance of a frequency in line with extensive colitis rather than the lesser 3–5-year repeats for adenoma alone.

Sclerosing cholangitis (see Chapter 6) is a marker of increased risk in almost all centres (see below), and should perhaps now be allowed to have an influence on intensity of surveillance strategy in borderline areas. The evidence is inadequate for firm recommendations, but my view has been to include in colonoscopic surveillance all patients with long-standing left-sided colitis and sclerosing cholangitis (who would not otherwise be colonoscoped at all) and to increase the frequency of colonoscopy from biennial to annual for those with extensive disease and cholangitis.

Groups at lower risk have not been identified with any confidence, but experience suggests that patients with inactive colitis, with virtually normal endoscopic appearances and persistently quiescent histology are under-represented amongst those with dysplasia and carcinomas. The Swedish data on lower risk in patients with three or more satisfactory colonoscopies[47] (see above) provide support for this stance. If this can be confirmed it would legitimize some relaxation of the intensity of surveillance in this subgroup. Prospective, controlled data are needed.

META-ANALYSIS AND MODELLING OF SURVEILLANCE STRATEGY IN ULCERATIVE COLITIS

Provenzale et al.[67] reviewed the literature and from it tried to determine the most cost-effective strategy. A decision analytical model was employed and costings were based on those thought reasonable for a health maintenance organization. Prophylactic colectomy at 10 years' extensive colitis was compared with surveillance colonoscopy at intervals of 1–5 years, with surgery subsequently performed for carcinoma or any grade of dysplasia, or only for carcinoma/high-grade dysplasia. Other than prophylactic colectomy, annual colonoscopy with colectomy for any dysplasia offered the most protection from malignancy, but this was also by far the most expensive option (US$247 200 per life-year gained) and gained on average a mere 4 additional days of expected life compared to bi-ennial colonoscopy, which was costed at US$159 500 per life-year gained. Interestingly, 5-yearly colonoscopy with colectomy for any dysplasia had the potential to be highly effective and was also cheaper than prophylactic colectomy (US$40 700 versus US$60 400 per life-year gained). The figure for 5-yearly surveillance is only a little higher than the costings for routine flexible sigmoidoscopy every 3–5 years as currently advocated for the general middle-aged population in both North America and Germany. Similarly muted conclusions come from other commentators, including Delco and Sonnenberg, who recognize that as decision analyses ultimately rely on medical evidence, they cannot provide a substitute for deficient clinical data.[68] They feel that the number of patient-years of follow-up still needed to clarify the issue statistically is prohibi-

tive. They finish by sanctioning surveillance, more or less as currently practised, with an emphasis placed on the search for new means of surveillance and cures!

Conclusions: ulcerative colitis

In macroscopically extensive ulcerative colitis there is an incidence of carcinoma or of dysplasia at about 0.5–1 per cent for each year of follow-up after 10 years of disease. For every 100 patients surveyed, one high-risk lesion or early cancer can be expected every 1–2 years (or approximately 1–2 per million population per year). A screening colonoscopy at 8–10 years is justified whether or not subsequent surveillance is intended, to check the extent of colitis (see Chapter 2) and because an important proportion of high-risk lesions is found at this index exami-nation in most surveillance series. DALMs and high- or low-grade dysplasias confirmed by two pathologists warrant colectomy. Up to 25 per cent of cancers will not be preceded (or detectable) by dysplasia, and tumours currently missed by surveillance are likely to be biologically different. Colonoscopic surveillance is expensive and, although of probable value, this is unproven, and there is a need for better markers of high- and low-risk patients. If it is to be done then it must be safe and proficiently performed. In the absence of controlled data, decisions are properly influenced by health economic issues. Colonoscopy every 2 years is a reasonable frequency for surveillance outside a trial setting. Additional procedures are advocated for the patient with sclerosing cholangitis and for the patient with borderline histology (indefinite for dysplasia). It is not clear at what age surveillance should stop if commenced, and what should be done for patients with less extensive disease; stop-ping at 75 years, and a rectal biopsy every 2 years from 10 years, respectively, are suggested.

Colorectal malignancy and surveillance in Crohn's disease

THE ANORECTUM

In extensive Crohn's colitis of more than 8–10 years' duration, regular clinical assessment of the anorectum is warranted (see below), with a high index of suspicion and a low threshold for examination and biopsy under anaesthetic if strictures are present. Those in whom the disease began in childhood or adolescence and those with chronic fistulae are probably at greatest risk. There are as yet no data which firmly justify more than clinically prompted investigations.

THE COLON

Many of the problems associated with surveillance in ulcerative colitis apply equally to Crohn's disease, but there are still fewer data. Dysplasia probably is a predictor of future malignancy, of similar robustness to dysplasia in ulcerative colitis, with a frequency of 80 per cent or more in published series once malignancy has supervened.[26]

To date fewer units have adopted a general policy of regular surveillance colonoscopy. A biennial colonoscopy surveillance programme commencing at 8 years in those with total or segmental Crohn's colitis began in New York in 1988, and provisional data have now been presented.[69] From the published abstract (yet to be followed by a full paper) it appears probable that the index colonoscopy was included as well as the subsequent true surveillance examinations. Dysplasia or frank malignancy was found in 6 per cent of cases, and these patients were generally older, with disease for longer, and more likely to have had previous partial colectomy. The colono-scopies were technically demanding and, even with paediatric endoscopes, were incomplete in 11 per cent. The authors nevertheless advocate surveillance for those with long-standing total or segmental colitis. Their arguments are supported by pathological data from Sweden,[24] but are weakened by the fact that 35 per cent of patients entered the programme because of new symptoms and accordingly represent a selected cohort, almost certainly at above-average risk of neoplasia. It is a pity that the difficulties in interpreting ulcerative colitis surveillance programmes were not tackled in Crohn's disease by a more controlled comparison of surveillance with normal clinical practice. Commentators are tending to be ambivalent in their views on the necessity for colonoscopy in chronic Crohn's colitis.[70]

Neoplasia in primary sclerosing cholangitis

COLORECTAL CARCINOMA

Several centres have considered whether primary sclerosing cholangitis (PSC) might increase the already elevated risk of colorectal carcinoma in patients with ulcerative colitis. The results are not entirely concordant, and the earlier reports are perhaps best discounted on the grounds of inadequate numbers and selection bias. There are only a few hundred reported cases of PSC, ulcerative colitis and colorectal carcinoma in the same patient. The Stockholm group[71] took advantage of their series which is almost population-based and yet one in which neither clinically overt PSC nor inflammatory bowel disease was likely to have been missed. A careful retrospective analysis was performed from contemporaneous records. A relatively high proportion of the patients with PSC lacked inflammatory bowel disease (18 of 58), but in other respects the clinical features were typical of those in other centres. Eighty controls with colitis but without PSC were paired with the 40 with both diseases, matching for age and for the extent and duration of colitis. During follow-up, 16 patients with PSC developed colonic dysplasia or carcinoma (40 per cent) compared with only 10 in the controls (12.5 per cent; $P < 0.001$). The cumulative risk of colorectal neoplasia was 9 per cent and 31 per cent, at 10 and 20 years, respectively, compared with only 2 per cent and 5 per cent in the controls without PSC. Interestingly, both colorectal and biliary neoplasia coincided in seven cases. Brentnall et al.[72] reported on a prospective series of 20 patients with extensive colitis and PSC, and saw nine patients with dysplasia (45 per cent), compared with only four in 25 patients matched for their colitis but without PSC (16 per cent). Recent retrospective data from the Cleveland Clinic indicate a 25 per cent risk of dysplasia or frank carcinoma (13 per cent) amongst 132 patients with both inflammatory conditions compared with only 5.6 per cent (2.5 per cent) in 196 with ulcerative colitis alone (RR: 3.15; CI: 1.3–7.3).[73] Neoplasia-free survival to 20 years was 79 per cent compared with 88 per cent. The 17 PSC-associated cancers were more often proximal (76 versus 20 per cent; $P < 0.04$), of worse grade (35 versus 0 per cent Dukes' C or D), and more likely to prove fatal. Three of the cancers and three additional dysplasia cases occurred in 26 patients who subsequently required liver transplantation. It is probable that the study is to some extent biased as the PSC patients were younger at colitis onset, had more extensive disease and had longer duration, introducing a degree of confounding. The Mayo Clinic, in a retrospective review of more than 170 patients with PSC, reached less compelling conclusions, with an adjusted OR for colorectal carcinoma with PSC of only 1.23 (CI: 0.62–2.42; NS).[74,75] The relative risk for colorectal neoplasia (excluding dysplasia alone) was elevated to 10.3 times

that of the general population of the USA, but this was not influenced by the presence or absence of PSC. The relative risk for colorectal neoplasia was numerically increased (though not significant) for patients with PSC without colitis, at 4.9, with confidence intervals between 0.1 and 27 times.

Perhaps an important key to understanding these differences of opinion lies in the report from The Johns Hopkins Hospital,[76] in which dysplasia or carcinoma was found in 37 per cent ($n = 35$), but in combination with a cumulative cancer incidence similar to historical controls. It is possible that PSC predisposes to dysplasia but not to invasive malignancy, and thus marks a group in whom dysplasia should be accorded lesser significance. Biological support for this contention is, however, entirely lacking, and we should continue to seek better data on which to base our clinical decisions.

Most commentators nonetheless agree that PSC is an independent risk factor for colonic neoplasia in patients with colitis, the magnitude of the risk remaining uncertain. A more intensive colonic surveillance strategy seems to me warranted for PSC patients: my patients are called for annual colonoscopy.

CHOLANGIOCARCINOMA

Cholangiocarcinoma affects at least 5 per cent of patients with PSC on a lifetime basis[71,74] and a regrettably high proportion are still diagnosed at autopsy. Progression from PSC to carcinoma is almost always difficult to identify, as the symptoms, signs and investigation results are so similar, but may be suspected in the patient whose condition suddenly deteriorates or becomes progressive rather than episodic. Cholangiocarcinoma is usually seen in patients with colitis rather than in those with PSC without inflammatory bowel disease[71,77] and is made substantially more likely by chronic alcohol excess.[78] There are no entirely reliable laboratory markers. Serological tumour markers are of limited value, as although CA19-9 is positively associated with cholangiocarcinoma,[78,79] it and CEA are frequently elevated in uncomplicated PSC.[80] It is, however, suggested that oncogene expression (K-*ras*), tumour suppressor gene mutation (p53), and evidence of increased cell proliferation (Ki-67) are present at an early stage in carcinogenesis and therefore of potential diagnostic value.[81] Positive cytological brushings or biliary biopsies obtained at ERCP are conclusive, but false negatives are frequent, in part because of the relatively fibrous nature of the tumours. Changes in the cholangiogram may sometimes help, especially when the axis of a strictured area of duct deviates from the general axis of the remainder of the duct; this strongly suggests neoplastic change. Conventional imaging with ultrasound and CT scanning has not proved sufficiently discriminatory, but endoscopic ultrasound (perhaps using intrabiliary probes) may make an increasingly useful contribution through its ability to demonstrate small mass lesions, themselves strongly indicative of malignant change. MRI scanning has proved itself superior to diagnostic ERCP in the generality of patients with cholangiocarcinoma,[82] but it remains to be seen whether that is true for the specific case of malignancy complicating PSC. There are newer data suggesting that positron emission tomography is particularly helpful but this promising technique is currently available in very few centres.[83] If surgery is contemplated, it needs to be radical if there is to be curative intent. Many transplant units have discontinued transplantation for pre-operatively diagnosed cholangiocarcinoma because of the near 100 per cent recurrence rate in the transplanted liver. This may, however, reflect the influence of the biliary 'field defect' in such patients and could perhaps be avoided if a porto-enteric anastomosis were insisted upon rather than the usual distal biliary join between donor and recipient tissues.

Cholangiocarcinoma is probably also over-represented in inflammatory bowel disease in the absence of PSC.[84]

SMALL BOWEL CANCER

Malignancy affecting the small bowel is almost certainly more common in Crohn's disease. The regional Copenhagen Crohn's cohort developed four small bowel tumours (from 374 patients followed for a median of 17 years).[13] Comparison with the Danish population data yielded a relative risk for small bowel tumours of 66.7 ($P < 0.0001$), a little higher than the relative risk of 50 ($P = 0.001$) quoted by the same centre a few years earlier.[85] These data reflect only tiny patient numbers but are consistent with an American cumulative incidence of 0.6 per cent, which is substantially higher than expected.[22] There were, however, no cases identified in the St Mark's series of 2500 patients with Crohn's.[23]

Data from collected series indicate a higher risk of Crohn's-related intestinal adenocarcinoma in males, and in those who have had Crohn's for 10 years or more; patients at most risk seem to be those with proximal and/or chronic unremitting disease. The diagnosis is often delayed and rarely made preoperatively.[16,22,86] The disease generally arises in areas involved by the Crohn's disease. Most cases in which this has been sought prove to have adjacent intestinal dysplasia. There does seem to be a dysplasia–carcinoma sequence as in the colon, but while K-*ras* and p53 mutations are seen in a majority, there is little evidence of other tumour gene defects.[87] The prognosis is very poor, with a median survival as short as 6 months after diagnosis.[16,22,86]

ANAL CARCINOMA

Carcinoma of the anal canal and the transitional zone leading to the rectum is seen more often in Crohn's disease than in the general population with (for example) no fewer than five anal tumours in the St Mark's series of 2500 Crohn's patients compared with an expected frequency of less than 1.[23] There were also seven tumours very low in the rectum, and in all 12 cases the patient had previously suffered from severe chronic anorectal disease. Although multimodality non-surgical therapy is now yielding good results for late-stage anal carcinoma, the awareness of this possible complication should lead to biopsy of any suspicious anorectal lesion that is not responding to medical therapy. This will usually require general anaesthetic to achieve adequate analgesia.

NEOPLASIA OF THE EXCLUDED/DEFUNCTIONED RECTUM?

It is probable that the rectum defunctioned for Crohn's disease is at a higher risk of neoplastic transformation than when the same diseased organ is in intestinal continuity. Amongst 23 Crohn's patients with rectal exclusion for a median of only 4 years who went on to interval proctectomy, dysplasia was found in 30 per cent of the proctectomy specimens.[88] In each case it was low grade and had not been anticipated (or especially sought) preoperatively. No invasive tumours were found. The authors reasonably enough recommend rectal surveillance in this context. Again, we lack a causal association but this seems to represent a high-risk group, unless those going on to completion proctectomy are especially unrepresentative of those with a defunctioned rectum. Rectoscopy and biopsy are readily enough accomplished, but more difficult to handle in the patient with defunction of a longer portion of the lower bowel, which may be difficult, or even impossible, to examine because of its disease. Virtual colonoscopy may help in the identification of mass lesions but will not provide histological advance warning. Much the same problems apply to the longer chronic fistula track.

OTHER NEOPLASIA IN PATIENTS WITH INFLAMMATORY BOWEL DISEASE

The regional Copenhagen Crohn's cohort ($n = 374$) has been carefully studied with long-term follow-up.[13] Despite the excess risk to the small bowel, colon and rectum discussed above, the lifetime gastrointestinal cancer risk was only 4.8 per cent versus 3.8 per cent in controls (NS). Non-gastrointestinal malignancies were recorded in 41 per cent versus 34.7 per cent in controls (NS). Likewise, ulcerative colitis patients appear prone to no more than background levels of neoplastic deaths overall (observed/expected 1.02, NS).[89]

There is new evidence that the risk of Hodgkin's disease is increased in ulcerative colitis. In an Italian population study between 1978 and 1992, 920 inflammatory bowel disease patients were followed for a median of 11 years. There were 64 new malignancies.[90] The overall cancer rate in this series equalled that in controls, although there was a slight excess in Crohn's disease. There was also a significant excess of Hodgkin's disease in ulcerative colitis patients, producing a standardized incidence rate of 9.3 (CI: 2.5–23.8). Respiratory tumours proved less frequent in ulcerative colitis and more frequent in Crohn's disease, probably because of smoking habits. The risk of lymphoma is a novel finding with no obvious explanation: it remains a very unusual association.

Iatrogenic malignancy in inflammatory bowel disease

Most of the excess malignancies in patients with inflammatory bowel disease are reasonably attributed to the disease process, but there have also been concerns that diagnostic and therapeutic interventions may play a part. Immunosuppressive drugs are particularly implicated, given their associations with malignancy when used for other indications, the best documented and most frequently observed examples occurring with immunosuppression for the prevention of rejection of solid organ transplants. Few data exist for the agents newer to inflammatory bowel disease, but some summarizing comments can be made for these and the more established drugs.

STEROIDS

It is unlikely that exogenous corticosteroids influence the risk of neoplasia in inflammatory bowel disease. As steroid use is deliberately minimized in accordance with other well-rehearsed arguments, and steroids are generally used for relatively short periods in active inflammatory bowel disease, they need be considered no further.

AMINOSALICYLATES

The aminosalicylate drugs probably have no important effects on systemic immune functioning, and no increased cancer risk has been attributed. On the contrary, several studies now indicate that their continuing use in ulcerative colitis reduces cancer risk. A 1994 population-derived, case–control study compared the pharmacological records of ulcerative colitis patients with complicating carcinoma to those of controls with no malignancy. There was a significant protective effect in those treated for at least 3 months with an aminosalicylate preparation, the relative risk for neoplasia being only 0.38 (CI: 0.20–0.69).[91] A subsequent case–control study from Leicester sought the OR for cancer risk, comparing 102 patients with colitis-related colorectal carcinoma and the same number of closely matched cancer-free colitics.[44] With appropriate adjustment for other variables, taking mesalazine in one of its forms (including sulphasalazine, olsalazine and balsalazide) reduced the apparent risk by 81 per cent (OR: 0.19; CI: 0.06–0.61; P = 0.006). Mesalazine needed to be taken at a daily dose of 1.2 g or more for full benefit, but lower doses were also protective. Daily doses of at least 2 g of sulphasalazine were required for benefit. This study failed to show significant benefit for other agents, other than, curiously, for systemic and topical steroids (OR: 0.26 and 0.44, respectively). The explanation for this effect may relate to effects of 5-ASA drugs on both intestinal apoptosis and proliferation.[92]

AZATHIOPRINE/MERCAPTOPURINE

Azathioprine is almost certainly genotoxic in man and its very cautious use around pregnancy has been discussed in Chapter 5. Additionally, non-Hodgkin's lymphoma, intestinal lymphoma, myeloma and skin cancers are over-represented in patients who have received azathioprine or 6-mercaptopurine for non-neoplastic disease.[93,94] Few patients with inflammatory bowel disease were included in the earlier studies, but a multiplicity of published case reports, and a review of 26 Crohn's patients with colorectal carcinoma, two of whom had earlier had azathioprine,[95] also suggested a greater than chance association.

The much larger reports of inflammatory bowel disease patients treated with immunosuppressants (723 in New York and 755 in London), which demonstrated no excess risk, were therefore especially reassuring.[96,97] The St Mark's patients were followed prospectively for a median of 9 years from the time of introduction of azathioprine.[96] A small overall increase in malignancies was detected, there being 31 malignancies compared with the 24.3 predicted by national mortality rates for the same age and sex distribution. This difference did not, however, reach statistical significance (P = 0.186). There were no lymphomas, but a significant excess of colorectal and anal tumours was found. The only other tumours to appear more commonly than expected were cervical and gastric carcinoma. It was thought likely that the excess of colorectal and anal tumours (15 observed versus 2.27 expected: $P < 0.00001$) represented an effect of the underlying disease rather than a complication of treatment, an interpretation supported by comparison with controls matched as nearly as possible for the nature of their disease but who had never received azathioprine. There were 86 azathioprine-treated patients with colitis of over 10 years' duration, for whom 180 colitis controls were identified. In the azathioprine group there were eight colorectal carcinomas (versus 0.26 expected) compared with 15 in the control group (versus 0.63 expected). The modest difference in relative risk (30.8 versus 23.8) was not significant ($P = 0.54$). It is highly probable that most of the increase in neoplasia in azathioprine-treated individuals is explained by more severe disease, those patients at this greater underlying risk of neoplasia being also those most likely to require immuno-suppression.

Reassuring though the St Mark's data are, it must be recognized that although the period of follow-up was substantial (median 9.0 years), the period of azathioprine usage was not, with a median of only 12.5 months. We have since seen one patient with gynaecological malignancy (probable cervical primary) presenting after 11 years of azathioprine therapy for otherwise intractable Crohn's disease, and another with breast cancer at 7 years (both initially treated elsewhere and therefore outside the St Mark's data-base). Clearly one should not be greatly influenced by anecdotes of this nature, but an increasing risk of neoplasia with greater durations of immuno-suppression is not illogical; reassuring data from long-term follow-up of short-term treatment should not be extrapolated to complacency about the safety of longer-term treatment. The apparent loss of benefit after more than 4 years of therapy lends further support to planned drug withdrawal at this stage.[98]

A comparable large study from Oxford is currently available only in abstract form, but yields the same message. Of 2205 (1350 ulcerative colitis) inflammatory bowel disease patients, 626 were treated with azathioprine between 1968 and 1999, to a mean total duration of 26.5 months. The mean follow-up was 13.7 years, including 6.9 years after azathioprine was started.[99] There were four colorectal carcinomas (including DALM and high-grade dysplasia) in 134 total colitics (3.0 per cent) and 3/165 left-sided colitics (1.8 per cent), compared with 12/294 (4.1 per cent) and 10/333 (3.0 per cent) of those who never received azathioprine. No cancers were found in 411 with proctitis alone. In Crohn's disease, there were seven colo-rectal carcinomas, three of whom had had azathioprine. The cumulative risk of cancer or dysplasia was 0.5, 1.3, 2.4 and 7.6 per cent at 10, 20, 30 and 40 years of ulcerative colitis, respectively. There were only 17 other cancers in the 619 azathioprine-treated patients (2.7 per cent) compared with 44 in 1586 non-exposed patients (2.8 per cent). Three of seven patients with lymphoma had received azathioprine and one of these also had rheumatoid arthritis.

A recent publication from Ireland describes four cases of non-Hodgkin's lymphoma amongst 782 patients with inflammatory bowel disease (238 of whom received immunosuppression).[100] Three of the tumours affected the intestine, one the mesentery, and the quoted incidence produces a standardized incidence ratio of 31 (CI: 2.0–85; $P = 0.0001$). Two patients had been on azathioprine and two on methotrexate, one of whom had also received cyclosporin, with an average of 20 months of immunosuppression preceding the diagnosis of malignancy. The very different modes of action of azathioprine, methotrexate and cyclosporin make one suspicious of a true drug effect, and there is considerable anxiety that their inflammatory bowel disease register was set up precisely because of the three lymphomas noted before its inception.

If we combine these datasets (New York, London, Oxford, Dublin) informally, there is a total of five cases of lymphoma amongst 2316 patients with inflammatory bowel disease exposed to azathioprine/6-mercaptopurine, one of whom had rheumatoid arthritis, which is a more definitely established association. The risk to our patients is unlikely to exceed 0.17 per cent, and extrapolation from Italian and the Oxford data suggests that inflammatory bowel disease itself might be a risk factor at about this level of magnitude.[90,99] The pragmatic response should be to suspect a (not necessarily causative) three-way association – severe inflammatory bowel disease, azathioprine, lymphoma – and to be vigilant. A formal surveillance strategy is difficult to conceptualize given the relatively inaccessible nature of the small bowel and the radiation doses that would be needed if serial follow-through or CT were to be performed.

CICLOSPORIN

There is evidence that ciclosporin increases the incidence of lymphoproliferative disorders and skin cancers after transplantation,[101–103] but few data particular to inflammatory bowel disease exist (the one Irish case is the only report other than in case report form).[100] It appears to be a dose-dependent phenomenon in transplant recipients and the risk of skin cancer is reduced if blood levels are maintained at 75–125 ng/mL rather than the traditional higher concentrations.[103] Continued monitoring is indicated, especially in patients treated for longer periods. It is disturbing[104] that colorectal carcinoma has occurred in no fewer than three of 27 patients with ulcerative colitis (and retained colons) within the first 14 months after liver transplantation for PSC. These patients were immunosuppressed (conventionally) with prednisolone, azathioprine and ciclosporin, and clearly represent a highly selected group, not least since sclerosing cholangitis may be a risk factor for colonic neoplasia (see above). It seems wise to enter such patients into an accelerated colonoscopic screening programme, but whether the increased risk is primarily related to drug, transplant, or disease remains unclear. Ciclosporin does appear exonerated from concerns of mutagenicity.[105]

METHOTREXATE AND OTHER IMMUNOSUPPRESSANTS

The risk of malignancy complicating long-term methotrexate therapy is thought to be low or absent, because methotrexate neither reacts with, nor becomes incorporated into, nucleic acid.[106] To date, no carcinogenic effect of the relatively low doses of methotrexate typically used for non-malignant indications has been demonstrated, background neoplasia rates remaining unaltered.[107,108] Again, data specific to inflammatory bowel disease are lacking, apart from the two Irish lymphoma cases, one of whom also received cyclosporin.[100] There is, however, a bizarre case report of reversible lymphoma of the skin in a patient treated for arthritis who also presented with hepatitis and lung cancer at the same time as the lymphoma.[109] Mycophenolate and tacrolimus have not yet been associated with neoplasia in inflammatory bowel disease, but their use has been very sparing and caution should be maintained.

INFLIXIMAB AND OTHER IMMUNOMODULATORS

There was great concern with the discovery of four lymphomas early on in the evaluation of infliximab, but in three cases there were other moderately strong risk factors (rheumatoid arthritis or AIDS). Lymphoma has been seen only twice in Crohn's disease, first in a 61-year-old man in the placebo limb of the follow-on multiple-dose study. He developed a duodenal B-cell lymphoma 9.5 months after his initial and sole infliximab infusion.[110] The second case was in the USA during general licensed use (Centocor data on file). Studies in rheumatoid and Crohn's, accumulating 1395 patient-years, yielded 14 malignancies (0.010 per patient per year, compared with a placebo rate of 0.0053 – NS). In the Crohn's disease patients in trials, there were 4/454 malignancies/patient-year versus 1/59 in controls (NS). Since licensing, and with total usage by more than 30 000 patients, Centocor's records (which may be incomplete) indicate a total of 16 malignancies with 12 different cancers. Data from Chicago on 202 carefully monitored patients suggest no differences from expected rates in control patients with Crohn's disease.[111] The two lymphomas now fall well within expected population frequencies given the wide overall use of the drug. There are no data in respect of neoplasia risk for any of the other immunomodulators in inflammatory bowel disease.

DIAGNOSTIC IMAGING AND RISK OF NEOPLASIA

Many patients with inflammatory bowel disease have repeated radiological examinations over many years, raising the possibility that medical exposure to ionizing radiation might contribute to risk of neoplasia. Ultrasound and MRI appear exonerated as far as can be told, and the exposure from scintigraphic imaging is reassuringly low (frequency and dosimetry), but conventional imaging (plain films, barium studies, fistulograms, etc.) and CT deserve attention. The average total annual radiation exposure in the UK and other Western nations has been about 2.5 mSv per person.[112] With approximately 500 radiological examinations for every 1000 individuals, at least 12 per cent of the total irradiation comes from medical sources (which in turn accounts for over 80 per cent of all man-made radiation).[113] Most of these examinations are of the chest or periphery, which expose the patient to a very low 'effective dose equivalent', when compared with a typical plain abdominal film at 1.14 mSv (10 mGy absorbed dose), a barium meal at 3.8 mSv, and a barium enema at 7.7 mSv.[114] The much greater figure for barium enema is a combined result of longer screening times as the flow of barium around the colon is monitored, the greater need for full-sized abdominal films and, to some extent, the greater energy required for the image in the lateral view. Accordingly, although barium enemas have accounted for only 0.9 per cent of all radiological procedures, they have contributed 14 per cent of the medical radiation dose in the UK.[112] It is highly probable that the above figures are outdated and exceeded by current practice and the much greater use of CT scanning of the abdomen and pelvis, which exposes the patient to higher radiation levels. Ironically, the newer techniques such as helical and ultra-thin slice scanning all increase irradiation.

Extrapolation from occupational exposure (as in uranium workers) predicts a roughly linear relationship between increasing radiation exposure and increasing risk of malignancy,[115] with no minimum radiation dose below which there is freedom from this increased risk. These assumptions lead to between 100 and 250 fatal cancers being attributed to medical radiation each year in the UK (1.8–4.5 per million population). The approximate lifetime risk that a given procedure induces a fatal malignancy can be calculated to lie between 20 and 60 per million for abdominal radiography, 50 and 170 per million for barium meal, 100 and 350 per million for barium enema, and at least 500 per million from abdominal CT scanning.[112,114] There is a probable additional risk of gonadal damage promoting childhood malignancy in the children of both males and females exposed to medical radiation during the reproductive period. The radiation dose from most nuclear scanning is much lower, and of proportionately lesser importance.

Could iatrogenic irradiation contribute to the

increased risk of colorectal carcinoma in ulcerative colitis? A lifetime's investigation might perhaps encompass three barium enemas and up to 20 plain abdominal films (more will usually have led to colectomy). Combining the additive risks of these procedures leads to an expected excess of roughly 1400 cancers per million patients ($3 \times 200 + 20 \times 40$). These radiation-induced cancers are unlikely to be colorectal, as occupational and atomic bomb data indicate that the gastrointestinal mucosa is a 'protected' site,[114,115] but even if all excess cancers resulting from radiological investigation of colitis were in the large bowel, then radiation would account for only about 0.14 per cent of colitis cancers – or around 1.5 per cent of the excess relative to the general population.

The situation is less easily modelled in Crohn's disease given less certainty as to the excess cancer rate, but a larger number of radiographic studies of the small bowel, and CT scans are typical. The relatively extreme case of a patient in whom 20 small bowel series, 2 barium enemas, and 10 CT scans had been performed would be at an increased risk of fatal malignancy in the region of 7400 per million. This lifetime risk of nearly 1 per cent should not be ignored when considering the need for radiological investigation, as Crohn's patients are usually young and likely to survive to be at risk, but can fairly readily be placed in perspective. Again, these excess malignancies can be expected to be extra-intestinal.

The epidemiological data are concordant with these predictions. The US National Cancer Institute has examined the pre-morbid radiographic history in over 1000 lymphoma, leukaemia and myeloma patients, in comparison with matched controls.[116] Only a small increase in the risk of myeloma (relative risk 1.14) could be clearly linked to prior radiation and, encouragingly, myeloma is not over-represented in inflammatory bowel disease-related neoplasia[1,116,117] (and see Chapter 2).

References

1 Ekbom A, Helmick CG, Zack M, Holmberg L, Adami HO. Survival and causes of death in patients with inflammatory bowel disease: a population-based study. *Gastroenterology* 1992; **103**: 954–60.

2 Persson P-G, Bernell O, Leijonmarck C-E, Farahmand BY, Hellers G, Ahlbom A. Survival and cause-specific mortality in inflammatory bowel disease: a population-based study. *Gastroenterology* 1996; **110**: 1339–45.

3 Langholz E, Munkholm P, Davidsen M, Binder V. Colorectal cancer risk and mortality in patients with ulcerative colitis. *Gastroenterology* 1992; **103**: 1444–51.

4 Nugent FW, Haggitt RC, Gilpin PA. Cancer surveillance in ulcerative colitis. *Gastroenterology* 1991; **100**: 1241–8.

5 Connell WR, Talbot IC, Harpaz N, *et al.* Clinicopathological characteristics of colorectal carcinoma complicating ulcerative colitis. *Gut* 1994; **35**: 1419–23.

6 Ekbom A, Helmick C, Zack M, Adami HO. Increased risk of large bowel cancer in Crohn's disease with colonic involvement. *Lancet* 1990; **336**: 357–9.

7 Binder V, Hendriksen C, Kreiner S. Prognosis in Crohn's disease – based on results from a regional patient group from the county of Copenhagen. *Gut* 1985; **26**: 146–50.

8 Kvist N, Jacobsen O, Norgaard P, *et al.* Malignancy in Crohn's disease. *Scand J Gastroenterol* 1986; **21**: 82–6.

9 Gollop JH, Phillips SF, Melton LJ, Zinsmeister AR. Epidemiological aspects of Crohn's disease: a population based study in Olmsted County, Minnesota, 1943–1982. *Gut* 1988; **29**: 49–56.

10 Fireman Z, Grossman A, Lilos P, *et al.* Intestinal cancer in patients with Crohn's disease: a population study in central Israel. *Scand J Gastroenterol* 1989; **24**: 346–50.

11 Mellemkjaer L, Johansen C, Gridley G, Linet MS, Kjaer SK, Olsen JH. Crohn's disease and cancer risk (Denmark). *Cancer Causes Control* 2000; **11**: 145–50.

12 Palli D, Trallori G, Saieva C, *et al.* General and cancer specific mortality of a population based cohort of patients with inflammatory bowel

disease: the Florence Study. *Gut* 1998; **42**: 175–9.

13 Jess T, Winther KV, Munkholm P, Langholz E, Binder V. Is there an increased risk of intestinal and extraintestinal cancer in patients with Crohn's disease? A population-based cohort followed from 1962 to 1997. *Gastroenterology* 2000; **118**: A254.

14 Korelitz BI. Carcinoma of the intestinal tract in Crohn's disease: results of a survey conducted by the National Foundation for Ileitis and Colitis. *Am J Gastroenterol* 1983; **78**: 44–6.

15 Weedon DD, Shorter RG, Ilstrup DM, Huizenga KA, Taylor WF. Crohn's disease and cancer. *N Engl J Med* 1973; **289**: 1099–103.

16 Greenstein AJ, Sachar DB, Smith H, Janowitz HD, Aufses AH. A comparison of cancer risk in Crohn's disease and ulcerative colitis. *Cancer* 1981; **48**: 2742–5.

17 Gyde SN, Prior P, McCartney JC, Thompson H, Waterhouse JAH, Allan RN. Malignancy in Crohn's disease. *Gut* 1980; **21**: 1024–9.

18 Stahl TJ, Schoetz DJ, Roberts PL, *et al.* Crohn's disease and carcinoma: increasing justification for surveillance? *Dis Colon Rectum* 1992; **35**: 850–6.

19 Gillen CD, Walmsley RS, Prior P, Andrews HA, Allan RN. Ulcerative colitis and Crohn's disease: a comparison of the colorectal cancer risk in extensive colitis. *Gut* 1994; **35**: 1590–2.

20 Cohen RD, Gordon DW, Argo CK, Hanauer SB. Risk factors for adenocarcinoma in ulcerative colitis and Crohn's disease: a retrospective, matched case-control study. *Gastroenterology* 1996; **110**: A505.

21 Mendelsohn RR, Korelitz BI, Gleim GW. Death from Crohn's disease. Lessons from a personal experience. *J Clin Gastroenterol* 1995; **20**: 22–6.

22 Michelassi F, Testa G, Pomidor WJ, Lashner BA, Block GE. Adenocarcinoma complicating Crohn's disease. *Dis Colon Rectum* 1993; **36**: 654–61.

23 Connell WR, Sheffield JP, Kamm MA, Ritchie JK, Hawley PR, Lennard-Jones JE. Lower gastrointestinal malignancy in Crohn's disease. *Gut* 1994; **35**: 347–52.

24 Rubio CA, Befrits R. Colorectal adenocarcinoma in Crohn's disease: a retrospective histologic study. *Dis Colon Rectum* 1997; **40**: 1072–8.

25 Ying LT, Hurlbut DJ, Depew WT, Boag AH, Taguchi K. Primary adenocarcinoma in an enterocutaneous fistula associated with Crohn's disease. *Can J Gastroenterol* 1998; **12**: 265–9.

26 Richards ME, Rickert RR, Nance FC. Crohn's disease-associated carcinoma. *Ann Surg* 1989; **209**: 764–73.

27 Rhodes JM. Mucins and inflammatory bowel disease. *Q J Med* 1997; **90**: 79–82.

28 Ryder SD, Jacyna MR, Levi AJ, Rizzi PM, Rhodes JM. Eating peanuts increases rectal proliferation in individuals with mucosal expression of peanut lectin receptor. *Gastroenterology* 1998; **114**: 44–9.

29 Yu L, Fernig DG, Smith JA, Milton JD, Rhodes JM. Reversible inhibition of proliferation of epithelial cell lines by *Agaricus bisporus* (edible mushroom) lectin. *Cancer Res* 1993; **53**: 4627–32.

30 Rhodes JM. Unifying hypothesis for inflammatory bowel disease and related colon cancer: sticking the pieces together with sugar. *Lancet* 1996; **347**: 40–4.

31 Evans RC Ashby D, Hackett A, Williams E, Rhodes JM. Consumption of peanuts, which contain a galactose-binding lectin, associates with increased risk for colorectal cancer whereas high non-starch polysaccharide galactose intake associates with a reduced risk. *Gut* 1997; **41**(Suppl 3): A124.

32 Jankowski JA, Bedford FK, Boulton RA, *et al.* Alterations in classical cadherins associated with progression in ulcerative and Crohn's colitis. *Lab Invest* 1998; **78**: 1155–67.

33 Ierardi E, Principi M, Noviello F, Passaro S, Burattini O, Francavilla A. Epithelial proliferation and *ras* p21 oncoprotein in the rectum of patients with ulcerative colitis. *Gut* 1999; **45**(Suppl V): A125.

34 Mouzas IA, Papavassiliou E, Koutroubakis I. Chemoprevention of colorectal cancer in inflammatory bowel disease? A potential role for folate. *Ital J Gastroenterol Hepatol* 1998; **30**: 421–5.

35 Babyatsky MW, Rossiter G, Podolsky DK. Expression of transforming growth factors α and β in colonic mucosa in inflammatory bowel disease. *Gastroenterology* 1996; **110**: 975–84.

36 Pokorny RM, Hofmeister A, Galandiuk S, Dietz AB, Cohen ND, Neibergs HL. Crohn's disease and ulcerative colitis are associated with the DNA repair gene *MLH1*. *Ann Surg* 1997; **225**: 718–23.

37 Crispin DA, Dziadon SM, Haggitt RC, *et al.* Chromosomal instability is associated with telomere shortening in UC patients with dysplasia or cancer. *Gastroenterology* 2000; **118**: A254.

38 Arai N, Mitomi H, Ohtani Y, Igarashi M, Kakita

A, Okayasu I. Enhanced epithelial cell turnover associated with p53 accumulation and high p21WAF1/CIP1 expression in ulcerative colitis. *Mod Pathol* 1999; **12**: 604–11.

39 Iwamoto M, Koji T, Makiyama K, Kobayashi N, Nakane PK. Apoptosis of crypt epithelial cells in ulcerative colitis. *J Pathol* 1996; **180**: 152–9.

40 Jenkins D, Seth R, Kummer JA, Scott BB, Hawkey CJ, Robins RA. Differential levels of granzyme B, regulatory cytokines, and apoptosis in Crohn's disease and ulcerative colitis at first presentation. *J Pathol* 2000; **190**: 184–9.

41 Perez-Machado MA, Espinosa LM, de la Madrigal EJ, Abreu L, Lorente GM, Alvarez-Mon M. Impaired mitogenic response of peripheral blood T cells in ulcerative colitis is not due to apoptosis. *Dig Dis Sci* 1999; **44**: 2530–7.

42 Boirivant M, Marini M, Di Felice G, *et al.* Lamina propria T cells in Crohn's disease and other gastrointestinal inflammation show defective CD2 pathway-induced apoptosis. *Gastroenterology* 1999; **116**: 557–65.

43 British Society of Gastroenterology. *Guidelines in Gastroenterology 4: Inflammatory Bowel Disease.* London: British Society of Gastroenterology, 1996.

44 Eaden JA, Abrams K, Ekbom A, Jackson E, Mayberry J. Colorectal cancer prevention in ulcerative colitis: a case-control study. *Aliment Pharmacol Ther* 2000; **14**: 145–53.

45 Axon ATR. Cancer surveillance in ulcerative colitis – a time for reappraisal. *Gut* 1994; **35**: 587–9.

46 Connell WR, Lennard-Jones JE, Williams CB, Talbot IC, Price AB, Wilkinson KH. Factors influencing the outcome of endoscopic surveillance for cancer in ulcerative colitis. *Gastroenterology* 1994; **107**: 934–44.

47 Karlén P, Broström O, Öst A, Tribukait B, Löfberg R. No mortality due to colorectal cancer during 23-year prospective colonoscopic surveillance for longstanding extensive ulcerative colitis. *Gut* 1999; **45**(Suppl V): A200.

48 Karlen P, Kornfeld D, Brostrom O, Lofberg R, Persson PG, Ekbom A. Is colonoscopic surveillance reducing colorectal cancer mortality in ulcerative colitis? A population based case control study. *Gut* 1998; **42**: 711–14.

49 Dixon MF, Brown LJR, Gilmour HM, *et al.* Observer variation in the assessment of dysplasia in ulcerative colitis. *Histopathology* 1988; **13**: 385–97.

50 Theodossi A, Spiegelhalter DJ, Jass J, *et al.* Observer variation and discriminatory value of biopsy features in inflammatory bowel disease. *Gut* 1994; **35**: 961–8.

51 Woolrich AJ, DaSilva MD, Korelitz BI. Surveillance in the routine management of ulcerative colitis: the predictive value of low grade dysplasia. *Gastroenterology* 1992; **103**: 431–8.

52 Bernstein CN, Shanahan F. Are we telling patients the truth about surveillance colonoscopy in ulcerative colitis? *Lancet* 1994; **343**: 71–4.

53 Schneider A, Stolte M. Differential diagnosis of adenomas and dysplastic lesions in patients with ulcerative colitis. *Z Gastroenterol* 1993; **31**: 653–6.

54 Engelsgjerd M, Farraye FA, Odze RD. Polypectomy may be adequate treatment for adenoma-like dysplastic lesions in chronic ulcerative colitis. *Gastroenterology* 1999; **117**: 1288–94.

55 Eaden JA, Ward BA, Mayberry JF. How gastroenterologists screen for colonic cancer in ulcerative colitis: an analysis of performance. *Gastrointest Endosc* 2000; **51**: 123–8.

56 Rubin CE, Haggitt RC, Burmer GC, *et al.* DNA aneuploidy in colonic biopsies predicts future development of dysplasia in ulcerative colitis. *Gastroenterology* 1992; **103**: 1611–20.

57 Befrits R, Hammarberg C, Rubio C, Jaramillo E, Tribukait B. DNA aneuploidy and histologic dysplasia in long-standing ulcerative colitis. A 10-year follow-up study. *Dis Colon Rectum* 1994; **37**: 313–19.

58 Ilyas M, Talbot IC. p53 expression in ulcerative colitis: a longitudinal study. *Gut* 1995; **37**: 802–4.

59 Brentnall TA, Crispin DA, Rabinovitch PS, *et al.* Mutations in the p53 gene: an early marker of neoplastic progression in ulcerative colitis. *Gastroenterology* 1994; **107**: 369–78.

60 Sato A, MacHinami R. p53 immunohistochemistry of ulcerative colitis-associated with dysplasia and carcinoma. *Pathol Int* 1999; **49**: 858–68.

61 Kullmann F, Fadaie M, Gross V, *et al.* Expression of proliferating cell nuclear antigen (PCNA) and Ki67 in dysplasia in inflammatory bowel disease. *Eur J Gastroenterol Hepatol* 1996; **8**: 371–9.

62 Thomas MG, Nugent KP, Forbes A, Williamson RC. Calcipotriol inhibits rectal epithelial cell production in ulcerative proctocolitis. *Gut* 1994; **35**: 1718–20.

63 Itzkowitz SH, Young E, Dubois D, *et al.* Sialosyl-Tn antigen is prevalent and precedes dysplasia in

ulcerative colitis: a retrospective case-control study. *Gastroenterology* 1996; **110**: 694–704.

64 Karlen P, Young E, Brostrom O, *et al.* Sialyl-Tn antigen as a marker of colon cancer risk in ulcerative colitis: relation to dysplasia and DNA aneuploidy. *Gastroenterology* 1998; **115**: 1395–404.

65 Rustgi AK. Hereditary gastrointestinal polyposis and nonpolyposis syndromes. *N Engl J Med* 1994; **331**: 1694–702.

66 Nuako KW, Ahlquist DA, Mahoney DW, Schaid DJ, Siems DM, Lindor NM. Familial predisposition for colorectal cancer in chronic ulcerative colitis: a case-control study. *Gastroenterology* 1998; **115**: 1079–83.

67 Provenzale D, Wong JB, Onken JE, Lipscomb J. Performing a cost-effectiveness analysis: surveillance of patients with ulcerative colitis. *Am J Gastroenterol* 1998; **93**: 872–80.

68 Delco F, Sonnenberg A. The unsolved problem of surveillance for colorectal cancer in ulcerative colitis. *Can J Gastroenterol* 1999; **13**: 655–60.

69 Rubin PH, Present DH, Chapman ML, Cortes JL, Harpaz N. Chronic Crohn's colitis: a 7 year experience with screening and surveillance colonoscopy in 113 patients. *Gastroenterology* 1996; **110**: A1005.

70 Jain SK, Peppercorn MA. Inflammatory bowel disease and colon cancer: a review. *Dig Dis* 1997; **15**: 243–52.

71 Broomé, U, Löfberg R, Veress B, Eriksson LS. Primary sclerosing cholangitis and ulcerative colitis: evidence for increased neoplastic potential. *Hepatology* 1995; **22**: 1404–8.

72 Brentnall TA, Haggitt RC, Rabinovitch PS, *et al.* Risk and natural history of colonic neoplasia in patients with primary sclerosing cholangitis and ulcerative colitis. *Gastroenterology* 1996; **110**: 331–8.

73 Shetty K, Rybicki L, Brzezinski A, Carey WD, Lashner BA. The risk for cancer or dysplasia in ulcerative colitis patients with primary sclerosing cholangitis. *Am J Gastroenterol* 1999; **94**: 1643–9.

74 Loftus EV Jr, Sandborn WJ, Tremaine WJ, *et al.* Risk of colorectal neoplasia in patients with primary sclerosing cholangitis. *Gastroenterology* 1996; **110**: 432–40.

75 Nuako KW, Ahlquist DA, Sandborn WJ, Mahoney DW, Siems DM, Zinsmeister AR. Primary sclerosing cholangitis and colorectal carci-noma in patients with chronic ulcerative colitis: a case-control study. *Cancer* 1998; **82**: 822–6.

76 Gurbuz AK, Giardiello FM, Bayless TM. Colorectal neoplasia in patients with ulcerative colitis and primary sclerosing cholangitis. *Dis Colon Rectum* 1995; **38**: 37–41.

77 Wiesner RH, Grambsch PM, Dickson ER, *et al.* Primary sclerosing cholangitis: natural history, prognostic factors and survival analysis. *Hepatology* 1989; **10**: 430–6.

78 Chalasani N, Baluyut A, Ismail A, *et al.* Cholangiocarcinoma in patients with primary sclerosing cholangitis: a multicenter case-control study. *Hepatology* 2000; **31**: 7–11.

79 Patel AH, Harnois DM, Klee GG, LaRusso NF, Gores GJ. The utility of CA 19-9 in the diagnoses of cholangiocarcinoma in patients without primary sclerosing cholangitis. *Am J Gastroenterol* 2000; **95**: 204–7.

80 Bjornsson E, Kilander A, Olsson R. CA 19-9 and CEA are unreliable markers for cholangiocarcinoma in patients with primary sclerosing cholangitis. *Liver* 1999; **19**: 501–8.

81 Boberg KM, Schrumpf E, Bergquist A, *et al.* Cholangiocarcinoma in primary sclerosing cholangitis: K-ras mutations and Tp53 dysfunction are implicated in the neoplastic development. *J Hepatol* 2000; **32**: 374–80.

82 Yeh TS, Jan YY, Tseng JH. Malignant perihilar biliary obstruction: magnetic resonance cholangiopancreatographic findings. *Am J Gastroenterol* 2000; **95**: 432–40.

83 Keiding S, Hansen SB, Rasmussen HH, *et al.* Detection of cholangiocarcinoma in primary sclerosing cholangitis by positron emission tomography. *Hepatology* 1998; **28**: 700–6.

84 Karlen P, Lofberg R, Brostrom O, Leijonmarck CE, Hellers G, Persson PG. Increased risk of cancer in ulcerative colitis: a population-based cohort study. *Am J Gastroenterol* 1999; **94**: 1047–52.

85 Munkholm P, Langholz E, Davidsen M, Binder V. Intestinal cancer risk and mortality in patients with Crohn's disease. *Gastroenterology* 1993; **105**: 1716–23.

86 Sigel JE, Petras RE, Lashner BA, Fazio VW, Goldblum JR. Intestinal adenocarcinoma in Crohn's disease: a report of 30 cases with a focus on coexisting dysplasia. *Am J Surg Pathol* 1999; **23**: 651–5.

87 Rashid A, Hamilton SR. Genetic alterations in sporadic and Crohn's-associated adenocarcinomas of the small intestine. *Gastroenterology* 1997; **113**: 127–35.

88 Leteurtre E, Kosydar P, Gambiez L, Colombel J-F, Quandalle P, Lecomte-Houcke M. Rectums exclus au cours de la maladie de Crohn: quel est le risque de dysplasie? *Gastroenterol Clin Biol* 1999; **23**: 477–82.

89 Katoh H, Iwane S, Munakata A, Nakaji S, Sugawara K. Long-term prognosis of patients with ulcerative colitis in Japan. *J Epidemiol* 2000; **10**: 48–54.

90 Palli D, Trallori G, Bagnoli S, *et al.* Hodgkin's disease risk is increased in patients with ulcerative colitis. *Gastroenterology* 2000; **119**: 647–53.

91 Pinczowski D, Ekbom A, Baron J, Yuen J, Adami HO. Risk factors for colorectal cancer in patients with ulcerative colitis: a case control study. *Gastroenterology* 1994; **107**: 117–20.

92 Reinacher-Schick A, Seidensticker F, Petrasch S, *et al.* Mesalazine changes apoptosis and proliferation in normal mucosa of patients with sporadic polyps of the large bowel. *Endoscopy* 2000; **32**: 245–54.

93 Kinlen LJ. Incidence of cancer in rheumatoid arthritis and other disorders after immunosuppressive treatment. *Am J Med* 1985; **78**(Suppl): 44–9.

94 Matteson EL, Hickey AR, Maguire L, Tilson HH, Urowitz MB. Occurrence of neoplasia in patients with rheumatoid arthritis enrolled in a DMARD registry. *J Rheumatol* 1991; **18**: 809–14.

95 Zelig MP, Choi PM. Azathioprine or 6-mercaptopurine therapy and colon carcinoma in Crohn's disease. *Gastroenterology* 1992; **102**: 1448 (letter).

96 Present DH, Meltzer ST, Krumholz MP, Wolke A, Korelitz BI. 6-Mercaptopurine in the management of inflammatory bowel disease: short- and long-term toxicity. *Ann Intern Med* 1989; **111**: 641–9.

97 Connell WR, Kamm MA, Dickson M, Balkwill AM, Ritchie JK, Lennard-Jones JE. Long-term neoplasia risk after azathioprine treatment in inflammatory bowel disease. *Lancet* 1994; **343**: 1249–52.

98 Bouhnik Y, Lémann M, Mary J-Y, *et al.* Long-term follow-up of patients with Crohn's disease treated with azathioprine or 6-mercaptopurine. *Lancet* 1996; **347**: 215–19.

99 Fraser AG, Jewell DP. Long-term risk of malignancy after treatment of inflammatory bowel disease with azathioprine – a 30 year study. *Gastroenterology* 2000; **118**: A254.

100 Farrell RJ, Ang Y, Kileen P, *et al.* Increased incidence of non-Hodgkin's lymphoma in inflammatory bowel disease patients on immunosuppressive therapy but overall risk is low. *Gut* 2000; **47**: 514–19.

101 Von Graffenried B. Sandimmun (cyclosporin) in autoimmune disease: overview on early clinical experience. *Am J Nephrol* 1989; **9**: 51–6.

102 Kurki PT. Safety aspects of long-term cyclosporin A therapy. *Scand J Rheumatol* 1992; **95**: 35–8.

103 Dantal J, Hourmant M, Cantarovich D., I Effect of long-term immunosuppression in kidney-graft recipients on cancer incidence: randomised comparison of two cyclosporin regimens. *Lancet* 1998; **351**: 623–8.

104 Bleday R, Lee E, Jessurun J, Heine J, Wong WD. Increased risk of early colorectal neoplasms after hepatic transplant in patients with inflammatory bowel disease. *Dis Colon Rectum* 1993; **36**: 908–12.

105 Olshan AF, Mattison DR, Zwanenburg TS. Cyclosporine A: review of genotoxicity and potential for adverse human reproductive and developmental effects. *Mutat Res* 1994; **317**: 163–73.

106 Turnbull C, Roach M. Is methotrexate carcinogenic? *Br Med J* 1980; **281**: 808.

107 Tishler M, Caspi D, Yaron M. Long-term experience with low dose methotrexate in rheumatoid arthritis. *Rheumatol Int* 1993; **13**: 103–6.

108 Weinblatt ME. Methotrexate for chronic diseases in adults. *N Engl J Med* 1995; **332**: 330–1.

109 Viraben R, Brousse P, Lamant L. Reversible cutaneous lymphoma occurring during methotrexate therapy. *Br J Dermatol* 1996; **135**: 116–18.

110 Rutgeerts P, D'Haens G, Targan S, *et al.* Efficacy and safety of retreatment with anti-tumor necrosis factor (infliximab) to maintain remission in Crohn's disease. *Gastroenterology* 1999; **117**: 761–9.

111 Hanauer SB, Schaible TF, DeWoody KL, *et al.* Long-term follow-up of patients treated with infliximab (anti-TNFα antibody) in clinical trials. *Gastroenterology* 2000; **118**(Suppl 2): A566.

112 National Radiation Protection Board. *Patient Dose Reduction in Diagnostic Radiology.* Documents of the NRPB. London: HMSO, 1990.

113 Mettler FA, Davis M, Kelsey CA, Rosenberg R, Williams A. Analytical modeling of worldwide

medical radiation use. *Health Phys* 1987; **52**: 133–41.

114 National Radiation Protection Board. *A National Survey of Doses to Patients undergoing a Selection of Routine X-ray Examinations in English Hospitals.* NRPB-R200. London: HMSO, 1986.

115 Sevc J, Kunz E, Tomasek L, Placek V, Horacek J. Cancer in man after exposure to Rn daughters. *Health Phys* 1988; **54**: 27–46.

116 Boice JD Jr, Morin MM, Glas AG, *et al.* Diagnostic X-ray procedures and risk of leukemia, lymphoma, and multiple myeloma. *J Am Med Assoc* 1991; **265**: 1290–4.

117 Sachar DB. Cancer in Crohn's disease: dispelling the myths. *Gut* 1994; **35**: 1507–8.

Appendix A: Scoring systems in inflammatory bowel disease

Crohn's disease

CROHN'S DISEASE ACTIVITY INDEX (CDAI)

The CDAI score is derived from summation of information culled from a diary card completed by the patient for the preceding 7 days, together with current clinical data as follows.

Days 1–7	Sum	×factor	Score
Number of liquid/very soft stools	. . .	2	. . .
Abdominal pain rating 0 = none; 1 = mild; 2 = moderate; 3 = severe	. . .	5	. . .
General well-being 0 = generally well; 1 = slightly under par; 2 = poor; 3 = very poor; 4 = terrible	. . .	7	. . .
Number of 6 listed categories now has: arthritis/arthralgia iritis/eveitis erythema nodosum/pyoderma gangrenosum/aphthous stomatitis anal fissure, fistula or abscess other fistular fever of > 37.0 °C in past week	. . .	20	. . .

	×factor	Score
Taking opioids for diarrhoea – No = 0; Yes = 30		. . .
Abdominal mass 0 = none; 20 = questionable; 50 = definite		. . .

	×factor	Score
Haematocrit (%)		
males: 47 – 'crit ❘	6	. . .
females: 42 – 'crit ❘		
Body weight (kg)		
percentage below standard weight for height		. . .
add if below standard weight; subtract if overweight		. . .

Total = CDAI

A score of <150 is usually taken to indicate a patient in remission. It can be seen that it is easily possible for a score in excess of 150 to be derived from the patient's symptoms alone without any more 'objective' evidence of disease.

Best WR, Becktel JM, Singleton JW, Kern F Jr. Development of a Crohn's disease activity index. National Cooperative Crohn's Disease Study. *Gastoenterology* 1976; **70**: 439–44.

THE MODIFIED/SIMPLIFIED CDAI

For day before visit:

X1   Number of soft or liquid stools
X2   Abdominal pain rating
        0 = none; 1 = mild; 2 = moderate; 3 = severe
X3   Well-being
        0 = well; 1 = slightly below par; 2 = poor; 3 = very poor; 4 = terrible
X4   Number of extra-intestinal manifestations (as for full CDAI)
X5   Abdominal mass
        0 = none; 2 = questionable; 5 = present

Score = $20[XI + 2(2 + X3 + X4 + X5)]$

The simplified index has the advantage that it permits scoring on the basis of the previous day's account only, and therefore is more applicable to regular clinic use. A score of <150 is taken as remission, 150–250 as mild, 251–400 as moderate, and >400 as severe disease activity.

Best WR, Beckett JM. The Crohn's disease activity index as a clinical instrument. In Pena A, Weterman IT, Booth CC, Strober W, eds. *Recent Advances in Crohn's Disease*. The Hague: Martinus Nijhoff, 1981: pp. 7–12.

HARVEY–BRADSHAW INDEX

A five point score based on:

A   General well-being   0 = very well; 1 = slightly below par; 2 = poor; 3 = very poor;
                                    4 = terrible
B   Abdominal pain   0 = none; 1 = mild; 2 = moderate; 3 = severe
C   Number of liquid stools per day

| D | Abdominal mass | 0 = none; 1 = dubious; 2 = definite; 3 = definite and tender |
| E | Complications | Score 1 for each of arthralgia, uveitis, erythema nodosum, pyoderma gangrenosum, aphthous ulcers, anal fissure, new fistula, abscess |

Comparison with the CDAI is good ($r = 0.93$; $P < 0.001$).

Approximate CDAI score	Approximate Harvey–Bradshaw score
100	2
150	4–5
200	6
250	7–8
300	9

Harvey RF, Bradshaw JM. A simple index of Crohn's disease activity. *Lancet* 1980; **1**: 514.

THE VAN HEES OR DUTCH INDEX OF CROHN'S DISEASE ACTIVITY

The score is derived from nine objective parameters each with its own multiplier, as follows:

Albumin (g/L)	×	−5.48
ESR (mm/h)	×	+0.29
Quettelet index (BMI x 10)	×	−0.22
Temperature (°C)	×	+16.4
Sex (1 for male; 2 for female)	×	−12.3
Previous resection (1 for no; 2 for yes)	×	−9.17
Extra-intestinal manifestations (1 for no; 2 for yes)	×	+10.7
Stool consistency (1 for normal; 2 for soft; 3 for watery)	×	+8.46
Abdominal mass (1 for no; 2 for possible; 3 for diameter < 6 cm; 4 for diameter 6–12 cm; 5 for diameter > 12 cm)	×	+7.83

Subtotal	A
Subtract constant	209
Final score	B

A score of <100 is considered normal; 100–150 represents mild activity; 150–210 represents moderate activity; and >210 represents severe disease.

Van Hees PAM, Van Elteren PH, Van Lier HJJ, Van Tongeren JHM. An index of inflammatory activity in patients with Crohn's disease. *Gut* 1980; **21**: 279–86.

ENDOSCOPIC SCORING SYSTEM FOR CROHN'S DISEASE – THE CROHN'S DISEASE ENDOSCOPIC INDEX OF SEVERITY (CDEIS)

Score for each segment of bowel involved as follows:
    rectum; sigmoid/L colon; transverse; R colon; ileum
Deep ulceration
    score 12 at each site present and summate (max = 60)   Total 1

Superficial ulceration

    score 6 at each site present and summate (max = 30) (can coexist with a 12 score)   Total 2

Surface involved by disease in cm for each site present and summate

    = linear measurements of diseased bowel but to a maximum of 10 (representing   Total 3

      100% of surface) (max overall therefore is 50)

Ulcerated surface area

    expressed in same way as surface involved (max = 50)   Total 4

Total A = Total 1 + 2 + 3 + 4

Number of segments fully examined (1 to 5) = n

Subtotal = Total A ÷ n = Total B

Add 3 if ulcerated stenosis anywhere

Add 3 if non-ulcerated stenosis anywhere

Total = CDEIS

CDEIS scores typically lie between 0 and 30. Further details in respect of definition of the various parameters are given in the full paper, but informal testing of experienced endoscopists indicates that consistent results may be achieved from a given operator's subjective interpretation of the criteria without special training.

    Mary JY, Modigliani R, for Groupe d'Etudes Thérapeutiques des Affections Inflammatoires du Tube Digestif (GET AID). Development and validation of an endoscopic index of the severity of Crohn's disease: a prospective multicentre study. *Gut* 1989; **30**: 983–9.

THE RUTGEERTS ILEITIS SCORE

A simpler endoscopic score, the Rutgeerts score is also in use for patients in whom the colon has been resected:

0   no lesion seen
1   fewer than 5 aphthous lesions
2   more than 5 aphthous lesions with normal mucosa between them, or skip areas of larger lesions or lesions confined to the ileocolic anastomosis (i.e. < 1 cm in length)
3   diffuse aphthous ileitis with diffusely inflamed mucosa
4   diffuse inflammation with larger ulcers, nodules, narrowing or both

    Rutgeerts P, Geboes K, Vantrappen G, Beyls J, Kerrenans R, Hiele M. Predictability of the postoperative course of Crohn's disease. *Gastroenterology* 1990; **99**: 956–63.

Ulcerative colitis

THE BARON SCORE

A four-point scale based on the sigmoidoscopic appearance, which is also used in modified form in the St Mark's score (see below).

0 = normal
1 = non-haemorrhagic – no bleeding spontaneously or on light touch
2 = haemorrhagic – bleeding to light touch but no spontaneous bleeding
3 = haemorrhagic – spontaneous bleeding proximal to the depth of insertion of the instrument

Baron JH, Connell AM, Lennard-Jones JE. Variation between observers in describing mucosal appearances in proctocolitis. *Br Med J* 1964; **1**: 89–92.

COLITIS ENDOSCOPIC INDEX

Mucosal membrane surface granulation
   diffuses reflected light

No	0
Yes	2

Vascular marking

Normal	0
Indistinct/deranged	1
Completely absent	2

Mucosal membrane sensitivity

None	0
Slightly increased (contact bleeding)	2
Greatly increased (spontaneous bleeding)	4

Coating on mucous membrane (mucus,
   fibrin, exudate, erosions, ulcers)

None	0
Slight	2
Marked	4

It is not entirely obvious that this more complex score adds substantially to the Baron scale, but it is preferred by some centres.

Rachmilewitz D. Coated mesalazine (5-aminosalicylic acid) vs sulphasalazine in the treatment of active ulcerative colitis: a randomised trial. *Br Med J* 1989; **298**: 82–6.

THE ST MARK'S SCORE

A four-item scale permitting a score between 0 and 9 for ulcerative colitis, which may also be extended to include the ESR (or an alternative biochemical marker of inflammation), derived from study of 10 parameters of potential clinical significance, including well-being, abdominal pain, stool frequency, consistency, bleeding, anorexia, nausea and vomiting, abdominal tenderness, extra-intestinal manifestations, and pyrexia.

A   Limitation of activities   0 = none; 1 = impaired but able to continue activities;
                                             2 = activity reduced; 3 = unable to work

B	Bowel frequency	0 = < 3 per day; 1 = 3–6 times; 2 = > 6 per day
C	Stool consistency	0 = normal; 1 = semiformed; 2 = liquid
D	Baron Sigmoidoscopy Score	0 = normal or grade 1; 1 = grade 2; 2 = grade 3

Powell-Tuck J, Day DW, Buckell NA, Wadsworth J, Lennard-Jones JE. Correlations between defined sigmoidoscopic appearances and other measures of disease activity in ulcerative colitis. *Dig Dis Sci* 1982; 27: 533–7.

SCHROEDER OR MAYO CLINIC SCORE – WIDELY KNOWN AS THE UCSS (ULCERATIVE COLITIS SCORING SYSTEM)

Stool frequency
    0 = normal number of stools for this patient
    1 = 1–2 stools/day more than usual
    2 = 3–4 stools/day more than usual
    3 = 5 or more extra stools each day

Rectal bleeding
    0 = none
    1 = streaks of blood with less than half the stools
    2 = obvious blood with most stools
    3 = blood alone passed

(Flexible) proctosigmoidoscopy findings
    0 = normal or inactive disease
    1 = mild disease (erythema/decreased vascular pattern/mild friability)
    2 = moderate disease (marked erythema/absent vascular pattern/friability/erosions)
    3 = severe disease (spontaneous bleeding/ulceration)

Physician's global assessment
    0 = normal (no symptoms of colitis and normal sigmoidoscopy)
    1 = mild disease (mild symptoms and mild abnormality at sigmoidoscopy)
    2 = moderate disease (moderate symptoms and sigmoidoscopy grade 1–2)
    3 = severe disease (severe needing steroids ± admission and sigmoidoscopy grade 2–3)

The suggested grouping then is into four groups – inactive disease, mild, moderate and severe disease.

	Inactive	Mild	Moderate	Severe
Symptoms	0–2	1–3	3–6	>/= 1
Endoscopy	0	1	1–2	>/= 2
Physician's score	0	1	2	3
Total	0–2	3–5	6–10	>/= 6

It may be argued that the UCSS is too heavily influenced by the physician's global assessment since this effectively determines the grouping, but the advantages yielded by a numerical score have led to its adoption in many clinical trials.

Schroeder KW, Tremaine WJ, Ilstrup DM. Coated oral 5-aminosalicylic acid therapy for mildly to moderately active ulcerative colitis. A randomized study. *N Engl J Med* 1987; **317**: 1625–9.

THE CAI OR COLITIS CLINICAL ACTIVITY INDEX

Number of stools per week	< 18	0
	18–35	1
	36–60	2
	> 60	3
Blood in stools (on weekly basis)	None	0
	Little	2
	Lot	4
General state of health	Good	0
	Impaired	1
	Poor	2
	Very poor	3
Abdominal pain/cramps	None	0
	Mild	1
	Moderate	2
	Severe	3
Temperature/fever as result of colitis (°C)	37–38	0
	> 38	3
Extra-intestinal manifestations	None	0
	Iritis	3
	Erythema nodosum	3
	Arthritis	3
Laboratory findings	ESR < 50 and Hb > 10.0 g/dL	0
	ESR > 50 mm in 1st 2 hours	1
	ESR > 50 mm in 1st hour	2
	Hb < 10.0 g/dL	4

A little like the CDAI, this has the disadvantage of requiring a week's data, and necessitates both clinical and laboratory data. It is no longer so widely used.

Rachmilewitz D. Coated mesalazine (5-aminosalicylic acid) vs sulphasalazine in the treatment of active ulcerative colitis: a randomised trial. *Br Med J* 1989; **298**: 82–6.

THE INTEGRATED DISEASE ACTIVITY INDEX (FOR ULCERATIVE COLITIS)

Variable	Score	Weighting
Bloody stool		× 60
Little or none	0	
Present	1	
Bowel movements/day		× 13
4 or fewer	1	
4–7	2	
8 or more	3	
ESR (mm/h)		× 0.5
Haemoglobin (g/dL)		× −4
Albumin (g/dL)		× −15
Constant		200

A weighted score including laboratory markers which is inevitably somewhat complex and suitable only for clinical trials purposes.

Seo M, Okada M, Yao T, *et al.* An index of disease activity in patients with ulcerative colitis. *Am J Gastroenterol* 1992; **87**: 971–6.

THE BIRMINGHAM/ROYAL FREE SIMPLE COLITIS INDEX

This took as its starting point the expanded Powell-Tuck index, together with additional criteria such as nocturnal defecation, and was then limited to the five most informative criteria. It has been internally validated, and has very good correlation with the Powell-Tuck score ($r = 0.959$; $P < 0.0001$), laboratory markers and the more complex Seo score. It may now be considered the first choice for regular documentation, still perhaps superseded by the more complex scores for clinical trial purposes.

Sympton	Score
Bowel frequency/day	
1–3	0
4–6	1
7–9	2
> 9	3
Bowel frequency/night	
1–3	1
4–6	2

Urgency of defecation	
Hurry	1
Immediately	2
Incontinence	3
Blood in stool	
Trace	1
Occasionally frank	2
Usually frank	3
General well-being	
Very well	0
Slightly below par	1
Poor	2
Very poor	3
Terrible	4
Extracolonic features	1 per manifestation

Walmsley RS, Ayres RCS, Pounder RE, Allan RN. A simple clinical colitis activity index. *Gut* 1998; 443: 29–32.

Histological scoring for ulcerative colitis

THE TRUELOVE AND RICHARDS SCORE

No significant inflammation	1
Mild to moderate inflammation	
Epithelium intact	2
Severe inflammation	
Ulceration and exudate	3

Truelove SC, Richards WRD. Biopsy studies in ulcerative colitis. *Br Med J* 1956; **1**: 1315.

THE BRISTOL (WARREN–BRADFIELD) SCORE

Acute	Score	Chronic	Score
PMN in lamina propria	1	Mild	1
PMN in crypt wall	2	Severe	2
Crypt abscesses	3		
Crypt destruction	4		
Maximum	4	2	
Total maximum		6	
PMN = polymorphonuclear cells			

Warren BF, Rigby HS, Neumann C, Hall M, Mountford RA, Bradfield JWB. The role of multiple colonoscopic biopsies in long-standing ulcerative colitis. *J Pathol* 1988; **155**: 347A.

POUCHITIS

Pouchitis scores have been devised on both sides of the Atlantic.

Moskowitz RL, Shepherd NA, Nicholls RJ. An assessment of inflammation in the reservoir after restorative proctocolectomy with ileoanal ileal reservoir. *Int J Colorectal Dis* 1986; **1**: 167–74.

Sandborn WJ, Tremaine WJ, Batts KP, Pemberton JH, Phillips SF. Pouchitis after ileal pouch–anal anastomosis: a pouchitis disease activity index. *Mayo Clin Proc* 1994; **69**: 409–15.

Crucially both include histological assessment. The Mayo Clinic score is now widely adopted.

Histological scoring for Crohn's disease

THE LEUVEN SCORE

D'Haens GR, Geboes K, Peeters M, Baaert F, Penninckx F, Rutgeerts P. Early lesions of recurrent Crohn's disease caused by infusion of intestinal contents in excluded ileum. *Gastroenterology* 1998; **114**: 262–7.

More general questionnaire formats for assessment are also in use. Probably the most relevant to inflammatory bowel disease are the following (discussed in Chapter 2):

Irvine EJ, Feagon B, Rochon J, *et al.* Quality of life: a valid and reliable measure of therapeutic efficacy in the treatment of inflammatory bowel disease. *Gastroenterolgy* 1994; **106**: 287–96.

Stewart AL, Hays RD, Ware JE Jr. The MOS short-form general health survey: reliability and validity in a patient population. *Med Care* 1988; **26**: 724–35.

The following may also be useful at times:

The American Society of Anesthetists or ASA score which benefits from its simplicity:

1 normal healthy person
2 mild-to-moderate systemic disease
3 severe systemic disease that is not incapacitating
4 incapacitating illness that is a constant threat to life
5 moribund patient who is not expected to survive with or without surgery

Saklad M. Grading of patients for surgical procedures. *Anesthesiology* 1941; **2**: 281–5.

The SIRS score (Bone *et al. Chest* 1992; **101**: 1644–55), and the MODS score (Marshall *et al. Crit Care Med* 95; **23**: 1638–52) also have their place.

Bone RC, Balk RA, Cerra FB, *et al.* Definitions for sepsis and organ failure and guidelines for the use of innovative therapies in sepsis. The ACCP/SCCM Consensus Conference Committee. American College of Chest Physicians/Society of Critical Care Medicine. *Chest* 1992; **101**: 1644–55.

Marshall JC, Cook DJ, Christou NV, Bernard GR, Sprung CL, Sibbald WJ. Multiple organ dysfunction score: a reliable descriptor of a complex clinical outcome. *Crit Care Med* 1995; **23**: 1638–52.

Appendix B: Useful addresses

Professional groups

American Gastroenterological Association
AGA National Office,
7910 Woodmont Avenue,
7th Floor,
Bethesda,
MD 20814, USA
www.gastro.org

American Society for Gastrointestinal Endoscopy
13 Elm Street,
Manchester,
MA 09144, USA
www.bsg.org.uk

British Society of Gastroenterology
3 St Andrew's Place,
Regent's Park,
London NW1 4LB, UK
bsg@mailbox.ulcc.ac.uk
www.bsg.org.uk

Crohn's and Colitis Foundation of America
386 Park Avenue South,
17th Floor,
New York,
NY 10016-8804, USA
www.ccfa.org

Crohn's in Childhood Research Appeal (CICRA)
Parkgate House,
356 West Barnes Lane,
Motspur Park,
Surrey KT3 6NB, UK
Tel: 020 8949 6209

Digestive Disorders Foundation
3 St Andrew's Place,
Regent's Park,
London NW1 4LB, UK
www.digestivedisorders.org.uk

IBD Library (Utah University)
www-medllib.med.utah.edu/WebPath/
TUTORIAL/IBD/IBD.html

IBDList Digest
http://128.248.251.136/
ibdlist@menno.com

IBD Forum
www.ibdforum.com

Self-help groups and sources of information for patients

Associacion de Enfermos de Crohn Y Colitis
Ulcerosa (ACCU)
Suriname 36,
El Atabal – Puerto de la Torre,
E-29190 Malaga, Espana

Association Français Aupetit (AFA)
Hôpital Rothschild,
33 Boulevard de Picpus,
F-75571,
Paris Cedex 12, France

Associazone per le Malattie Infiammatorie
Croniche dell'Intestino (AMICI)
Via Adolfo Wildt 19/4,
I-20138 Milano, Italia

Australian Crohn's and Colitis Association
PO Box 201,
Moorolbark,
VIC 3138, Australia

Canadian Foundation for Ileitis and Colitis
387 Bloor Street East,
Suite 402,
Toronto,
ON M4W 1H7, Canada

Colitis-Crohn-Foreningen (CCF)
Lyngevej 116,
DK-3450 Allerod,
Denmark

Crohn's and Colitis Foundation of America
386 Park Avenue South,
17th Floor,
New York,
NY 10016-8804, USA
www.ccfa.org

Deutsche Morbus Crohn/Colitis ulcerosa
  Vereingung (DCCV) eV
Paracelsusstrasse 15,
D-51375 Leverkusen,
Deutschland

European Federation of Crohn's and Ulcerative
  Colitis Associations (EFCCA)
Düstere-Eichen-Weg 24,
D-37073 Göttingen,
Deutschland

Health management guides on Ulcerative colitis
  & Crohn's disease from
www.whatshouldido.com/ibd
Tel: 023 8022 9041

Ileostomy Association now known as:
  ia (the ileostomy & internal pouch support
  group)
PO Box 132,
Scunthorpe DN15 9YW, UK
Tel: 0800 0184724

Insurance Ombudsman Bureau
135 Park Street,
London SE1 1EA, UK

Irish Society for Colitis and Crohn's Disease
  (ISCCD)
58 Limekiln Green,
Dublin, Eire

National Association for Colitis and Crohn's
  disease (NACC)
4 Beaumont House,
Sutton Road,
St Alban's,
Herts AL1 5HH, UK
Tel: 01727 844296/830038
www.nacc.org.uk
e-mail: nacc@nacc.org.uk

National Digestive Diseases Information
  Clearinghouse
Box NDDIC,
9000 Rockville Pike,
Bethesda,
MD 20892, USA

Organisation Crohn
Mrs Tsaketa
Notara 53,
Piraeus,
Greece 18532
Tel: 42 27 276

Organ før Riksføbundet før Mag- & Tarmsjuka
  (RMT)
Box 9514,
S-10274 Stockholm, Sweden

Red Lion Group (Ileo-anal pouch support group)
20 The Maltings,
Green Lane,
Ashwell,
Herts SG7 5LW, UK

South African Crohn's Disease Association
PO Box 2638,
Cape Town 8000,
South Africa

NACC produce two excellent brief booklets: *Ulcerative Colitis* and *Crohn's Disease* (15 and 20 pages respectively) which are available from the NACC office or via their website (see above). DDF have an excellent leaflet on ulcerative colitis and Crohn's disease available from DDF, PO Box 251, Edgware, Middlesex, HA8 6HG. Also *A Patient Guide to IBD* (Cambridge), which is particularly good on therapeutic enteral regimens, is available from SHS International, Wavertree Boulevard, Liverpool, L7 9PT. Arguably the best single book for the patient seeking a more detailed account is *Inflammatory Bowel Disease: a Guide for Patients and their Families*, 2nd edn, eds Stein SH, Rood RP. Philadelphia: Lippincott Raven, 1999, 235 pp, US$22.

Index

Note: the abbreviation IBD = inflammatory bowel disease.